Quality Improvement in Neurosurgery

Editors

JOHN D. ROLSTON
SEUNGGU J. HAN
ANDREW T. PARSA

NEUROSURGERY
CLINICS OF NORTH AMERICA

www.neurosurgery.theclinics.com

Consulting Editors
RUSSELL LONSER
ISAAC YANG

April 2015 • Volume 26 • Number 2

ELSEVIER

1600 John F. Kennedy Boulevard • Suite 1800 • Philadelphia, Pennsylvania, 19103-2899

http://www.theclinics.com

NEUROSURGERY CLINICS OF NORTH AMERICA Volume 26, Number 2
April 2015 ISSN 1042-3680, ISBN-13: 978-0-323-35978-8

Editor: Jennifer Flynn-Briggs
Developmental Editor: Colleen Viola

Neurosurgery Clinics of North America (ISSN 1042-3680) is published quarterly by Elsevier Inc., 360 Park Avenue South, New York, NY 10010-1710. Months of issue are January, April, July, and October. Business and Editorial Offices: 1600 John F. Kennedy Blvd., Suite 1800, Philadelphia, PA 19103-2899. Customer Service Office: 11830 Westline Industrial Drive, St. Louis, MO 63146. Periodicals postage paid at New York, NY, and additional mailing offices. Subscription prices are $380.00 per year (US individuals), $572.00 per year (US institutions), $415.00 per year (Canadian individuals), $711.00 per year (Canadian institutions), $525.00 per year (international individuals), $711.00 per year (international institutions), $185.00 per year (US students), and $255.00 per year (international and Canadian students). International air speed delivery is included in all *Clinics* subscription prices. All prices are subject to change without notice. **POSTMASTER:** Send address changes to *Neurosurgery Clinics of North America*, Elsevier Periodicals Customer Service, 11830 Westline Industrial Drive, St. Louis, MO 63146. **Customer Service: 1-800-654-2452 (US and Canada). From outside the US and Canada, call: 1-314-453-7041. Fax: 1-314-453-5170. E-mail: JournalsCustomerService-usa@elsevier.com (for print support) and journalsonlinesupport-usa@elsevier.com (for online support).**

Reprints. For copies of 100 or more, of articles in this publication, please contact the Commercial Reprints Department, Elsevier Inc., 360 Park Avenue South, New York, NY 10010-1710. Tel. 212-633-3874; Fax: 212-633-3820; E-mail: reprints@elsevier.com.

Neurosurgery Clinics of North America is covered in *MEDLINE/PubMed (Index Medicus), EMBASE/Excerpta Medica, and Current Contents/Clinical Medicine (CC/CM).*

Contributors

CONSULTING EDITORS

RUSSELL LONSER, MD
Professor and Chair, Department of
Neurological Surgery, The Ohio State
University Wexner Medical Center, Columbus,
Ohio

ISAAC YANG, MD
Attending Neurosurgeon, Assistant Professor
Department of Neurosurgery, Director of
Medical Student Education, David Geffen
School of Medicine at UCLA, Jonsson
Comprehensive Cancer Center, University of
California Los Angeles, Los Angeles, California

EDITORS

JOHN D. ROLSTON, MD, PhD
Department of Neurological Surgery, University
of California, San Francisco, San Francisco,
California

SEUNGGU J. HAN, MD
Department of Neurological Surgery, University
of California, San Francisco, San Francisco,
California

ANDREW T. PARSA, MD, PhD
Michael J. Marchese Professor and Chair,
Department of Neurological Surgery,
Northwestern University Feinberg School of
Medicine, Chicago, Illinois

AUTHORS

NASIM AFSAR-MANESH, MD
Department of Neurological Surgery, University
of California Los Angeles, Los Angeles,
California

JORDAN P. AMADIO, MD, MBA
Neurosurgery Resident Physician, Department
of Neurosurgery, Emory University School of
Medicine, Atlanta, Georgia

ANTHONY L. ASHER, MD
Department of Neurological Surgery, Carolina
Neurosurgery and Spine Associates, Carolinas
HealthCare System Neuroscience Institute,
Charlotte, North Carolina

BERNARD R. BENDOK, MD
Professor of Neurological Surgery, Radiology,
and Otolaryngology, Northwestern University
Feinberg School of Medicine, Chicago, Illinois

MITCHEL S. BERGER, MD
Department of Neurological Surgery, University
of California, San Francisco, San Francisco,
California

MARK BERNSTEIN, MD, MHSc, FRCSC
Division of Neurosurgery, Toronto Western
Hospital; Joint Centre for Bioethics, University
of Toronto, Toronto, Ontario, Canada

JONATHAN T. CARTER, MD, FACS
Associate Professor of Clinical Surgery,
Department of Surgery, University of
California, San Francisco, San Francisco,
California

HUGO QUINNY CHENG, MD
Clinical Professor of Medicine, Division of
Hospital Medicine, University of California, San
Francisco, San Francisco, California

SAMUEL J. CHEWNING Jr, MD
Carolina Neurosurgery and Spine Associates,
Charlotte, North Carolina

WINWARD CHOY, BA
Department of Neurological Surgery, University
of California Los Angeles, Los Angeles,
California

LAWRANCE K. CHUNG, BS
Department of Neurological Surgery, University
of California Los Angeles, Los Angeles,
California

JASON M. DAVIES, MD, PhD
Department of Neurological Surgery, University
of California, San Francisco, San Francisco,
California

KYLE M. FARGEN, MD, MPH
Resident, Department of Neurological Surgery,
University of Florida, Gainesville, Florida

**MICHAEL G. FEHLINGS, MD, PhD, FRCSC,
FACS**
Vice Chair of Research, Department of
Surgery, Halbert Chair in Neural Repair and
Regeneration; Co-Director Spinal Program,
University Health Network, University of
Toronto, Toronto, Ontario, Canada

GEORGE M. GHOBRIAL, MD
Department of Neurological Surgery, Thomas
Jefferson University Hospital, Philadelphia,
Pennsylvania

RACHEL GROMAN, MPH
Vice President, Clinical Affairs and Quality
Improvement, Hart Health Strategies, Inc,
Madison, Wisconsin

YOUSSEF J. HAMADE, MD
Department of Neurological Surgery,
Northwestern University Feinberg School of
Medicine, Chicago, Illinois

SEUNGGU J. HAN, MD
Department of Neurological Surgery, University
of California, San Francisco, San Francisco,
California

JAMES S. HARROP, MD
Professor of Neurological Surgery and
Orthopedics, Department of Neurological
Surgery, Thomas Jefferson University Hospital,
Philadelphia, Pennsylvania

JAMES G. KAHN, MD, MPH
Professor, Philip R. Lee Institute for
Health Policy Studies, Global Health
Economics Consortium, University of
California, San Francisco, San Francisco,
California

CATHERINE Y. LAU, MD
Division of Hospital Medicine, Department
of Medicine and Neurological Surgery,
University of California, San Francisco;
Assistant Clinical Professor, Director
Patient Safety and Quality, Department
of Neurological Surgery, San Francisco,
California

MICHAEL T. LAWTON, MD
Department of Neurological Surgery, University
of California, San Francisco, San Francisco,
California

NEIL A. MARTIN, MD
Department of Neurological Surgery, University
of California Los Angeles, Los Angeles,
California

MATTHEW J. McGIRT, MD
Department of Neurological Surgery,
Carolina Neurosurgery and Spine
Associates, Carolinas HealthCare System
Neuroscience Institute, Charlotte,
North Carolina

J. MOCCO, MD, MS
Associate Professor, Department of
Neurological Surgery, Vanderbilt
University School of Medicine, Nashville,
Tennessee

DANIEL T. NAGASAWA, MD
Department of Neurological Surgery, University
of California Los Angeles, Los Angeles,
California

ANICK NATER, MD
Division of Neurosurgery, Department of
Surgery, Institute of Medical Science,
University of Toronto, Toronto, Ontario,
Canada

VINITRA NATHAN
Division of Neurosurgery, Toronto Western
Hospital, University of Toronto, Toronto,
Ontario, Canada

NELSON M. OYESIKU, MD, PhD
Director, Neurosurgery Residency Program;
Professor, Neurosurgery and Medicine
(Endocrinology); Editor-in-Chief, Al Lerner
Chair and Vice-Chairman, Department of
Neurosurgery, Emory Pituitary Center, Emory
University School of Medicine, Atlanta, Georgia

ALP OZPINAR, BS
Oregon Health Sciences University, School of
Medicine, Portland, Oregon

SCOTT L. PARKER, MD
Department of Neurological Surgery,
Vanderbilt University Medical Center,
Nashville, Tennessee

PANAYIOTIS PELARGOS, MD
Department of Neurological Surgery, University
of California Los Angeles, Los Angeles,
California

ANDREW J. RINGER, MD
Professor of Neurosurgery, Department of
Neurosurgery, Mayfield Clinic, University of
Cincinnati, Cincinnati, Ohio

JOHN D. ROLSTON, MD, PhD
Department of Neurological Surgery, University
of California, San Francisco, San Francisco,
California

NATHAN R. SELDEN, MD, PhD
Department of Neurological Surgery, Oregon
Health and Science University, Portland,
Oregon

PHILIP V. THEODOSOPOULOS, MD
Professor and Vice Chair, Department of
Neurological Surgery, University of California,
San Francisco, San Francisco, California

KIM THILL, BA
Department of Neurological Surgery, University
of California Los Angeles, Los Angeles,
California

NOLAN UNG, BS
Department of Neurological Surgery, University
of California Los Angeles, Los Angeles,
California

BRITTANY VOTH, BA, MPH
Department of Neurological Surgery, University
of California Los Angeles, Los Angeles,
California

CHRISTOPHER D. WITIW, MD
Division of Neurosurgery, Toronto Western
Hospital, University of Toronto, Toronto,
Ontario, Canada

ISAAC YANG, MD
Attending Neurosurgeon, Assistant Professor
Department of Neurosurgery, Director of
Medical Student Education, David Geffen
School of Medicine at UCLA, Jonsson
Comprehensive Cancer Center, University of
California Los Angeles, Los Angeles, California

JOHN E. ZIEWACZ, MD, MPH
Carolina Neurosurgery and Spine Associates,
Charlotte, North Carolina

SCOTT L. ZUCKERMAN, MD
Resident, Department of Neurological Surgery,
Vanderbilt University School of Medicine,
Nashville, Tennessee

CORINNA C. ZYGOURAKIS, MD
Department of Neurological Surgery, University
of California, San Francisco, San Francisco,
California

Contents

Preface: Quality Improvement in Neurosurgery   xiii

John D. Rolston, Seunggu J. Han, and Andrew T. Parsa

Improving Patient Safety in Neurologic Surgery   143

Seunggu J. Han, John D. Rolston, Catherine Y. Lau, and Mitchel S. Berger

> The delivery of safe healthcare is one of the fundamental tenets of medicine, but the study of patient safety has lagged in neurosurgery. Patients are at high risk for medical errors, adverse events, and complications. To prevent and mitigate these risks, it is not enough to shame and blame individual practitioners for mistakes or errors. Complete health care delivery systems should be evaluated for ways to reduce adverse events and errors, and restrict the harm they cause. This article reviews the context of patient safety in history, and outlines the ways in which patient safety is being improved.

Errors in Neurosurgery   149

John D. Rolston and Mark Bernstein

> Medical errors are common and dangerous, estimated to cause over 400,000 deaths per year in the United States alone. The field of neurosurgery is not immune to these errors, and many studies have begun analyzing the frequency and types of errors that neurosurgical patients experience, along with their effects and causes. Fortunately, these data are guiding new innovations to reduce and prevent errors, like checklists, computerized order entry, and an increased appreciation for volume–outcome relationships. This article describes the epidemiology of errors, their classification, methods for identifying and discovering errors, and new strategies for error prevention.

Adverse Events in Neurosurgery and Their Relationship to Quality Improvement   157

John E. Ziewacz, Matthew J. McGirt, and Samuel J. Chewning Jr

> Adverse events are common in neurosurgery. Their reporting is inconsistent and widely variable due to nonuniform definitions, data collection mechanisms, and retrospective data collection. Historically, neurosurgery has lagged behind general and cardiac surgical fields in the creation of multi-institutional prospective databases allowing for benchmarking and accurate adverse event/outcomes measurement, the bedrock of evidence used to guide quality improvement initiatives. The National Neurosurgery Quality and Outcomes Database has begun to address this issue by collecting prospective, multi-institutional outcomes data in neurosurgical patients. Once reliable outcomes exist, various targeted quality improvement strategies may be used to reduce adverse events and improve outcomes.

The Relationship Between National Health Care Policies and Quality Improvement in Neurosurgery   167

Rachel Groman

> Although federal programs aimed at improving the overall value of health care are well intentioned, most remain fundamentally flawed in terms of their metrics, their

methodologies, and the pace at which they are being implemented. Without a serious reevaluation of these strategies, these programs will, at best, have limited effectiveness, and, at worst, lead to critical deteriorations in patient quality, safety, and access to care.

Quality Improvement Tools and Processes   177

Catherine Y. Lau

The Model for Improvement and the Plan-Do-Study-Act cycle is a popular quality improvement (QI) tool for health care providers to successfully lead QI projects and redesign care processes. This tool has several distinct components that must be addressed in sequence to organize and critically evaluate improvement activities. Unlike other health sciences clinical research, QI projects and research are based on dynamic hypotheses that develop into observable, serial tests of change with continuous collection and feedback of performance data to stakeholders.

Cost-Effectiveness Research in Neurosurgery   189

Corinna C. Zygourakis and James G. Kahn

Cost and value are increasingly important components of health care discussions. Despite a plethora of cost and cost-effectiveness analyses in many areas of medicine, there has been little of this type of research for neurosurgical procedures. This scarcity is vexing because this specialty represents one of the most expensive areas in medicine. This article discusses the general principles of cost-effectiveness analyses and reviews the cost- and cost-effectiveness-related research to date in neurosurgical subspecialties. The need for standardization of cost and cost-effectiveness measurement and reporting within neurosurgery is highlighted and a set of metrics for this purpose is defined.

Economics, Innovation, and Quality Improvement in Neurosurgery   197

Christopher D. Witiw, Vinitra Nathan, and Mark Bernstein

Innovation to improve patient care quality is a priority of the neurosurgical specialty since its beginnings. As the strain on health care resources increases, the cost of these quality improvements is becoming increasingly important. The aims of this article are to review the available tools for assessing the cost of quality improvement along with the willingness to pay and to provide a conceptual framework for the assessment of innovations in terms of quality and economic metrics and provide examples from the neurosurgical literature.

Volume-Outcome Relationships in Neurosurgery   207

Jason M. Davies, Alp Ozpinar, and Michael T. Lawton

For a variety of neurosurgical conditions, increasing surgeon and hospital volumes correlate with improved outcomes, such as mortality, complication rates, length of stay, hospital charges, and discharge disposition. Neurosurgeons can improve patient outcomes at the population level by changing practice and referral patterns to regionalize care for select conditions at high-volume specialty treatment centers. Individual practitioners should be aware of where they fall on the volume spectrum and understand the implications of their practice and referral habits on their patients.

Neurosurgical Checklists: A Growing Need   219

Scott L. Zuckerman, Kyle M. Fargen, and J. Mocco

The US health care system is currently undergoing a paradigm shift from pay-for-service toward pay-for-performance reimbursement, with a focus on quality measures and patient satisfaction. An important tool gaining increasing emphasis during the quality revolution is the surgical checklist. What was once perceived as an invasion of the practitioner's integrity is now a mainstay in all operating rooms, mandated by several national organizations. Although other fields have pioneered the checklist revolution, neurosurgery is now beginning to follow suit. The authors review the available published neurosurgical checklists and their early results on patient safety.

Quality Improvement in Neurological Surgery Graduate Medical Education   231

Scott L. Parker, Matthew J. McGirt, Anthony L. Asher, and Nathan R. Selden

There has been no formal, standardized curriculum for neurosurgical resident education in quality improvement. There are at least 2 reasons to integrate a formalized quality improvement curriculum into resident education: (1) increased emphasis on the relative quality and value (cost-effectiveness) of health care provided by individual physicians, and (2) quality improvement principles empower broader lifelong learning. An integrated quality improvement curriculum should comprise specific goals and milestones at each level of residency training. This article discusses the role and possible implementation of a national program for quality improvement in neurosurgical resident education.

Technology and Simulation to Improve Patient Safety   239

George M. Ghobrial, Youssef J. Hamade, Bernard R. Bendok, and James S. Harrop

Improving the quality and efficiency of surgical techniques, reducing technical errors in the operating suite, and ultimately improving patient safety and outcomes through education are common goals in all surgical specialties. Current surgical simulation programs represent an effort to enhance and optimize the training experience, to overcome the training limitations of a mandated 80-hour work week, and have the overall goal of providing a well-balanced resident education in a society with a decreasing level of tolerance for medical errors.

Electronic Medical Records and Quality Improvement   245

Jonathan T. Carter

Widespread adoption of electronic medical records (EMRs) in the United States is transforming the practice of medicine from a paper-based cottage industry into an integrated health care delivery system. Most physicians and institutions view the widespread use of EMRs to be inevitable. But the transformation has not been painless. Many have questioned whether the substantial investment in electronic health records has really been justified by improved patient outcomes or quality of care. This article describes historical and recent efforts to use EMRs to improve the quality of patient care, and provides a roadmap of EMR uses for the foreseeable future.

Using Clinical Registries to Improve the Quality of Neurosurgical Care   253

Anthony L. Asher, Scott L. Parker, John D. Rolston, Nathan R. Selden, and Matthew J. McGirt

Despite rising and unsustainable US health care costs, many stakeholders feel that the quality of medical services is limited and inconsistent. Value-based reforms are touted as the key to achieving health care system sustainability. Health care value is defined as quality delivered divided by cost incurred. Unfortunately, quality in health care is difficult to accurately define, and methods to reliably assess and report health care quality are often lacking. Clinical registries have emerged as important mechanisms to define, measure, and promote health care quality. The purpose of this article is to describe the role of registries in neurosurgical quality improvement.

Measuring Outcomes for Neurosurgical Procedures   265

Philip V. Theodosopoulos and Andrew J. Ringer

Health care evolution has led to focused attention on clinical outcomes of care. Surgical disciplines are increasingly asked to provide evidence of treatment efficacy. As the technological advances push the surgical envelope further, it becomes imperative that postoperative outcomes are studied in a prospective fashion to assess the quality of care provided. In this article, the authors present their experience from a multiyear implementation of an outcomes initiative and share lessons learned, emphasizing the important structural elements of such an endeavor.

Development and Implementation of Guidelines in Neurosurgery   271

Michael G. Fehlings and Anick Nater

Although it is intuitive that any neurosurgeon would seek to consistently apply the best available evidence to patient management, the application of evidence-based medicine (EBM) principles and clinical practice guidelines (CPGs) remains variable. This article reviews the origin and process of EBM, and the development, assessment, and applicability of EBM and CPGs in neurosurgical care, aiming to demonstrate that CPGs are one of the valid available options that exist to improve quality of care. CPGs are not intended to define the standard of care but to compile dynamic advisory statements, which need to be updated as new evidence emerges.

The Role of Neurosurgery Journals in Evidence-Based Neurosurgical Care   283

Jordan P. Amadio and Nelson M. Oyesiku

Neurosurgery journals have played an active role in improving the quality of the neurosurgical literature. This role has expanded to improve the quality of care by incorporating an evidence-based view of neurosurgery practice. Neurosurgery journals have facilitated the organization of knowledge into clinically useful forms via the publication of meta-analyses and dissemination of clinical practice guidelines. Peer review continues to be a core feature of neurosurgery publishing, with attendant ethical and procedural safeguards. Finally, neurosurgery journals have spearheaded innovative responses to cultural and technological changes, including initiatives to deliver high-quality research in electronic formats and support the education of future neurosurgery investigators.

Comanagement Hospitalist Services for Neurosurgery   295

Hugo Quinny Cheng

Neurosurgeons and hospitalists are turning to comanagement arrangements to address medical problems in surgical patients. Compared with traditional medical consultation, comanagement lets the hospitalist share authority and responsibility for patient care. It is associated with improved provider satisfaction and more efficient care, but impact on clinical outcomes is uncertain. Shared responsibility for patient care requires careful planning to avoid conflicts and fragmentation of care.

Recent Advances in the Patient Safety and Quality Initiatives Movement: Implications for Neurosurgery   **301**

Isaac Yang, Nolan Ung, Daniel T. Nagasawa, Panayiotis Pelargos, Winward Choy, Lawrance K. Chung, Kim Thill, Neil A. Martin, Nasim Afsar-Manesh, and Brittany Voth

The US health care system is fragmented in terms of quality care, costs, and patient satisfaction. With the passage of the Affordable Care Act, national attention has been placed on the health care system, but effective change has yet to be observed. Unnecessary costs, medical errors, and uncoordinated efforts contribute to patient morbidity, mortality, and decreased patient satisfaction. In addition to national efforts, local initiatives within individual departments must be implemented to improve overall satisfaction without the sacrifice of costs. In this article, the current issues with the health care system and potential initiatives for neurosurgery are reviewed.

Index   **317**

NEUROSURGERY CLINICS OF NORTH AMERICA

FORTHCOMING ISSUES

July 2015
Endoscopic Endonasal Skull Base Surgery
Daniel M. Prevedello, *Editor*

October 2015
Chiari Malformation
Jeffrey Leonard and David Limbrick, *Editors*

January 2016
Epilepsy
Kareem Zaghloul and Edward Chang, *Editors*

RECENT ISSUES

January 2015
Central Neurocytomas
Dong Gyu Kim and Isaac Yang, *Editors*

October 2014
Pain Management
Andre Machado, Milind Deogaonkar, and Ashwini Sharan, *Editors*

July 2014
Endovascular Management of Cerebrovascular Disease
Ricardo Hanel, Ciaran Powers, and Eric Sauvageau, *Editors*

April 2014
Minimally Invasive Spine Surgery
Zachary A. Smith and Richard G. Fessler, *Editors*

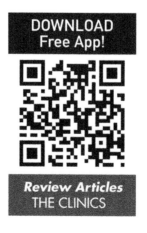

Preface

Quality Improvement in Neurosurgery

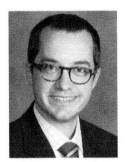
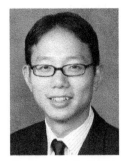
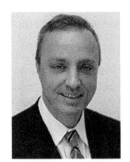

John D. Rolston, MD, PhD   Seunggu J. Han, MD   Andrew T. Parsa, MD, PhD

Editors

Health care workers want to provide the best care they can, and patients demand it. Moreover, our society wishes this care to be safe, efficient, and economically sustainable. Achieving these goals is the subject of quality improvement (QI), an ever-growing collection of systems and studies targeted at improving patient outcomes and the processes that achieve them. The recognized need for QI in health care is not new, appearing at various key moments first described in Ernest Codman's "End Result System,"[1] later with the formation of the Joint Commission in 1952,[2] and more recently the publication of *To Err is Human* by the Institute of Medicine in 1999.[3] But the scope of quality studies is steadily growing, most recently with an increasingly sharp focus on health economics and the idea of value-based purchasing.[4]

Unlike many other disciplines in medicine, QI is intimately associated with governing and regulatory systems. Drivers of QI have long included physician-led systems like the American Medical Association and the American College of Surgeons, but the US Federal Government is also highly invested, predominantly after the creation of Medicare and Medicaid in 1965 made it economically critical to do so.[5,6] More recently, with the passage of the Affordable Care Act in 2010, the importance of QI has been repeatedly reiterated.[7]

In a 2012 report to Congress,[8] the "Triple Aim" was outlined by the Department of Health and Human Services to define the goals for modern health care QI:

1. "Better Care: Improve the overall quality of care, by making health care more patient-centered, reliable, accessible, and safe."
2. "Healthy People/Healthy Communities: Improve the health of the US population by supporting proven interventions to address behavioral, social, and environmental determinants of health in addition to delivering higher-quality care."
3. "Affordable Care: Reduce the cost of quality health care for individuals, families, employers, and government."

Because of the government's involvement, engagement in QI initiatives is no longer optional for providers of health care. Reimbursements are being tied to quality measures through Value-Based Purchasing, Pay-for-Performance, and the creation of Accountable Care Organizations. Data on quality of care provided by individuals and institutions are becoming available to patients. Participation in registries and QI programs is also now tied to reimbursements from the Centers for Medicare and Medicaid Services.

Because of these changes, it is more important than ever for neurosurgeons to understand the process of QI, to see how it can ultimately improve the health of their patients, and to engage in critically evaluating the evidence behind quality measures and processes. This issue of *Neurosurgery*

Neurosurg Clin N Am 26 (2015) xiii–xiv
http://dx.doi.org/10.1016/j.nec.2015.01.001
1042-3680/15/$ – see front matter © 2015 Published by Elsevier Inc.

Clinics of North America is an attempt to gather much of this information in a single resource, with a focus on QI as it relates to neurosurgeons and neurosurgery departments. Our hope is that the following articles provide concise starting points on the primary issues of QI in neurosurgery.

The editors would like to acknowledge Catherine Y. Lau, MD for her contributions to this article.

John D. Rolston, MD, PhD
Department of Neurological Surgery
University of California, San Francisco
San Francisco, CA 94143, USA

Seunggu J. Han, MD
Department of Neurological Surgery
University of California, San Francisco
San Francisco, CA 94143, USA

Andrew T. Parsa, MD, PhD
Department of Neurological Surgery
Northwestern University Feinberg School of Medicine
Chicago, IL 60611, USA

E-mail addresses:
rolstonj@neurosurg.ucsf.edu (J.D. Rolston)
hansj@neurosurg.ucsf.edu (S.J. Han)
aparsa@nmff.org (A.T. Parsa)

REFERENCES

1. Donabedian A. The end results of health care: Ernest Codman's contribution to quality assessment and beyond. Milbank Q 1989;67:233–56 [discussion: 257–67].
2. Roberts JS, Coale JG, Redman RR. A history of the Joint Commission on Accreditation of Hospitals. JAMA 1987;258:936–40.
3. Kohn LT, Corrigan J, Donaldson MS. To err is human: building a safer health system. Washington, DC: National Academy Press; 2000.
4. Rowe JW. Pay-for-performance and accountability: related themes in improving health care. Ann Intern Med 2006;145:695–9.
5. United States Congress House Committee on Ways and Means. Subcommittee on Health. Medicare quality of care, and outcomes and effectiveness research: hearing before the Subcommittee on Health of the Committee on Ways and Means, House of Representatives, One Hundred Second Congress, first session, April 30, 1991. Washington, DC: U.S. G.P.O.: For sale by the U.S. G.P.O., Supt. of Docs., Congressional Sales Office; 1991.
6. United States Congress Senate Committee on Finance. Subcommittee on Medicare and Long-Term Care. Medicare quality assurance: hearing before the Subcommittee on Medicare and Long-Term Care of the Committee on Finance, United States Senate, One Hundred Second Congress, first session, February 22, 1991. Washington, DC: U.S. G.P.O.: For sale by the U.S. G.P.O., Supt. of Docs., Congressional Sales Office; 1991.
7. Butler PD, Chang B, Britt LD. The Affordable Care Act and academic surgery: expectations and possibilities. J Am Coll Surg 2014;218:1049–55.
8. Annual Progress Report to Congress. National Strategy for Quality Improvement in Health Care. Available at: http://www.ahrq.gov/workingforquality/nqs/nqs2012annlrpt.pdf. Accessed August 1, 2014.

Improving Patient Safety in Neurologic Surgery

Seunggu J. Han, MD*, John D. Rolston, MD, PhD, Catherine Y. Lau, MD, Mitchel S. Berger, MD

KEYWORDS

- Patient safety • Surgical safety • Neurosurgery patient safety

KEY POINTS

- Health care is performed by conscientious but fallible people. Errors inevitably occur.
- To ensure patient safety, clinicians must incorporate systems thinking, in which the responsibility of patient safety is placed on all parts of the health care team and infrastructure, from hospital administrators to bedside nurses.
- Effective and uninhibited communication between team members is essential for increasing patient safety, although this has been difficult to achieve in medicine, given the prominent hierarchies among different staff.
- There are many avenues to pursue in improving patient safety, from patient registries and databases to the study of volume-outcome relationships and the establishment of centers of excellence; to maximize the safety of neurosurgical patients, all these strategies should be pursued.

INTRODUCTION

Because of its high level of complexity, neurosurgery is a high-risk specialty, and improving patient outcomes has remained central in its spectrum of academic pursuits. However, only recently has there been a growing recognition of the need for a systematic approach for improving the safety and reducing adverse events for patients. This change has been in part caused by growing recognition of the pervasive nature of medical errors, adverse events, and complications that reduce patient safety, along with the growth in the body of literature describing their impacts, as well as economic and regulatory pressures from health care governing bodies. Independent of these pressures, neurosurgery clinicians have always taken pride in being providers who carry a strong sense of personal responsibility for their patients. With any errors or bad outcomes being considered as personal failings, it has frequently been considered that the solution to these problems is simply to work harder, believing that if clinicians do their best not to make a mistake, mistakes would not occur. However, it has become clear that this is not the case, and that the only way to deliver safe care is to place fallible but conscientious people in systems of care that support them with the knowledge and the tools to identify and anticipate adverse events and prevent them before they can harm patients. At the root of this is the need to change the neurosurgical culture: to practice medicine with patient safety as a priority within systems that help clinicians understand, identify, and prevent errors in a systematic fashion, with a focus on solutions rooted in systems-based approaches (**Fig. 1**).

MODERN PATIENT SAFETY MOVEMENT

In the past, it was a common belief that American health care was very safe. Although high-profile cases of adverse events in health care were widely

Department of Neurological Surgery, University of California, San Francisco, 505 Parnassus Avenue, San Francisco, CA 94143-0112, USA
* Corresponding author. Department of Neurological Surgery, University of California, San Francisco, 505 Parnassus Avenue, M-779, San Francisco, CA 94143-0112.
E-mail address: hansj@neurosurg.ucsf.edu

Neurosurg Clin N Am 26 (2015) 143–147
http://dx.doi.org/10.1016/j.nec.2014.11.007
1042-3680/15/$ – see front matter © 2015 Elsevier Inc. All rights reserved.

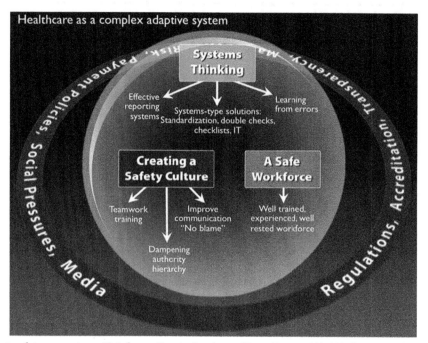

Fig. 1. Patient safety ecosystem. IT, information technology. (*From* Berger MS, Wachter RM, Greysen SR, et al. Changing our culture to advance patient safety: the 2013 AANS presidential address. J Neurosurg 2013;119(6):1361; with permission.)

reported, such as the cases of Libby Zion and Betsy Lehman, they were frequently seen as rare failures by individual practitioners. However, reports such as the Harvard Medical Practice Study in 1991 showed that adverse events in health care were more common than was ever anticipated.[1] In addition, early leaders in the field, such as Lucian Leape,[2] introduced the concept that errors in medicine were systems-based problems, and not just individual failings. Then a landmark moment in health care safety came with the Institute of Medicine (IOM) report in 1999, estimating that up to 100,000 patients die every year as a direct result of medical errors,[3] and that this was equivalent to a jumbo jet crashing every day of the year. The IOM's report was shocking, and it became clear that errors and adverse events were more common and their impact larger than had previously been realized.

ERRORS AND ADVERSE EVENTS

With widespread sentiment that something needed to be done, tackling the problem first required a systematic effort to identify, categorize, and analyze adverse events and health care errors. Within neurosurgery, a recent review from Gawande's group systematically reviewed the literature to describe the patterns of adverse events encountered within neurosurgery.[4–8] Looking across different subspecialties, their report categorized adverse events based on their contributing factors, including surgical technique, technology, and communication.[4] For errors in neurosurgery, Oremakinde and Bernstein[9] reported on their experience of prospective collecting errors that occurred around operative cases. They confirmed that errors occurred much more frequently than was previously thought, with at least 1 error in almost every case. Furthermore, they described a method of organizing errors into types of errors, which include those that are technical, involving contamination, equipment failure, or caused by communication, with errors further characterized by their severity and clinical impact.[10] These studies show the complexity of the factors contributing to patient safety and the adverse events that threaten patients.

ECONOMIC CONSIDERATIONS

There is now a growing economic case for promoting patient safety. The economic cost of errors and adverse events is estimated to be US$17 billion to $29 billion.[5] In addition, the list of never events reported by The National Quality Foundation was recently adopted by The Centers for Medicare and Medicaid Services (CMS) as a basis for withholding payments from hospitals. In addition to these patient safety outcomes being tied to reimbursement structures, accreditation of hospitals and care organizations is also being based on quality measures of patient safety and adherence to best-practice guidelines.

CHECKLISTS

The most important innovation in the modern patient safety movement has arguably been the introduction of checklists.[11] There are now many examples of the powerful impact checklists can have on enhancing patient safety. Pronovost and colleagues[12] designed a checklist to reduce central line infections in Michigan intensive care units and successfully reduced the rates of central line infections by half. The same checklist was adopted by the Agency for Healthcare Research, and this resulted in a reduction of central line infections by 30% to 40% across the country. Another powerful example is the surgical safety checklist developed by the World Health Organization (WHO), and the implementation of the checklist at centers worldwide greatly decreased rates of complications, surgical site infections, unplanned returns to the operating room, and even perioperative deaths.[13] Application of the surgical checklist to the neurosurgical setting has also been evaluated and reported by several groups. One such example comes from the department at the Mayo Clinic in Arizona, which implemented an operative checklist across 8 years of study, and there was a nearly 100% compliance without a single case of wrong-site, wrong-procedure, or wrong-patient events.[14] That study shows a key factor as to why checklists work to prevent errors: compliance on the part of all stakeholders.

A FOCUS ON COMMUNICATION AND TEAMWORK

Implementation of checklists also seems to promote enhanced perception of teamwork and an attitude that prioritizes patient safety among members of a multidisciplinary surgical team.[15] Lessons taken from the experience of the aviation industry have stressed the importance of optimizing teamwork and communication, and it became evident that degraded teamwork conditions with steep authority gradients could easily lead to adverse outcomes for passengers and patients alike. To test these concepts in neurosurgery, Sexton and colleagues[16] asked pilots and surgeons whether they would object to someone else in the team speaking up if they thought something was not right. Almost all the pilots said they would not mind, but only half of the surgeons answered that they would not mind. In addition,

the investigators asked members of the operating room team about their assessment of level of teamwork; nearly all the surgeons replied that the teamwork was excellent, but most other members did not share the sentiment. Together, this shows the steep authority gradient that traditionally exists in many operating room settings.

Deconstructing this steep authority gradient and improving communication between team members first requires recognition of the gradient's existence and the potential harmful impact it can have on patient safety. Second, through continued teamwork training, all members of the care team should be encouraged to speak up if they have any concerns about the course of the care, and hence work to gradually shift the culture so that all members are active participants effectively working together to provide safe and high-quality patient care. These opportunities should ideally be constructed around a framework, such as checklists and time-outs. Another example of this effort is provided by the development and implementation of a perioperative safety video introduced by our group.[17] The goal of the video was to outline the standard but critical safety checks and multidisciplinary team communication practices that are fundamental for every operative procedure. The target audience included all members of the multidisciplinary staff, including attending surgeons and anesthesiologists, trainees, perioperative and operating room nursing staff, and other members such as neurophysiologic monitoring specialists. Thus, at all stages of development, the video included active input from a champion taskforce that included representatives from each discipline.

VOLUME OUTCOMES IN NEUROSURGERY

Another potential strategy to improve patient safety is to consider regionalization of care for certain types of operative procedures. There is a growing body of evidence that the same procedure performed at high-volume centers is associated with lower rates of complications and improved outcomes. This relationship has been shown to be true in varying degrees across all subspecialties within neurosurgery.[18–26]

DATABASES

A further key to the quality puzzle is the continual need to assess the ever-changing landscape of patient safety in neurosurgery, as well as to track the impact that quality improvement interventions are having. In addition, there is a need for benchmarking so that individuals and groups can compare their results and outcomes in a nonpunitive setting, and this is how the National Neurosurgery Quality and Outcomes Database (N2QOD) will play a fundamental role.[27] N2QOD provides the ability to compare an individual's performance with the expected outcomes based on national data, and thus in turn provides feedback throughout continuous measurement of outcomes, which will directly serve as a powerful tool for identifying errors and areas in need of improvement. However, the success of this effort, like the checklist, depends on participation of all stakeholders, and clinicians must change their culture to be more transparent and increase the reporting of outcomes, including adverse events and complications.

BUILDING A PATIENT SAFETY PROGRAM

Building a successful patient safety program requires a shared vision to prioritize providing the safest and highest quality care possible for patients.[11] This vision requires a fundamental change in the culture that starts at the leadership level. The focus of the American Association of Neurological Surgeons (AANS) during the 2012 to 2013 year was centered on advancing patient safety, and the presidential address of the 2013 AANS annual meeting outlined the history of patient safety and quality improvement, summarized the efforts of the field's leaders, and detailed the direction neurosurgery needs to take to continue advancing patient safety.[11] This improvement requires adopting and consistently applying systematic approaches to improving the safety of patients; approaches that occur within a broad safety ecosystem (see **Fig. 1**). External forces, such as new governmental regulations, will influence this ecosystem, but clinicians owe it to their patients to treat these problems with the care and seriousness they deserve.

REFERENCES

1. Brennan TA, Leape LL, Laird NM, et al. Incidence of adverse events and negligence in hospitalized patients. Results of the Harvard Medical Practice Study I. N Engl J Med 1991;324(6):370–6.
2. Leape LL. Error in medicine. JAMA 1994;272(23): 1851–7.
3. Kohn LT, Janet CJ, Donaldson MS. To err is human: building a safer health system. Washington, DC: National Academy Press; 2000.
4. Wong JM, Bader AM, Laws ER, et al. Patterns in neurosurgical adverse events and proposed strategies for reduction. Neurosurg Focus 2012;33(5):E1.
5. Wong JM, Panchmatia JR, Ziewacz JE, et al. Patterns in neurosurgical adverse events: intracranial neoplasm surgery. Neurosurg Focus 2012;33(5): E16.
6. Wong JM, Ziewacz JE, Ho AL, et al. Patterns in neurosurgical adverse events: cerebrospinal fluid shunt surgery. Neurosurg Focus 2012;33(5):E13.
7. Wong JM, Ziewacz JE, Ho AL, et al. Patterns in neurosurgical adverse events: open cerebrovascular neurosurgery. Neurosurg Focus 2012;33(5):E15.
8. Wong JM, Ziewacz JE, Panchmatia JR, et al. Patterns in neurosurgical adverse events: endovascular neurosurgery. Neurosurg Focus 2012;33(5):E14.
9. Oremakinde AA, Bernstein M. A reduction in errors is associated with prospectively recording them. J Neurosurg 2014;121(2):297–304.
10. Stone S, Bernstein M. Prospective error recording in surgery: an analysis of 1108 elective neurosurgical cases. Neurosurgery 2007;60(6):1075–80 [discussion: 1080–2].
11. Berger MS, Wachter RM, Greysen SR, et al. Changing our culture to advance patient safety: the 2013 AANS Presidential Address. J Neurosurg 2013; 119(6):1359–69.
12. Pronovost P, Needham D, Berenholtz S, et al. An intervention to decrease catheter-related bloodstream infections in the ICU. N Engl J Med 2006; 355(26):2725–32.
13. Haynes AB, Weiser TG, Berry WR, et al. A surgical safety checklist to reduce morbidity and mortality in a global population. N Engl J Med 2009;360(5):491–9.
14. Lyons MK. Eight-year experience with a neurosurgical checklist. Am J Med Qual 2010;25(4):285–8.
15. Haynes AB, Weiser TG, Berry WR, et al. Changes in safety attitude and relationship to decreased postoperative morbidity and mortality following implementation of a checklist-based surgical safety intervention. BMJ Qual Saf 2011;20(1):102–7.
16. Sexton JB, Thomas EJ, Helmreich RL. Error, stress, and teamwork in medicine and aviation: cross sectional surveys. BMJ 2000;320(7237):745–9.
17. Lau CY, Greysen SR, Mistry RI, et al. Creating a culture of safety within operative neurosurgery: the design and implementation of a perioperative safety video. Neurosurg Focus 2012;33(5):E3.
18. Barker FG 2nd. Craniotomy for the resection of metastatic brain tumors in the U.S., 1988-2000: decreasing mortality and the effect of provider caseload. Cancer 2004;100(5):999–1007.
19. Barker FG 2nd, Amin-Hanjani S, Butler WE, et al. In-hospital mortality and morbidity after surgical treatment of unruptured intracranial aneurysms in the United States, 1996-2000: the effect of hospital and surgeon volume. Neurosurgery 2003;52(5): 995–1007 [discussion: 1007–9].
20. Barker FG 2nd, Curry WT Jr, Carter BS. Surgery for primary supratentorial brain tumors in the United

States, 1988 to 2000: the effect of provider caseload and centralization of care. Neuro Oncol 2005;7(1): 49–63.

21. Barker FG 2nd, Klibanski A, Swearingen B. Transsphenoidal surgery for pituitary tumors in the United States, 1996-2000: mortality, morbidity, and the effects of hospital and surgeon volume. J Clin Endocrinol Metab 2003;88(10):4709–19.

22. Curry WT, McDermott MW, Carter BS, et al. Craniotomy for meningioma in the United States between 1988 and 2000: decreasing rate of mortality and the effect of provider caseload. J Neurosurg 2005; 102(6):977–86.

23. Englot DJ, Ouyang D, Wang DD, et al. Relationship between hospital surgical volume, lobectomy rates, and adverse perioperative events at US epilepsy centers. J Neurosurg 2013;118(1):169–74.

24. Hoh BL, Rabinov JD, Pryor JC, et al. In-hospital morbidity and mortality after endovascular treatment of unruptured intracranial aneurysms in the United States, 1996-2000: effect of hospital and physician volume. AJNR Am J Neuroradiol 2003;24(7):1409–20.

25. Smith ER, Butler WE, Barker FG 2nd. Craniotomy for resection of pediatric brain tumors in the United States, 1988 to 2000: effects of provider caseloads and progressive centralization and specialization of care. Neurosurgery 2004;54(3):553–63 [discussion: 563–5].

26. Smith ER, Butler WE, Barker FG 2nd. In-hospital mortality rates after ventriculoperitoneal shunt procedures in the United States, 1998 to 2000: relation to hospital and surgeon volume of care. J Neurosurg 2004;100(2 Suppl Pediatrics):90–7.

27. Asher AL, McCormick PC, Selden NR, et al. The National Neurosurgery Quality and Outcomes Database and NeuroPoint Alliance: rationale, development, and implementation. Neurosurg Focus 2013;34(1):E2.

Errors in Neurosurgery

John D. Rolston, MD, PhD[a],*, Mark Bernstein, MD, MHSc[b]

KEYWORDS

- Medical error • Surgical error • Quality improvement • Patient safety • Wrong-sided surgery
- Sentinel event

KEY POINTS

- Medical errors are common and serious, leading to an estimated 440,000 deaths annually in the United States.
- For neurosurgery patients, prospective studies found errors in 25% to 85% of all cases.
- Only 25% of recorded errors are caused by surgical technique; most errors involve the whole health care team, highlighting the importance of systems thinking.
- A wide range of tools has been developed to help reduce the frequency and impact of errors, such as the World Health Organization's Surgical Safety Checklist, computerized order entry, and surgical navigation systems.

INTRODUCTION

Despite their training and intentions, health care workers will inevitably make mistakes when caring for patients. Some of these errors can be serious and life threatening, while others are near misses, identified early and fixed before they cause harm. Understanding the frequency and danger posed by medical errors, and offering strategies to prevent them, forms the basis of the modern patient safety movement.

Neurosurgery is far from immune to these errors. The complexity of neurosurgical patients and the interdisciplinary teams required to manage their conditions expose these patients to the same errors found in other medical and surgical specialties, along with errors unique to neurosurgery.

DEFINITION AND CLASSIFICATION OF ERRORS

Medical errors have been defined in various ways, but at their core, they are acts of omission or commission that cause harm or have the potential to cause harm to patients.[1,2] This definition was elaborated in the neurosurgical literature by Stone and Bernstein as any act of omission or commission resulting in deviation from a perfect course for the patient. A perfect course was defined as one in which nothing went wrong, from the smallest detail (such as dropping a sponge) to the most obvious example (that is, one that every neurosurgeon would easily recognize, like wrong-sided surgery).[3,4]

Importantly, patient safety studies differentiate errors from adverse events (**Fig. 1**), which are inadvertent injuries resulting from medical care, or the failure to deliver medical care.[5–7] Errors have the potential to cause harm, while adverse events are harm. In other words, errors can lead to adverse events if they are not caught first (ie, a near miss[8]), but adverse events can also occur without errors (ie, a nonpreventable adverse event, such as a hemorrhage following a perfectly executed external ventricular drain placement).

Disclosures: The authors have no conflicts of interest to disclose. J.D. Rolston was supported in part by a fellowship from the Congress of Neurological Surgeons.
[a] Department of Neurological Surgery, University of California, 505 Parnassus Avenue, M779, San Francisco, CA 94143-0112, USA; [b] Division of Neurosurgery, Toronto Western Hospital, University of Toronto, University Health Network, 399 Bathurst Street, 4W451, Toronto, Ontario M5T 2S8, Canada
* Corresponding author.
E-mail address: rolstonj@neurosurg.ucsf.edu

Neurosurg Clin N Am 26 (2015) 149–155
http://dx.doi.org/10.1016/j.nec.2014.11.011
1042-3680/15/$ – see front matter © 2015 Elsevier Inc. All rights reserved.

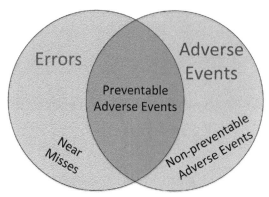

Fig. 1. Relationship of errors to adverse events. Errors are acts of omission or commission that cause harm or have the potential to cause harm to patients. Adverse events are inadvertent injuries resulting from medical care, or the failure to deliver medical care, and can be classified further as preventable or nonpreventable. Near misses are errors that are caught before they can cause injury to a patient.

Errors are further divided into active errors (or sharp-end errors) and latent errors (or blunt-end errors).[9] Active errors are the most recognizable, usually involving a frontline health care worker directly interacting with a patient, such as a surgeon injuring the carotid artery during an aneurysm clipping, or an anesthesiologist connecting the incorrect gas anesthetic, isoflurane in place of oxygen, to an anesthesia machine.[10] Latent errors, on the other hand, refer to errors within the system makeup itself (including bureaucracy, facilities, equipment, or organization) that permit other errors to occur. In the specific case of anesthesia gases noted previously, modern anesthesia machines have specialized connectors (the pin index safety system) that allow only the correct gas cylinder to be hooked up (eg, only oxygen canisters can link to the oxygen intake), which have almost eliminated this type of error.[11]

Active errors are frequently studied in psychology, and classifications have been proposed to subdivide errors and identify common error-generating mechanisms. Perhaps the best known is James Reason's classification of active errors into slips and mistakes.[12] Slips occur when planned actions are not executed correctly—as in literally slipping with a scalpel. Mistakes occur when an incorrect action is selected, even if executed perfectly, such as wrong-sided surgery.

An example of a more complex classification of errors is the National Coordinating Council (NCC) for Medication Error Reporting and Prevention, which separates errors into 9 classes (A through I) according to how much harm was caused, where class A is no error and class I is an error potentially contributing to a patient's death.[9] Notably, the NCC classification divides errors by their effects; Reason's classification divides errors by their mechanisms.

EPIDEMIOLOGY OF ERRORS

The modern patient safety movement arguably began with the publication of the Institute of Medicine's (IOM's) *To Err is Human*, in 1999.[9,13] This study, relying on the Harvard Medical Practice Study,[7] estimated that between 44,000 and 98,000 Americans were killed each year by medical errors.[13] This figure led to the alarming jumbo jet comparison, where the number of deaths caused by medical errors was likened to 1 passenger jet crashing daily.[9] The mortality estimates from the IOM's report have since been revised still higher, with up to 440,000 deaths caused by medical errors per year.[14] The conservative economic cost of such errors is estimated at $17 billion to $29 billion.[15]

Errors affect all aspects of the medical system, from medication administration to surgical procedures. In the perioperative period, an estimated 3% of patients suffer an adverse event, half of which are preventable.[16] Over 14% of neurosurgical patients, in particular, suffer one or more perioperative complications, many of which are preventable.[17] Wrong-side or wrong-patient procedures occur in roughly 1 case out of every 100,000 operations, and in 2.2 cases of every 10,000 craniotomies.[18] Surveys of neurosurgeons show that 25% of physicians have made an incision on the wrong side of the head, and 35% admitted to wrong-level lumbar surgery in their careers.[19] Unintentionally retained equipment (eg, instruments and sponges) mar about 1 of every 5500 to 10,000 operations.[9]

Only a few studies have analyzed errors specifically in neurosurgical patients. Stone and Bernstein reported on the prospective collection of error data in neurosurgery patients over a 7-year period from 2000 to 2006[4] and Oremakinde and Bernstein incorporated data from the prior study,[3] and reported their experience cataloging errors from 2000 to 2013, where all errors were prospectively logged by the senior author for 2082 of his cases.[3] Errors occurred in 85.3% of cases; 24.2% were due to contamination. Twenty-four percent were due to technical errors, and 22.4% equipment failure or missing equipment. The remainder were due to delays, nursing, anesthesia, or other sources[3]; 54.2% of these errors had no or minimal clinical significance.

Bostrom and colleagues[20] also prospectively cataloged errors from neurosurgical procedures and logged errors in 25% of 756 cases. Their classification showed that 37.3% of errors were caused by missing equipment or equipment failure; 33.1% were caused by errors in medical judgment or management, and 23.7% were technical or procedural errors.[20] In both this study and the study by Oremakinde and Bernstein,[3] American Society of Anesthesiologists (ASA) classification correlated with the presence of errors, and cranial cases had a higher proportion of errors than spinal cases. This increased error rate in cranial cases parallels data looking at raw complications in neurosurgical cases, including nonpreventable adverse events, and showing that cranial cases have higher morbidity.[17]

The economic burden of surgical errors is great. The National Practitioner Data Bank shows $1.3 billion in settlements alone between 1990 and 2010.[21] These data do not include the 90% of patients not receiving payments, but who still filed suit. Wrong-site surgeries have an average payout of $127,159, and retained foreign bodies average $86,247.[22] The number of these events seems to be increasing over time, despite changes in policies and practices, perhaps due to increased reporting.[23]

Neurosurgical patients are attended to by the complete health care system, exposing them to the full spectrum of medical errors, not just those directly related to surgery. Medication errors are well studied in medicine as a whole, and adverse drug events are unfortunately common; at least 5% of inpatients suffer at least 1 adverse drug event,[24] and roughly 5% of hospital admissions stem from adverse medication events.[9] Medication errors cost $16.4 billion yearly for hospitalized patients,[9,25] and $5 billion for outpatients.[26]

Infections are other harmful complications, and often are caused by errors. According to the Centers for Disease Control and Prevention (CDC), up to 10% of patients will suffer from an iatrogenic infection.[9,27] Deaths from iatrogenic infections number an estimated 100,000 annually.[9,27] The costs of iatrogenic infections are around $40 billion.[9,27] Again, neurosurgery patients suffer from these events as well, with 1.0% suffering a superficial surgical site infection, 1.5% developing postoperative pneumonia, and 2.3% developing a urinary tract infection.[17]

IDENTIFYING ERRORS

Before errors can be tracked, they must first be identified. Many strategies have been developed to accomplish this, with varying degrees of sensitivity and investment. The Global Trigger Tool uses a set of adverse events with a high probability of being associated with errors, like intraoperative deaths and unplanned returns to the operating room. When one of these events occurs (setting off the trigger), the case is flagged and manually analyzed for errors. The ability of the global trigger tool to detect errors is exquisite (94.9% sensitivity and 100% specificity), although the process requires a large investment of time and personnel to carry out, making it often impractical.[28]

Morbidity and mortality conferences are among the most common methods of monitoring errors in the neurosurgical field.[25,29,30] The costs are low, and the conferences are typically geared toward education. However, most errors are self-reported by the involved surgeon, and near misses are rarely presented. Physicians also tend to focus on their own performance and that of other individuals, rather than examining the system in which the error occurred.

Incident reports are the typically unstructured event summaries by doctors, nurses, and other health care workers via paper or computerized systems. These reports are not standardized, and different health care workers will have different thresholds for reporting errors. Further, these reports are predominantly driven by nursing and support staff, with unfortunately few physicians participating.[31]

Claims data, like that found in the Nationwide Inpatient Sample (NIS), and prospective registries, like the American College of Surgeons (ACS) National Surgical Quality Improvement Program (NSQIP),[32,33] National Neurosurgery Quality and Outcomes Database (N2QOD),[34] and the International Spine Study Group (ISSG),[35,36] are frequent sources of data for publications in the neurosurgical literature. They have contributed a great deal of information about complication and adverse event frequencies, but do not track errors specifically. That is, they do not specifically state whether the events they report were preventable or caused by human or system error. Furthermore, claims databases rely on data entered by staff not directly affiliated with the health care team (eg, billing and coding departments), which raises worries about inadequate or inaccurate data. These databases ultimately have high specificity (98.5%) but very low sensitivity (5.8%).[28]

STRATEGIES TO REDUCE ERRORS

One of the first steps in reducing errors relies on culture.[37] All team members must feel that it is acceptable and desirable to openly discuss and prospectively track errors.[3,4,20,37] This has not been a common practice in neurosurgery, but it is clearly the right thing to do. In fact, the prospective recording of error may actually be associated with their reduction over time due to a number of factors.[3] There is no financial barrier to changes in culture, and patients have proven to be open to conversations about errors.[38] Yet clearly there may remain hospital and societal barriers to widespread adoption of this approach of openness in discussing individual and institutional errors.

On a more widespread level, a patchwork of error prevention strategies has developed within medicine, and many are now being adopted by neurosurgical services. The use of checklists is one prominent example. The World Health Organization (WHO) created the Surgical Safety Checklist in 2007 to improve team communication and ensure key preoperative steps were conducted.[39,40] A multisite pilot of the WHO checklist found a 4% reduction in complications and 0.7% reduction in mortality.[39] Subsequently, many neurosurgical programs have adopted similar checklists and time out procedures,[3,41] and have reported a consequent reduction in wrong-site surgeries[42] and errors in general.[3] These improvements are critical for neurosurgery programs; neurosurgery is the third most likely specialty to perform a wrong-site or wrong-level surgery, after orthopedic and general surgery,[18] and most of these events appear to arise following breakdowns in communication.[18] Embracing checklist procedures appears to address some of these problems, and will almost certainly continue to be an integral part of surgical programs in the future.

Another prominent method for decreasing errors in medicine and surgery has been the engineering of new technologies to eliminate or reduce the chance of errors, like barcode-enabled medication administration,[43] the pin safety system for anesthesia gases,[11] and computerized order entry.[44] An example in neurosurgery is the widely adopted introduction of image-guided surgery, such as frameless stereotactic navigation systems[45] and intra-operative imaging[46] for cranial neurosurgery. Not only does image-guidance make the finding of brain lesions faster and safer, but important normal structures like venous sinuses can be accurately localized prior the creation of craniotomy bone cuts. Moreover, these technologies can help nearly eliminate the chance of wrong-sided surgery.

Other methods to reduce errors include the performance of select procedures in high-volume centers specializing in those procedures. There is an often-noted reduction of morbidity and mortality in centers with higher volumes of procedures compared with lower-volume centers, which is typically attributed to higher quality care and likely a reduced number of errors. Such volume-outcome

effects have been documented in aneurysm surgery,[47] carotid endarterectomy,[48] epilepsy surgery,[49] transsphenoidal surgery,[50] endovascular therapy,[51] and spine surgery.[52,53] Improvement in technical skills is well documented following repetitive performance. Surgeons performing laparoscopic cholecystectomies have a 1.7% chance of causing injuries during their first surgery, reduced to a 0.17% chance on their 50th surgery.[54] This is also seen in transforaminal lumbar interbody fusions,[55] skull base surgeries,[56] and transsphenoidal surgeries.[57] Yet the volume–outcome relationships are also likely due in part to procedure familiarity on behalf of the entire system—nurses, anesthesiologists, sterile processing departments, radiology, and others. All participants in a procedure contribute to patient safety, and all have learning curves.

ETHICAL ISSUES

There are 2 main ethical issues inherent in a discussion of errors: (1) the failure of modern health care—and neurosurgeons in particular—to embrace, discuss, and study errors in an effort to improve patient safety; and (2) the disclosure of errors to patients and their families.

Regarding the study of error, neurosurgeons have dedicated countless hours of work and financial expenditures in clinical and research activity to improve the outcome of every disease they treat. So why have they been so slow to discuss and study an issue that relates to the care of every single patient they treat, irrespective of disease? The main answers to this question are obvious and have been touched on previously. Gladly, this trend is changing, particularly over the last 20 years. It will generally not be considered unethical for a neurosurgeon or team to commit an error, since this is inherent in being human; however, it is unethical to not study and reduce errors and to put systems in place to prevent errors and to prevent committed errors from injuring the patient. The authors respectfully recommend that, at the individual level, every neurosurgeon should participate in some form of prospective error tracking, whether this is through a formalized registry, or simply a personal database kept by the physician. It is not enough to participate in departmental morbidity and mortality conferences. This engagement with tracking follows the tradition of many of the founders of surgery and neurosurgery, such as Codman's "end results" hospital[58] and Harvey Cushing's meticulous documentation of errors and adverse events.[59]

Regarding disclosure, it has become clear that from an ethical and legal perspective, immediate disclosure of error to a patient and family is imperative. It is clear that any reasonable person would want to know about the occurrence of an error that has injured the patient or has the potential to do so. Not only does this respect the patient's dignity and autonomy, but from a practical perspective, it is recognized that full and immediate disclosure of errors will likely decrease the chance of medicolegal action, or reduce the size of the financial settlement.[60] There are guidelines on how, when, and how much to disclose, and most hospitals have risk management teams to help guide clinicians.[61]

SUMMARY

Medical errors are common, dangerous, and an understudied component of neurosurgery. Depending on the report, they occur in anywhere from 25% to 85% of all neurosurgical cases. Importantly, only an estimated 25% of these errors are related to surgical technique. Most errors occur within the context of the complete health care system: nurses, physicians, technicians, administrators, and patients themselves. Fortunately, there is an increasing emphasis on quality improvement and patient safety in medicine that recognizes the importance of the health care team.

To best serve patients, there are several goals that must be accomplished. First, errors must be prospectively tracked, whether at the departmental[20] or individual level,[3,4] so that trends, predictors, and the efficacy of interventions can be studied. Second, the culture of neurosurgery needs to accommodate frank and open discussion of errors. Errors are inevitable in human-driven systems. If one can discuss errors openly, one can better seek ways to prevent them in the future.[9,37] Lastly, innovations must continuously be sought to mitigate and eliminate errors. Advances like stereotactic guidance, computerized order entry, and barcode medication administration are examples of indispensible tools used to engineer the safety of patients.

These goals of tracking, openness, and innovation are intertwined. Innovations to reduce or prevent errors must be tested empirically, which requires prospective analysis of errors. And prospective analysis requires a willingness to admit errors and a tolerance from the community when hearing about errors.

Ultimately, medical errors are a scourge on neurosurgical patients, as important as any particular disease. Just as there are cancer registries and clinical trials for brain tumors, medical error must be treated with the same seriousness. Eliminating errors, like eliminating cancer, often seems an impossible goal. But advances are steadily being made, and to truly care for patients, one cannot ignore these issues.

REFERENCES

1. Grober ED, Bohnen JM. Defining medical error. Can J Surg 2005;48:39–44.
2. Leape LL. Error in medicine. JAMA 1994;272:1851–7.
3. Oremakinde AA, Bernstein M. A reduction in errors is associated with prospectively recording them. J Neurosurg 2014;121(2):297–304.
4. Stone S, Bernstein M. Prospective error recording in surgery: an analysis of 1108 elective neurosurgical cases. Neurosurgery 2007;60:1075–80 [discussion: 1080–2].
5. Brennan TA, Hebert LE, Laird NM, et al. Hospital characteristics associated with adverse events and substandard care. JAMA 1991;265:3265–9.
6. Brennan TA, Leape LL. Adverse events, negligence in hospitalized patients: results from the Harvard Medical Practice Study. Perspect Healthc Risk Manage 1991;11:2–8.
7. Brennan TA, Leape LL, Laird NM, et al. Incidence of adverse events and negligence in hospitalized patients. Results of the Harvard Medical Practice Study I. N Engl J Med 1991;324:370–6.
8. Barach P, Small SD. Reporting and preventing medical mishaps: lessons from non-medical near miss reporting systems. BMJ 2000;320:759–63.
9. Wachter RM. Understanding patient safety. 2nd edition. New York: McGraw Hill Medical; 2012.
10. Petty WC. AANA journal course: update for nurse anesthetists—medical gases, hospital pipelines, and medical gas cylinders: how safe are they? AANA J 1995;63:307–24.
11. Dorsch JA, Dorsch SE. Understanding anesthesia equipment. 5th edition. Philadelphia: Wolters Kluwer Health/Lippincott Williams & Wilkins; 2008.
12. Reason JT. Human error. Cambridge (United Kingdom); New York: Cambridge University Press; 1990.
13. Kohn LT, Corrigan J, Donaldson MS. To err is human: building a safer health system. Washington, DC: National Academy Press; 2000.
14. James JT. A new, evidence-based estimate of patient harms associated with hospital care. J Patient Saf 2013;9:122–8.
15. Thomas EJ, Studdert DM, Newhouse JP, et al. Costs of medical injuries in Utah and Colorado. Inquiry 1999;36:255–64.
16. Thomas EJ, Studdert DM, Burstin HR, et al. Incidence and types of adverse events and negligent care in Utah and Colorado. Med Care 2000;38:261–71.
17. Rolston JD, Han SJ, Lau CY, et al. Frequency and predictors of complications in neurological surgery: national trends from 2006 to 2011. J Neurosurg 2014;120:736–45.

18. Cohen FL, Mendelsohn D, Bernstein M. Wrong-site craniotomy: analysis of 35 cases and systems for prevention. J Neurosurg 2010;113:461–73.

19. Jhawar BS, Mitsis D, Duggal N. Wrong-sided and wrong-level neurosurgery: a national survey. J Neurosurg Spine 2007;7:467–72.

20. Bostrom J, Yacoub A, Schramm J. Prospective collection and analysis of error data in a neurosurgical clinic. Clin Neurol Neurosurg 2010;112:314–9.

21. Mehtsun WT, Ibrahim AM, Diener-West M, et al. Surgical never events in the United States. Surgery 2013;153:465–72.

22. Mehtsun WT, Weatherspoon K, McElrath L, et al. Assessing the surgical and obstetrics–gynecology workload of medical officers: findings from 10 district hospitals in Ghana. Arch Surg 2012;147:542–8.

23. Rydrych D. Success in preventing wrong-site procedures in Minnesota with the Minnesota Time Out. Pennsylvania Patient Safety Advisory 2011;8:150–2.

24. Bates DW, Cullen DJ, Laird N, et al. Incidence of adverse drug events and potential adverse drug events. Implications for prevention. ADE Prevention Study Group. JAMA 1995;274:29–34.

25. National Priorities Partnership and National Quality Forum. Preventing Medication errors: A $21 billion opportunity. 2010. Available at: http://psnet.ahrq.gov/resource.aspx?resourceID=20529.

26. Berwick DM, Winickoff DE. The truth about doctors' handwriting: a prospective study. BMJ 1996;313:1657–8.

27. Scott, RD. The direct medical costs of healthcare-associated infections in U.S. hospitals and the benefits of prevention. Centers for Disease Control and Prevention, March 2009. Available at: http://www.cdc.gov/HAI/pdfs/hai/Scott_CostPaper.pdf.

28. Classen DC, Resar R, Griffin F, et al. 'Global trigger tool' shows that adverse events in hospitals may be ten times greater than previously measured. Health Aff 2011;30:581–9.

29. Seiler RW. Principles of the morbidity and mortality conference. Acta Neurochir Suppl 2001;78:125–6.

30. Houkin K, Baba T, Minamida Y, et al. Quantitative analysis of adverse events in neurosurgery. Neurosurgery 2009;65:587–94 [discussion: 594].

31. Wild D, Bradley EH. The gap between nurses and residents in a community hospital's error reporting system. Jt Comm J Qual Patient Saf 2005;31:2725–32.

32. Khuri SF, Daley J, Henderson W, et al. The Department of Veterans Affairs' NSQIP: the first national, validated, outcome-based, risk-adjusted, and peer-controlled program for the measurement and enhancement of the quality of surgical care. National VA surgical quality improvement program. Ann Surg 1998;228:491–507.

33. Khuri SF. The NSQIP: a new frontier in surgery. Surgery 2005;138:837–43.

34. McGirt MJ, Speroff T, Dittus RS, et al. The national neurosurgery quality and outcomes database (N2QOD): general overview and pilot-year project description. Neurosurg Focus 2013;34:E6.

35. Tang JA, Scheer JK, Smith JS, et al. The impact of standing regional cervical sagittal alignment on outcomes in posterior cervical fusion surgery. Neurosurgery 2012;71:662–9 [discussion: 669].

36. Schwab FJ, Blondel B, Bess S, et al. Radiographical spinopelvic parameters and disability in the setting of adult spinal deformity: a prospective multicenter analysis. Spine 2013;38:E803–12.

37. Berger MS, Wachter RM, Greysen SR, et al. Changing our culture to advance patient safety: the 2013 AANS Presidential Address. J Neurosurg 2013;119:1359–69.

38. Holliman D, Bernstein M. Patients' perception of error during craniotomy for brain tumour and their attitudes towards pre-operative discussion of error: a qualitative study. Br J Neurosurg 2012;26:326–30.

39. Haynes AB, Weiser TG, Berry WR, et al. A surgical safety checklist to reduce morbidity and mortality in a global population. N Engl J Med 2009;360:491–9.

40. Weiser TG, Haynes AB, Dziekan G, et al. Effect of a 19-item surgical safety checklist during urgent operations in a global patient population. Ann Surg 2010;251:976–80.

41. McLaughlin N, Winograd D, Chung HR, et al. University of California, Los Angeles, surgical time-out process: evolution, challenges, and future perspective. Neurosurg Focus 2012;33:E5.

42. Oszvald A, Vatter H, Byhahn C, et al. "Team time-out" and surgical safety—experiences in 12,390 neurosurgical patients. Neurosurg Focus 2012;33:E6.

43. Young J, Slebodnik M, Sands L. Bar code technology and medication administration error. J Patient Saf 2010;6:115–20.

44. Ammenwerth E, Schnell-Inderst P, Machan C, et al. The effect of electronic prescribing on medication errors and adverse drug events: a systematic review. J Am Med Inform Assoc 2008;15:585–600.

45. Sommer B, Grummich P, Hamer H, et al. Frameless stereotactic functional neuronavigation combined with intraoperative magnetic resonance imaging as a strategy in highly eloquent located tumors causing epilepsy. Stereotact Funct Neurosurg 2014;92:59–67.

46. Elhawary H, Liu H, Patel P, et al. Intraoperative real-time querying of white matter tracts during frameless stereotactic neuronavigation. Neurosurgery 2011;68:506–16 [discussion: 516].

47. Zacharia BE, Bruce SS, Carpenter AM, et al. Variability in outcome after elective cerebral aneurysm repair in high-volume academic medical centers. Stroke 2014;45:1447–52.

48. Cowan JA Jr, Dimick JB, Thompson BG, et al. Surgeon volume as an indicator of outcomes after carotid endarterectomy: an effect independent of specialty practice and hospital volume. J Am Coll Surg 2002;195:814–21.

49. Englot DJ, Ouyang D, Wang DD, et al. Relationship between hospital surgical volume, lobectomy rates, and adverse perioperative events at US epilepsy centers. J Neurosurg 2013;118:169–74.

50. Barker FG 2nd, Klibanski A, Swearingen B. Transsphenoidal surgery for pituitary tumors in the United States, 1996-2000: mortality, morbidity, and the effects of hospital and surgeon volume. J Clin Endocrinol Metab 2003;88:4709–19.

51. Brinjikji W, Rabinstein AA, Lanzino G, et al. Patient outcomes are better for unruptured cerebral aneurysms treated at centers that preferentially treat with endovascular coiling: a study of the national inpatient sample 2001-2007. AJNR Am J Neuroradiol 2011;32:1065–70.

52. Dasenbrock HH, Clarke MJ, Witham TF, et al. The impact of provider volume on the outcomes after surgery for lumbar spinal stenosis. Neurosurgery 2012;70:1346–53 [discussion: 1353–4].

53. Taylor HD, Dennis DA, Crane HS. Relationship between mortality rates and hospital patient volume for Medicare patients undergoing major orthopaedic surgery of the hip, knee, spine, and femur. J Arthroplasty 1997;12:235–42.

54. Moore MJ, Bennett CL. The learning curve for laparoscopic cholecystectomy. The Southern Surgeons Club. Am J Surg 1995;170:55–9.

55. Silva PS, Pereira P, Monteiro P, et al. Learning curve and complications of minimally invasive transforaminal lumbar interbody fusion. Neurosurg Focus 2013; 35:E7.

56. Wang AY, Wang JT, Dexter M, et al. The vestibular schwannoma surgery learning curve mapped by the cumulative summation test for learning curve. Otol Neurotol 2013;34:1469–75.

57. Chi F, Wang Y, Lin Y, et al. A learning curve of endoscopic transsphenoidal surgery for pituitary adenoma. J Craniofac Surg 2013;24:2064–7.

58. Kaska SC, Weinstein JN. Historical perspective. Ernest Amory Codman, 1869-1940. A pioneer of evidence-based medicine: the end result idea. Spine 1998;23: 629–33.

59. Latimer K, Pendleton C, Olivi A, et al. Harvey Cushing's open and thorough documentation of surgical mishaps at the dawn of neurologic surgery. Arch Surg 2011;146:226–32.

60. Kraman SS, Hamm G. Risk management: extreme honesty may be the best policy. Ann Intern Med 1999;131:963–7.

61. Bernstein M, Hebert PC, Etchells E. Patient safety in neurosurgery: detection of errors, prevention of errors, and disclosure of errors. Neurosurg Q 2003; 13:125–37.

Adverse Events in Neurosurgery and Their Relationship to Quality Improvement

John E. Ziewacz, MD, MPH*, Matthew J. McGirt, MD,
Samuel J. Chewning Jr, MD

KEYWORDS

- Adverse events • Neurosurgery • "Never events" • Quality improvement • N2QOD

KEY POINTS

- Adverse events in neurosurgery are common and their reporting is nonuniform and variable across reports and institutions; retrospective data tend to underestimate the rate of adverse events.
- The National Neurosurgery Quality and Outcomes Database (N2QOD) is a prospective, multi-institutional database in its pilot form that allows the generation of national normative data for outcomes and adverse events and allows for interinstitutional benchmarking.
- The results of primary research should be synthesized to guide the formation of standards and guidelines that can serve as the evidence basis for targeted quality improvement initiatives.
- Targeted quality improvement initiatives can reduce adverse events and improve outcomes; quality improvement initiatives differ based on the nature of the adverse event targeted and range from technical education to systems-based protocols and checklists.

INTRODUCTION

Adverse events are the sine qua non of quality improvement initiatives. They serve as the prime motivator behind systematic efforts to improve outcomes and to reduce error and associated harm. Adverse events in neurosurgery can be defined as both the unexpected perioperative complications as well as the anticipated neurologic or general deterioration related to surgical approach or other known causative factors. In addition to factors that result in actual harm to patients, it is also important to recognize those events that result in "near misses": events that are unexpected and/or dangerous, but that are caught in time or for various reasons do not result in patient harm. It is important to capture these events in any reporting because these "near misses" are often harbingers of actual patient harm if the proximate systemic causes continue without remedy. Furthermore, those events that are "expected" due to surgical approach, for instance, may still be targets of interventions that may reduce the rate of approach-related morbidity. Examples of this include awake craniotomy for lesions in eloquent cortex and minimally invasive approaches for certain pathologies of the spine.[1,2]

Avoiding, or mitigating the effects of adverse events, with resultant reduced harm and improved outcomes, requires multiple simultaneous efforts. These include defining adverse events, collecting standardized data, targeting systematic improvement initiatives, and studying the results of those initiatives, feeding back again to the collection of primary data. The field of neurosurgery has been

Carolina Neurosurgery and Spine Associates, 225 Baldwin Avenue, Charlotte, NC 28204, USA
* Corresponding author. 110 Lake Concord Road Northeast, Concord, NC 28025.
E-mail address: jziewacz@gmail.com

Neurosurg Clin N Am 26 (2015) 157–165
http://dx.doi.org/10.1016/j.nec.2014.11.014
1042-3680/15/$ – see front matter © 2015 Elsevier Inc. All rights reserved.

neurosurgery.theclinics.com

historically slow to adopt robust data collection of adverse events compared with general and cardiac surgery disciplines,[3,4] although this is rapidly changing. The collection of these data and the resultant benchmarking this allows is paramount to being able to target initiatives aimed at reducing adverse events. This article reviews the role of adverse events in neurosurgery in relation to their role in quality improvement, taking into account what is known of the patterns of adverse events, the collection of data related to adverse events, and current and future quality improvement initiatives aimed at reducing adverse events and subsequent patient harm.

ADVERSE EVENTS IN NEUROSURGERY: DATA COLLECTION

Any effort to reduce adverse events requires comprehensive data capturing such events. Historically, the broad collection of these data has been sparse. Additionally, it is important to capture patient-centered outcomes, as adverse events are materially related to these outcomes. This is particularly important because adverse events and complications in neurosurgery are not rare.[5] Previous work by Wong and colleagues[6-10] aimed at describing patterns of adverse events in 4 major realms of neurosurgery:

1. Intracranial neoplasm surgery
2. Cerebrospinal fluid shunt surgery
3. Open cerebrovascular neurosurgery
4. Endovascular neurosurgery

Reported adverse event rates for these subspecialties were common, and variable. Reported rates for the most common complications in these specialties, respectively, were (1) 9% to 40% for intracranial neoplasm surgery (all adverse events); (2) 8% to 64% for mechanical shunt malfunction and 3% to 12% shunt infection for cerebrospinal fluid shunt surgery; (3) 27% to 71% hemorrhage-related hyperglycemia for open cerebrovascular neurosurgery, with the estimated rate of new infarct associated with subarachnoid hemorrhage (SAH) being 40% and technical adverse events (eg, incomplete clipping or infarct due to major vessel occlusion) occurred 3% to 18% of the time; and (4) 2% to 61% for endovascular neurosurgery (all adverse events).[6-10] These data highlight a number of important features of adverse events in neurosurgery:

1. Adverse events are not rare.
2. Adverse events are variable between institutions and reports.

3. Adverse events differ between subspecialties and patient condition and can be categorized into technical adverse events and nontechnical adverse events.

These data demonstrating such variability between adverse event rates in differing reports likely represents both a true difference in occurrence rates among institutions and inconsistency in reporting. Factors influencing these differences include nonuniform definitions of adverse events, nonstandardized collection techniques, and retrospective collection of adverse event data.[11,12] Accordingly, other studies have demonstrated that prospective data collection aimed specifically at the collection of adverse events identify higher rates of adverse events than retrospective studies.[13-16] A prospective study of 942 consecutive patients undergoing major adult spinal surgery who were part of a cohort analyzed prospectively using an adverse event collection tool demonstrated that 87% of patients experienced at least one adverse event (including major and minor, surgical and medical), with 39% of those adversely impacting length of stay.[15] Before the introduction of the prospective adverse evaluation tool, the authors' documented perioperative morbidity rate had been 23%.[15] Similarly, a prospective study of 1000 consecutive pediatric neurosurgical procedures at a single institution focused on adverse events documented 229 complications in 202 procedures and an overall complication rate of 20.2%, with an unplanned return to the operating room occurring in 52% of procedures associated with an adverse event.[13] These data from prospective studies highlight the need for prospective data collection aimed specifically at identifying adverse events in the perioperative period. It is important for this data collection to be standardized across institutions to make an "apples-to-apples" comparison of adverse event rates and to therefore learn from institutions that are performing well in studied areas, and those that are performing poorly. In concert, overall outcomes data, which includes adverse event data, must be collected, as this will inform development of practice standards and guidelines that can function as the evidence basis for quality improvement initiatives aimed at reducing adverse events, the results of which can cycle back to inform further primary data collection (**Fig. 1**).

Historically, such concerted efforts at large-scale, interinstitutional data collection lagged in neurosurgery. Recently, however, organized neurosurgery has attempted to address this lack of standardized, prospectively collected outcomes data. The most comprehensive project to acquire this

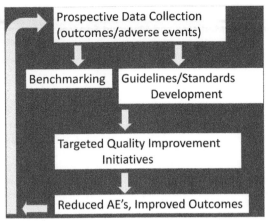

Fig. 1. Schematic diagram illustrating the cyclical relationship among data collection, benchmarking/standards development, and quality improvement initiatives aimed at decreasing adverse events and improving outcomes.

type of data is the National Neurosurgery Quality and Outcomes Database (N2QOD).[17]

NATIONAL NEUROSURGERY QUALITY AND OUTCOMES DATABASE

As a result of a shifting health care climate with increasing focus on the delivery of high-value care, the American Association of Neurologic Surgeons launched N2QOD with the accrual of patients beginning in Spring 2012.[18] N2QOD is a prospectively collected, multi-institutional data registry that in its current pilot stage collects perioperative data for 5 common lumbar degenerative disorders: (1) symptomatic lumbar disc herniation, (2) symptomatic recurrent lumbar disc herniation, (3) lumbar spondylolisthesis, (4) lumbar stenosis, and (5) lumbar adjacent segment disease. The initial goal of the pilot project is to prospectively collect data at both academic and private settings in a real-world practice environment. These data are currently collected by a full-time equivalent (FTE) data collector and include neurosurgically relevant perioperative risk factors for risk adjustment, standardized adverse event/complication profiles, occupational outcome, and validated patient outcomes measures (EuroQol-5D [EQ-5D], oswestry disability index [ODI], and numeric pain rating scale [NRS]).[18] The goal of the pilot is to establish initial risk-adjusted, validated data across institutions with 1-year follow-up. This allows for the development of national norms and allows for institutional benchmarking against these national norms. This variation between institutions then can be the starting point for examining proximate causes for the differences in

outcome and provide the basis for quality improvement initiatives aimed at improving outcomes and reducing adverse events, particularly for those institutions that are underperforming.

One of the main current drawbacks of N2QOD is that it includes only a subset of patients undergoing lumbar spine surgery, which is not representative of the entire neurosurgical patient population. However, the lumbar spine pilot is a "proof of principle" project in a common set of neurosurgical patients. If successful, the plan is to expand N2QOD to a cervical module and then a cranial module. A second potential challenge to N2QOD is that data collection requires an FTE data collector. This limits the ability of some institutions/neurosurgical practices to participate in N2QOD. One of the future goals is to identify non-FTE data extraction via automated electronic medical record (EMR) extraction and other means.[18] Although N2QOD is not without limitations, it represents the first large-scale, organized attempt at multi-institutional, validated, patient-centered outcomes data in neurosurgery, and is a step forward in providing the data necessary to improve outcomes and reduce adverse events.

"NEVER EVENTS" AND NEUROSURGERY

In 2006, in response to the 2005 Deficit Reduction Act, the Centers for Medicare and Medicaid Services (CMS) was tasked with identifying conditions that were either high cost, high volume, or both, that resulted in diagnosis-related groups that were more costly as a secondary diagnosis, and that were thought to reasonably be preventable by evidence-based practices.[19–21] CMS targeted serious reportable events, or "never events," originally described by the National Quality Forum as being a compilation of events that are "serious, largely preventable, and result in clinical harm."[22] Stemming from this work, CMS developed a list of hospital-acquired conditions (HACs) for which hospitals would no longer receive additional reimbursement if the conditions were not present on admission (**Box 1**).[19,20] This policy began in 2008 and since that time the list of HACs for which additional reimbursement would not be provided has undergone multiple iterations, with additions to the list on a frequent basis. **Box 1** includes the list of HACs for 2013, 2014, and 2015.

In addition to HACs for which CMS will not reimburse as secondary diagnoses, there are some "never events" for which CMS will not reimburse for a primary diagnosis. These include wrong site, wrong procedure, and wrong patient errors (WSPEs).[21] Importantly, these WSPEs include wrong-level spine operations.[21]

Box 1
Hospital-acquired conditions not covered by the Centers for Medicare and Medicaid Services as secondary diagnoses

- Foreign object retained after surgery
- Air embolism
- Blood incompatibility
- Stage III and IV pressure ulcers
- Falls and trauma
  - Fractures
  - Dislocations
  - Intracranial injuries
  - Crushing injuries
  - Burn
  - Other injuries
- Manifestations of poor glycemic control
  - Diabetic ketoacidosis
  - Nonketotic hyperosmolar coma
  - Hypoglycemic coma
  - Secondary diabetes with ketoacidosis
  - Secondary diabetes with hyperosmolarity
- Catheter-associated urinary tract infection
- Vascular catheter-associated infection
- Surgical site infection, mediastinitis, after coronary artery bypass graft
- Surgical site infection after bariatric surgery for obesity
  - Laparoscopic gastric bypass
  - Gastroenterostomy
  - Laparoscopic gastric restrictive surgery
- Surgical site infection after certain orthopedic procedures
  - Spine
  - Neck
  - Shoulder
  - Elbow
- Surgical site infection after cardiac implantable electronic device
- Deep vein thrombosis/pulmonary embolism after certain orthopedic procedures:
  - Total knee replacement
  - Hip replacement
- Iatrogenic pneumothorax with venous catheterization

From Centers for Medicare and Medicaid Services: hospital acquired conditions. Available at: http://www.cms.gov/Medicare/Medicare-Fee-for-Service-Payment/HospitalAcqCond/Hospital-Acquired_Conditions.html. Accessed August 29, 2014.

A review of surgical "never events" in the United States estimated that 4082 surgical never-event malpractice claims were registered every year and that malpractice payments for surgical never events between 1990 and 2010 totaled $1.3 billion.[23] Furthermore, rates of patient harm were high, with mortality occurring in 6.6% of patients, permanent injury in 32.9%, and temporary injury in 59.2%.[23]

An initial Agency for Healthcare Research and Quality–funded study of wrong-site surgery that included 2,826,367 nonspine operations found that 1 wrong-site operation occurred in every 112,994 operations, suggesting that most hospitals would experience a wrong-site surgery once in every 5 to 10 years.[21,24] Interestingly, the investigators noted that only 62% of cases would have been prevented by The Joint Commission Universal Protocol. However, it appears that in neurosurgery, wrong-site surgery is more frequent than this, particularly when including wrong-level spine surgeries, which importantly is included in non-reimbursed never events for primary diagnoses.[25]

Although the overall rate of all HACs in neurosurgical patients is unknown, recent work has begun to address HACs in the neurosurgical patient population. A single-institution study of HACs in a neurosurgical patient population comprising 1289 procedures found a 2% rate of HACs that were all wound infections.[26] Length of stay and readmission rates were significantly higher for those who experienced an HAC.[26] Importantly, nonpayment for rehospitalization and reoperation for HACs and nonreimbursement for index procedures resulted in significant reductions in reimbursement at this tertiary care institution.[26]

In 2 studies reporting the prevalence of patient safety indicators (PSI) and HACs in unruptured and ruptured aneurysm care demonstrated that for those who underwent treatment for unruptured cerebral aneurysms documented in the National Inpatient Sample between 2002 and 2010 (54,589 hospitalizations), PSIs or HACs were documented in 14.6% of patients who underwent surgical clipping (1492/8314) and 10.9% of those who underwent endovascular coiling (1353/9916).[27] For ruptured aneurysm treatment (62,972 hospitalizations for subarachnoid hemorrhage), patients who underwent clipping experienced a rate of PSI/HAC of 47.9% (6547/10,274) and those who underwent coiling experienced a rate of PSI/HAC of 51.0% (5623/8248).[28] These data are from an administrative database and it is possible that with prospectively collected data, rates could be even higher. Importantly, patient age and comorbidities are strong independent predictors of the occurrence of "never events" in cerebrovascular neurosurgery, suggesting that a focus on individual patient characteristics may be fruitful in reducing HACs and that risk adjustment for reimbursement schemes attached to HACs may be appropriate.[29] A study of HACs in intracranial neoplasm surgery found a 5.4% incidence in this sample of 310,133 patients undergoing surgical treatment for neoplasm.[30] In accordance with the results in cerebrovascular neurosurgery, medical comorbidities were significantly associated with the development of an HAC. Furthermore, those who experienced an HAC experienced a significantly higher in-hospital mortality rate and total hospital costs.[30] Those at urban teaching hospitals and hospitals with higher surgical volume experienced significantly more HACs than those at rural nonteaching hospitals or those with lower volume.[30] This may have profound consequences for patient treatment in light of the payment model linking HACs to reimbursement.

Specifically focusing on WSPEs, neurosurgery seems to have a relatively high rate compared with other specialties.[25,31] As compared with an initial study demonstrating a rate of wrong-site operation of 1 in 112,994, a national survey of neurosurgeons including 4695 lumbar surgeries, 2649 cervical surgeries, and 10,203 craniotomies noted that the incidence of wrong-level lumbar surgery, cervical spine surgery, and wrong-site craniotomy were 12.8 of 10,000, 7.6 of 10,000, and 2.0 of 10,000, respectively.[25] Associated factors were found to be surgeon fatigue, emergent operations, unusual time pressure, unusual anatomy, and failure to use radiography to verify the operative site.[25]

There are a number of factors that render wrong-site (wrong-level) surgery in the spine more likely than for other procedures.[32] Among these are similar anatomy of vertebral segments and anomalous vertebral anatomy, such as 6 lumbar vertebrae or variable rib anatomy.[33] Accordingly, studies of wrong-level surgery of the spine identify higher rates for wrong-site surgery than other specialities.[25,32,34] One survey study noted that almost 50% of spinal surgeon respondents had operated on the wrong level of the spine at least once in their careers, and the estimated prevalence of wrong-level spine surgery was 1 of 3110 procedures.[34] A second study also reiterated that nearly 50% of spine surgeons reported operating on the wrong level at least once, and more than 10% of surgeons had operated on the wrong side of the spine.[32] Additionally, 20% of reporting surgeons had been the subject of a wrong-level lawsuit.[32] The relatively high rates of wrong-level surgery indicate the unique challenges in spine surgery as opposed to other fields regarding WSPEs. Given the high costs in patient harm, financial expenses, and legal activity, concerted efforts must be made to reduce the rate of WSPEs in spinal surgery. Accordingly, multiple strategies have been proposed for reducing WSPEs in spinal surgery.[31,32,34–36] Among these include (1) The Joint Commission time out/universal protocol, (2) intraoperative imaging, (3) placement of fiducials preoperatively, particularly in the thoracic spine, (4) direct communication between the patient and surgeon preoperatively, (5) site marking, and (6) the use of surgical checklists.[31,32,34–36] There is some evidence that wrong-level surgery was reduced after introduction of The Joint Commission universal protocol[37]; however, it is noted that a significant number of wrong-level surgeries occur despite the universal protocol[32,38] and that strategies aimed at preventing wrong-level surgery are inconsistently adopted and applied.[32,34] Further research into the best practices for localization for spinal surgery is required, as well as studies tracking adherence to existing protocols, to reduce the rate of wrong-level spinal surgery.

STRATEGIES FOR REDUCING ADVERSE EVENTS IN NEUROSURGERY

Quality improvement initiatives aimed at reducing adverse events and improving outcomes in neurosurgery must focus on the specific types of adverse events and their root causes. Although there is considerable overlap, adverse events can be categorized into technical and nontechnical events. Examples of technical adverse events would include clipping a parent vessel during open aneurysm surgery or perforating the bowel during shunt surgery. These types of events are best addressed by efforts aimed at education, specialization, and regionalization. Indeed, there is evidence that some procedures, such as carotid endarterectomy and intracranial tumor surgery, are associated with lower complication and mortality rates when performed at higher-volume centers.[39–41] Coordinated efforts should be made to ensure that appropriate referrals for certain procedures are made to referral centers with high volumes and resources available to aid in preventing or mitigating adverse events. For certain subspecialties within neurosurgery, an effort toward certification of "centers of excellence" is being promoted to further regionalize and subspecialize care with the goal of improving outcomes.[42]

Other efforts to reduce technical error include increased subspecialization and fellowship training. Although further subspecialization and fellowship training at face value seem to be valuable in improving technical skill, particularly given the increasing breadth of neurosurgical procedures (e.g., scoliosis correction on one hand and endovascular neurosurgery on the other), there is a lack of evidence demonstrating improved outcomes owed to fellowship training. However, some evidence suggests that increasing subspecialization in surgery results in decreased technical complications.[43] Also, increased subspecialization may come at the cost of a loss of general knowledge and ability.

A further manner to address technical errors in neurosurgery is through simulation. Simulation is standard in other fields, such as aviation and nuclear power; however, it has been relatively underrepresented in medicine and neurosurgery. Initial studies of simulation aimed at improving performance in certain situations such as operating room crises have demonstrated favorable initial results. Participants noted the simulations were sufficiently authentic and perceived to be useful.[44,45] In neurosurgery, the use of simulation is in its infancy, although one study of a simulation curriculum including simulations with physical models, cadaver dissections, and haptic/computerized sessions demonstrated that junior and senior residents reported proficiency improvements and regarded simulation favorably.[46] A study of a haptic ventriculostomy simulator found that the simulation platform was realistic in terms of visual, tactile, and handling characteristics as judged by neurosurgical faculty and residents.[47] It is likely that as technology expands and the drive to maximize outcomes continues, simulation will play an important role in neurosurgical education, aimed at reducing technical adverse events.

Nontechnical adverse events, such as transfusing non–cross-matched blood, catheter-based urinary tract infections, and postoperative deep vein thrombosis/pulmonary embolism are typically the result of multiple individual and system-related errors, such as breakdowns in communication and failure to adhere to evidence-based practices. For these adverse events, a range of quality improvement tools may be used in an effort to reduce errors and improve outcomes. Momentum recently has focused on surgical checklists. After the publication of 2 seminal studies demonstrating significant reduction of morbidity and mortality in both developed and developing countries, surgical checklists have gained a foothold in surgery.[48,49] To date, their use in neurosurgery has been limited, but their use is increasing and initial results indicate favorable outcomes.[50–53] A by-product of checklist use is that it may improve team dynamics and communication, further reinforcing behaviors that are known to affect adverse events and patient outcome.[51,54,55]

Further quality improvement initiatives include targeted "plan-do-study-act" cycles, wherein iterative small-scale testing of evidence-based protocols or bundles is used to both study and refine quality improvement initiatives (**Fig. 2**). In these cycles, an evidence-based protocol is enacted after tailoring to a local environment, typically after a baseline data collection period. The protocol is then enacted and both outcomes and adherence are measured. A cyclical feedback loop is created

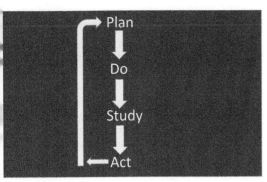

Fig. 2. Illustration of the "plan-do-study-act" cycle: a tool for implementation of quality improvement initiatives.

wherein collected data are analyzed and changes are instituted. New results are then analyzed and the cycle continues as adverse events decrease and outcomes improve.[56] Recently, evidence-based small-scale (ie, single-unit–based) interventions based on this concept have recently been enacted in neurosurgical settings and have demonstrated significant reductions in adverse events.[57,58]

SUMMARY

Adverse events are common in neurosurgery. Their causes are multifactorial and to date their study has been variable, largely retrospective, and uncoordinated. Recent efforts at rigorous, co-ordinated, nationwide prospective data collection will begin to provide the solid evidence basis for targeted quality improvement initiatives aimed at reducing adverse events and improving outcomes. This momentum to use quality improvement initiatives to reduce adverse events and improve outcomes will only gain in importance considering their relatively high incidence in neurosurgery and trends toward linking reimbursement and incentives to decreased adverse events and improved outcomes.

REFERENCES

1. Ibrahim GM, Bernstein M. Awake craniotomy for supratentorial gliomas: why, when and how? CNS Oncol 2012;1(1):71–83.
2. Barbagallo GM, Yoder E, Dettori JR, et al. Percutaneous minimally invasive versus open spine surgery in the treatment of fractures of the thoracolumbar junction: a comparative effectiveness review. Evid Based Spine Care J 2012;3(3):43–9.
3. Shahian DM, Jacobs JP, Edwards FH, et al. The Society of Thoracic Surgeons national database. Heart 2013;99(20):1494–501.
4. Rowell KS, Turrentine FE, Hutter MM, et al. Use of national surgical quality improvement program data as a catalyst for quality improvement. J Am Coll Surg 2007;204(6):1293–300.
5. Houkin K, Baba T, Minamida Y, et al. Quantitative analysis of adverse events in neurosurgery. Neurosurgery 2009;65(3):587–94.
6. Wong JM, Bader AM, Laws ER, et al. Patterns in neurosurgical adverse events and proposed strategies for reduction. Neurosurg Focus 2012;33(4):E1.
7. Wong JM, Panchmatia JR, Ziewacz JE, et al. Patterns in neurosurgical adverse events: intracranial neoplasm surgery. Neurosurg Focus 2012;33(5):E16.
8. Wong JM, Ziewacz JE, Ho AL, et al. Patterns in neurosurgical adverse events: cerebrospinal fluid shunt surgery. Neurosurg Focus 2012;33(5):E13.
9. Wong JM, Ziewacz JE, Ho AL, et al. Patterns in neurosurgical adverse events: open cerebrovascular neurosurgery. Neurosurg Focus 2012;33(5):E15.
10. Wong JM, Ziewacz JE, Panchmatia JR, et al. Patterns in neurosurgical adverse events: endovascular neurosurgery. Neurosurg Focus 2012;33(5):E14.
11. Lebude B, Yadla S, Albert T, et al. Defining "complications" in spine surgery: neurosurgery and orthopedic spine surgeons' survey. J Spinal Disord Tech 2010;23(8):493–500.
12. Landriel Ibanez FA, Hem S, Ajler P, et al. A new classification of complications in neurosurgery. World Neurosurg 2011;75(5–6):709–15.
13. van Lindert EJ, Delye H, Leonardo J. Prospective review of a single center's general pediatric neurosurgical intraoperative and postoperative complication rates. J Neurosurg Pediatr 2014;13(1):107–13.
14. Kelly AM, Batke JN, Dea N, et al. Prospective analysis of adverse events in surgical treatment of degenerative spondylolisthesis. Spine J 2014;14(12):2905–10.
15. Street JT, Lenehan BJ, DiPaola CP, et al. Morbidity and mortality of major adult spinal surgery. A prospective cohort analysis of 942 consecutive patients. Spine J 2012;12(1):22–34.
16. Dea N, Versteeg A, Fisher C, et al. Adverse events in emergency oncological spine surgery: a prospective analysis. J Neurosurg Spine 2014;21:698–703.
17. Neuropoint Alliance Projects. N2QOD: The National Neurosurgery Quality and Outcomes Database. Available at: http://www.neuropoint.org/NPA%20N2QOD.html. Accessed August 29, 2014.
18. McGirt MJ, Speroff T, Dittus RS, et al. The National Neurosurgery Quality and Outcomes Database (N2QOD): general overview and pilot-year project description. Neurosurg Focus 2013;34(1):E6.
19. Sand H, Owen M, Amin A. CMS' hospital-acquired conditions for the neurohospitalist. Neurohospitalist 2012;2(1):18–27.

20. Centers for Medicare and Medicaid Services: Hospital acquired conditions. Available at: http://www.cms.gov/Medicare/Medicare-Fee-for-Service-Payment/HospitalAcqCond/Hospital-Acquired_Conditions.html. Accessed August 29, 2014.

21. AHRQ Patient Safety Network: Wrong site, wrong procedure, and wrong patient surgery. Available at: http://psnet.ahrq.gov/primer.aspx?primerID=18. Accessed August 29, 2014.

22. National Quality Forum. Serious reportable events. Available at: http://www.qualityforum.org/Topics/SREs/Serious_Reportable_Events.aspx. Accessed August 29, 2014.

23. Mehtsun WT, Ibrahim AM, Diener-West M, et al. Surgical never events in the United States. Surgery 2013;153(4):465–72.

24. Kwaan MR, Studdert DM, Zinner MJ, et al. Incidence, patterns, and prevention of wrong-site surgery. Arch Surg 2006;141(4):353–7 [discussion: 357–8].

25. Jhawar BS, Mitsis D, Duggal N. Wrong-sided and wrong-level neurosurgery: a national survey. J Neurosurg Spine 2007;7(5):467–72.

26. Teufack SG, Campbell P, Jabbour P, et al. Potential financial impact of restriction in "never event" and periprocedural hospital-acquired condition reimbursement at a tertiary neurosurgical center: a single-institution prospective study. J Neurosurg 2010;112(2):249–56.

27. Fargen KM, Rahman M, Neal D, et al. Prevalence of patient safety indicators and hospital-acquired conditions in those treated for unruptured cerebral aneurysms: establishing standard performance measures using the Nationwide Inpatient Sample database. J Neurosurg 2013;119(4):966–73.

28. Fargen KM, Neal D, Rahman M, et al. The prevalence of patient safety indicators and hospital-acquired conditions in patients with ruptured cerebral aneurysms: establishing standard performance measures using the Nationwide Inpatient Sample database. J Neurosurg 2013;119(6):1633–40.

29. Wen T, He S, Attenello F, et al. The impact of patient age and comorbidities on the occurrence of "never events" in cerebrovascular surgery: an analysis of the Nationwide Inpatient Sample. J Neurosurg 2014;121:580–6.

30. Zacharia BE, Deibert C, Gupta G, et al. Incidence, cost, and mortality associated with hospital-acquired conditions after resection of cranial neoplasms. Neurosurgery 2014;74(6):638–47.

31. Neily J, Mills PD, Eldridge N, et al. Incorrect surgical procedures within and outside of the operating room: a follow-up report. Arch Surg 2011;146(11):1235–9.

32. Groff MW, Heller JE, Potts EA, et al. A survey-based study of wrong-level lumbar spine surgery: the scope of the problem and current practices in place to help avoid these errors. World Neurosurg 2013;79(3–4):585–92.

33. Hsu W, Kretzer RM, Dorsi MJ, et al. Strategies to avoid wrong-site surgery during spinal procedures. Neurosurg Focus 2011;31(4):E5.

34. Mody MG, Nourbakhsh A, Stahl DL, et al. The prevalence of wrong level surgery among spine surgeons. Spine (Phila Pa 1976) 2008;33(2):194–8.

35. Devine J, Chutkan N, Norvell DC, et al. Avoiding wrong site surgery: a systematic review. Spine (Phila Pa 1976) 2010;35(9 Suppl):S28–36.

36. Mayer JE, Dang RP, Duarte Prieto GF, et al. Analysis of the techniques for thoracic- and lumbar-level localization during posterior spine surgery and the occurrence of wrong-level surgery: results from a national survey. Spine J 2014;14(5):741–8.

37. Vachhani JA, Klopfenstein JD. Incidence of neurosurgical wrong-site surgery before and after implementation of the universal protocol. Neurosurgery 2013;72(4):590–5.

38. Longo UG, Loppini M, Romeo G, et al. Errors of level in spinal surgery: an evidence-based systematic review. J Bone Joint Surg Br 2012;94(11):1546–50.

39. Cowan JA, Dimick JB, Leveque JC, et al. The impact of provider volume on mortality after intracranial tumor resection. Neurosurgery 2003;52(1):48–54.

40. Curry WT, McDermott MW, Carter BS, et al. Craniotomy for meningioma in the United States between 1988 and 2000: decreasing rate of mortality and the effect of provider caseload. J Neurosurg 2005;102(6):977–86.

41. Hannam JA, Glass L, Kwon J, et al. A prospective, observational study of the effects of implementation strategy on compliance with a surgical safety checklist. BMJ Qual Saf 2013;22(11):940–7.

42. McLaughlin N, Laws ER, Oyesiku NM, et al. Pituitary centers of excellence. Neurosurgery 2012;71(5):916–24 [discussion: 924–6].

43. Howell AM, Panesar SS, Burns EM, et al. Reducing the burden of surgical harm: a systematic review of the interventions used to reduce adverse events in surgery. Ann Surg 2014;259(4):630–41.

44. Ziewacz JE, Arriaga AF, Bader AM, et al. Crisis checklists for the operating room: development and pilot testing. J Am Coll Surg 2011;213(2):212–7.

45. Arriaga AF, Bader AM, Wong JM, et al. Simulation-based trial of surgical-crisis checklists. N Engl J Med 2013;368(3):247–53.

46. Gasco J, Holbrook TJ, Patel A, et al. Neurosurgery simulation in residency training: feasibility, cost, and educational benefit. Neurosurgery 2013;73(Suppl 1):39–45.

47. Lemole GM Jr, Banerjee PP, Luciano C, et al. Virtual reality in neurosurgical education: part-task ventriculostomy simulation with dynamic visual and haptic feedback. Neurosurgery 2007;61(1):142–8.

48. Haynes AB, Weiser TG, Berry WR, et al. A surgical safety checklist to reduce morbidity and mortality in a global population. N Engl J Med 2009;360(5): 491–9.

49. de Vries EN, Prins HA, Crolla RM, et al. Effect of a comprehensive surgical safety system on patient outcomes. N Engl J Med 2010;363(20):1928–37.

50. Da Silva-Freitas R, Martin-Laez R, Madrazo-Leal CB, et al. Establishment of a modified surgical safety checklist for the neurosurgical patient: initial experience in 400 cases. Neurocirugia (Astur) 2012;23(2): 60–9.

51. Oszvald A, Vatter H, Byhahn C, et al. "Team time-out" and surgical safety-experiences in 12,390 neurosurgical patients. Neurosurg Focus 2012;33(5):E6.

52. McConnell DJ, Fargen KM, Mocco J. Surgical checklists: a detailed review of their emergence, development, and relevance to neurosurgical practice. Surg Neurol Int 2012;3:2.

53. Fargen KM, Velat GJ, Lawson MF, et al. Enhanced staff communication and reduced near-miss errors with a neurointerventional procedural checklist. J Neurointerv Surg 2013;5(5):497–500.

54. Lepanluoma M, Takala R, Kotkansalo A, et al. Surgical safety checklist is associated with improved operating room safety culture, reduced wound complications, and unplanned readmissions in a pilot study in neurosurgery. Scand J Surg 2014;103(1): 66–72.

55. Lau CY, Greysen SR, Mistry RI, et al. Creating a culture of safety within operative neurosurgery: the design and implementation of a perioperative safety video. Neurosurg Focus 2012;33(5):E3.

56. Plesk E. Quality improvement methods in clinical medicine. Pediatrics 1999;103(1 Suppl E):203–14.

57. Titsworth WL, Hester J, Correia T, et al. Reduction of catheter-associated urinary tract infections among patients in a neurological intensive care unit: a single institution's success. J Neurosurg 2012;116(4):911–20.

58. Titsworth WL, Hester J, Correia T, et al. The effect of increased mobility on morbidity in the neurointensive care unit. J Neurosurg 2012;116(6):1379–88.

The Relationship Between National Health Care Policies and Quality Improvement in Neurosurgery

CrossMark

Rachel Groman, MPH

KEYWORDS

• Quality • Value • Mandate • Measure • Federal • Legislation

KEY POINTS

- Physicians face an unprecedented level of accountability for factors often outside their control and of questionable significance.
- Neurosurgeons and other largely hospital-based specialties face pressure to comply with often overlapping and conflicting federal mandates on multiple fronts.
- Rapid implementation of these programs has resulted in misguided strategies and, in many cases, may be causing more harm than good.
- It is critical that policy makers first establish the data infrastructure needed to most accurately identify and most appropriately target gaps in care.

INTRODUCTION

As US policymakers continue to grapple with unacceptable rates of medical errors, unsubstantiated variations in practice patterns, and potentially avoidable spending, physicians are finding themselves in the center of a perfect storm. Today's physician faces not only multiple, often conflicting, regulatory requirements that interfere with the daily practice of medicine but also an unprecedented level of accountability for factors often outside their control and of questionable significance. These misguided mandates, aimed at improving US health care system performance, have produced little evidence to date of actually raising the bar on anything but confusion and frustration.

Despite significant financial investments, the United States remains one of the least efficient health care delivery systems in the developed world.[1,2] US physicians also have one of the lowest rates of job satisfaction.[3] Frustrations are likely to increase as patient-centered care is further eroded, and physicians are forced to divert an increasing portion of their attention to administrative compliance with one-size-fits-all care mandates.

Although many reforms are being implemented in the private sector and at the local and state level, most are driven by policies enacted at the federal level. Recent federal regulatory actions have shepherded in a new era of health care delivery and payment reforms that has fundamentally restructured incentives and revolutionized information sources that drive clinical decision making. These reforms were heavily influenced by the findings of the Institute of Medicine,[4,5] which not only identified dramatic deficiencies in the quality of US health care, but demanded that the nation aggressively address these problems.

As early as 2006, President Bush issued an executive order "to ensure that health care programs

Clinical Affairs and Quality Improvement, Hart Health Strategies, Inc, 310 North Pinckney Street, Madison, WI 53703, USA
E-mail address: rgroman@hhs.com

Neurosurg Clin N Am 26 (2015) 167–175
http://dx.doi.org/10.1016/j.nec.2014.11.006
1042-3680/15/$ – see front matter © 2015 Elsevier Inc. All rights reserved.

administered or sponsored by the Federal Government promote quality and efficient delivery of health care through the use of health information technology, transparency regarding health care quality and price, and better incentives for program beneficiaries, enrollees, and providers."[6] The Tax Relief and Health Care Act of 2006 was enacted soon after, establishing the Physician Quality Reporting Initiative (now known as the Physician Quality Reporting System or PQRS). The Medicare Improvements for Patients and Providers Act of 2008 made the PQRS a permanent feature of the Medicare program and authorized financial incentives and penalties for electronic prescribing. The groundbreaking American Reinvestment and Recovery Act of 2009, which included the Health Information Technology for Economic and Clinical Health (HITECH) Act, subsequently authorized a more than $19 billion investment in the nation's health information technology (HIT) infrastructure and federal incentives to encourage physicians and hospitals to use HIT in a meaningful manner. The Patient Protection and Affordable Care Act (ACA) of 2010 went one step further by transforming these largely voluntary, incentive-only initiatives into mandates with increasing penalties. The ACA also heavily emphasized value over volume, holding health care providers accountable for not only the quality of their care, but their ability to control costs.

DISCUSSION

Whether in private practice or academics, part of a large integrated system, or largely independent, few neurosurgeons will remain untouched by these increasingly complex and punitive policies. Those policies and programs most likely to have impacted the daily practice of neurosurgeons recently or in the coming years are summarized below.

Hospital Inpatient Quality Reporting Program

Under the Hospital Inpatient Quality Reporting (IQR) Program, originally mandated under the Medicare Prescription Drug, Improvement, and Modernization Act of 2003, hospitals that do not successfully report to the Centers for Medicare and Medicaid Services (CMS) on a designated set of quality measures will see a reduction in their annual payment increase.

The Hospital IQR Program measure set has grown from a starter set of 10 quality measures to a set of more than 60 measures for the fiscal year (FY) 2017 payment determination. These measures include both chart-abstracted and claims-based clinical process of care measures,

including 8 new stroke measures and 8 venous thromboembolism measures; outcomes measures focusing on mortality, surgical complications, health care–associated infections, and readmissions; survey-based patient experience measures; cost measures that evaluate all Medicare Part A and B spending on specific episodes (eg, pneumonia and heart failure) and broader episodes spanning 3 days before admission to 30 days before discharge; and structural measures that assess features of hospitals to assess their capacity to improve quality of care, such as participation in a clinical data registry.

Starting with the FY 2015 payment determination, the penalty for the Hospital IQR will increase to one-quarter of a hospital's annual payment update. As a result of growing penalties and separate efforts to further tie hospital payment to performance on a subset of these measures (described below), neurosurgeons and other largely hospital-based specialists have likely experienced a recent surge in institutional pressure to comply with these metrics.

Hospital Value-Based Purchasing Program

Expanding on the IQR, the Hospital Value-Based Purchasing Program (VBP), a separate ACA-authorized program, redistributes reductions made to hospitals' Medicare Diagnosis-Related Group payments based on a hospital's performance on a subset of the IQR measures. In FY 2015, hospitals stand to lose up to 1.5% of their Medicare diagnosis-related group payments under this program and up to 2.0% by FY 2017. To date, more hospitals have received penalties than bonuses, and the average penalty amount continues to increase.[7]

For FY 2015, 20% of a hospital's performance score will be based on clinical processes of care, such as removing urinary catheters from surgery patients within 2 days and administering prophylactic antibiotics within 1 hour before surgery to decrease the risk of infection. Thirty percent of a hospital's performance score will be based on patient satisfaction, such as whether the physicians and nurses communicated well. Another 30% will be based on outcomes, including mortality rates for heart attacks, heart failure, or pneumonia that occurred in the hospital or within a month after discharge, as well as select hospital-acquired infections, such as central line–associated blood stream infections. The remaining 20% will be based on how well a hospital manages costs for each admission from the 3 days before each admission to 30 days after discharge. Because post–acute care spending in the first 30 days after discharge costs Medicare just as much as the initial inpatient episode, and is one of the fastest growing categories of Medicare spending,[8] hospital-based physicians will experience unprecedented pressure to more effectively manage the post–acute care of each patient.

Although the inpatient setting is the guinea pig of federal value-based payment reforms, the ACA calls for similar programs for physicians, skilled nursing facilities, home health agencies, and ambulatory surgical centers.

Readmission Reduction Program

Also authorized under the ACA, this program reduces Medicare payments that would have otherwise been paid to hospitals to account for excess (ie, preventable) hospital readmissions. The Readmission Reduction penalty comes on top of the VBP and other hospital-based payment cuts described below.

Over the last 2 years, this program has resulted in a two-thirds reduction in payments to hospitals. Recently released data regarding the third year, in which up to 3.0% of a hospital's Medicare payments are at risk for excess readmissions, revealed that Medicare is fining a record number of hospitals, or 2,610, which is 433 more than last year and represents more than three-quarters of hospitals eligible for the program. Even though the nation's readmission rate is decreasing, Medicare's average fines will be higher, with 39 hospitals receiving the largest penalty allowed.[9] Part of this has to do with the fact that in FY 2015, the number of conditions on which the assessment is based—originally heart attack, heart failure, and pneumonia—has been expanded to include readmissions related to chronic obstructive pulmonary disease and total hip and knee replacement.

The program has been widely criticized, most notably for insufficient mechanisms to adjust for patient case mix and patient noncompliance with discharge orders. The Medicare Payment Advisory Commission, in particular, has recommended changes in the way this penalty is calculated and the method for adjusting readmission rates based on socioeconomic factors.[10] The program also fails to reward hospitals with lower-than-average readmission rates or those that made improvements over time.

Hospital-Acquired Condition Reduction Program

Although hospitals are already held accountable for specific hospital-acquired conditions (HACs) under the Hospital VBP Program, the ACA mandates the implementation of a separate HAC reduction penalty program that takes an additional 1.0% of payments away from hospitals with the most patients who suffered injury or infection during their stay. This program begins with October 1, 2014 discharges and affects FY 2015 hospital payment adjustments. One-quarter of hospitals deemed to have the worst performance with regard to HACs will automatically see a reduction in inpatient payments. Measures focus on central line–associated blood stream infection rates, catheter-associated urinary tract infection rates, and a composite of other measures that includes postoperative pulmonary embolism and deep vein thrombosis rates, wound dehiscence rates, and accidental puncture and laceration rates. Like the Readmission Reduction Program, these penalties come on top of other federal quality mandates, and there is no credit for improvement over time.

Under a separate and seemingly duplicative program known as the Hospital-Acquired Conditions/Present on Admission (POA) Reporting Program, which was authorized under the Deficit Reduction Act of 2005, since 2007 hospitals have been required to submit information on Medicare claims specifying whether diagnoses were POA. Starting with 2008 discharges, hospitals no longer receive payment for secondary diagnoses—such as vascular catheter-associated infections, surgical site infections, and deep vein thromboses—that were not POA.

Since 2009, CMS also has used Medicare National Coverage Determinations to target serious and largely preventable "never events." As a result of these policies, Medicare no longer pays hospitals for what it characterizes as wrong procedures, correct procedures on the wrong body part, and correct procedures on the wrong patient.

Physician Quality Reporting System

Although neurosurgeons may feel indirect pressure from their institutions as a result of these hospital-level quality initiatives, they also face a handful of physician-level mandates that will more directly impact reimbursement and care delivery. These programs are not only adding to the administrative burden of compliance, but they are also placing a growing portion of Medicare Part B payments at risk.

Most notable is the PQRS. Since 2007, the PQRS has been a voluntary reporting program, offering only Medicare incentive payments to physicians who reported quality measure data to CMS. However, the ACA phases out these incentives and replaces them with penalties, essentially making the program a mandate. Starting with the 2015 reporting year, physicians who fail to satisfy PQRS reporting requirements will lose 2.0% of their total annual Medicare Part B payments. Also starting in 2015, select physicians will be subject to additional payment adjustments based partially on PQRS measure performance as described below. Simultaneously, CMS has rapidly upped the ante for successful reporting in ways that limit meaningful participation for many specialists. Doubt about the value of the measures and the ability of this program to have a positive impact on quality, as well as frustration over constantly changing and cumbersome reporting requirements, have kept participation among physicians relatively low.

In the most current data available (2012), only 36% of all eligible professionals participated in the PQRS. The number was only slightly higher within neurosurgery, with participation rates at 40% of all eligible neurosurgeons.[11] Although physicians traditionally have had the luxury of deciding whether the cost and burden of PQRS participation outweighed any benefit, impending penalties and broadening implications of PQRS compliance will make this decision much more challenging going forward.

Physician Value-Based Payment Modifier

Keeping with the theme of value-based purchasing, the ACA also requires CMS to adjust Medicare physician payments based on quality and cost measure performance. CMS is required to apply a value-based payment modifier (VBM) to select physicians by 2015, based on 2013 reporting, and to all physicians by 2017, based on 2015 reporting. With its discretionary authority, CMS has opted to apply the modifier rapidly, holding group practices with 100 or more eligible professionals accountable in the first year and quickly transitioning to group practices with 10 or more eligible professionals in the second year. CMS also has chosen to double the penalty every year. Although group practices with 100 or more eligible professionals are subject to a 1.0% penalty in 2015, smaller practices and solo practitioners may be subject to a penalty as high as 4.0% in 2017 (as proposed in the 2015 Medicare Physician Fee Schedule proposed rule, pending finalization).

Concern over the rapid and arbitrary application of penalties is heightened by the program's reliance on measures that are often meaningless to specialists. In terms of quality, performance-based payment adjustments are based largely on PQRS measures reported by physicians, which as described in more detail below, are often poor indicators of quality. In terms of cost, CMS

continues to rely on broad-based cost measures (such as total per capita cost measures and the Medicare spending per beneficiary measure, similar to those used in the inpatient hospital quality reporting programs), which assess the total amount billed per patient and not the cost of the specific care provided by the individual physician. CMS claims that it relies on these measures for lack of a better available alternative but continues to work to develop more specifically defined episode-based cost measures that evaluate resource use related to specific diagnoses or procedures, including lumbar fusions.

Electronic Health Record Incentive Program (Meaningful Use)

The HITECH Act provides more than $19 billion in federal dollars to encourage the use of Electronic Health Records (EHR) among health professionals and to build the nation's HIT infrastructure. Since 2011, CMS has provided incentive payments to physicians and hospitals that proved to be meaningful users of federally certified EHR technology. However, 2014 marks the last year that incentives are available under this program. Starting in 2015, this traditionally voluntary program becomes a mandate as physicians and hospitals that fail to comply with meaningful use face reductions in their overall Medicare reimbursement starting at 1.0% and increasing to as high as 5.0% by 2020.

To satisfy meaningful use, a physician must demonstrate that he or she is using certified EHR technology to meet specific quality objectives and to report on specific clinical quality measures. Over time, physicians and hospitals must comply with higher stages of meaningful use, showing that the EHR is not only used for simple data capture and sharing but for increasingly advanced clinical processes, more rigorous information exchange (including sharing data with patients), and eventually improved outcomes.

As of 2013, more than 50% of eligible professionals (mostly physicians) and more than 80% of hospitals have demonstrated meaningful use[12] and have received more than $16 billion in incentive payments.[13]

Recent surveys of physicians have found that EHRs fail to support efficient and effective clinical workflows[14] and have actually worsened physician satisfaction. Although physicians find value in the ability of EHRs to provide data and perform certain analytics, they also find that in their current state, they are typically not cost effective, do not support care coordination, and do not save time.[15]

The EHR Incentive Program itself also has been widely criticized as relying on core requirements that are not relevant to specialists, containing confusing and constantly changing requirements that are challenging to keep up with and do not align with other quality reporting programs, and having metrics that are outside the control of physicians, such as whether patients accessed their medical records. Furthermore, weak federal certification standards often fail to ensure that EHR vendor products can be used in a meaningful manner to satisfy program requirements.

Center for Medicare and Medicaid Innovation

Alongside these more targeted reforms, the ACA also authorized the creation of a new Center for Medicare and Medicaid Innovation, (CMMI) which was allocated $10 billion over 10 years to test and evaluate different payment structures and methodologies to reduce program expenditures in Medicare and Medicaid while maintaining or improving quality of care. Models that improve quality and reduce the rate of cost growth could be expanded and made a permanent feature of these federal programs.

In 2013, the Congressional Budget Office released a report concluding that CMS's demonstrations aimed at enhancing the quality of health care and improving the efficiency of health care delivery in Medicare's fee-for-service programs have not reduced Medicare spending. In nearly every program involving disease management and care coordination, spending was either unchanged or increased relative to the spending that would have occurred in the absence of the program when the fees paid to the participating organizations were considered. Despite these concerns, Center for Medicare and Medicaid Innovation initiatives are moving forward full speed, although some in Congress are pressing for more oversight and details about funded projects.

Alongside the Innovation Center, the ACA mandated the testing of other innovative Bundled Payments for Care Improvement Initiative, a pilot to test 4 different models that link payments for multiple services that beneficiaries receive during an episode of care. It also created the Shared Savings Program, which recognizes accountable care organizations (ACOs) or networks of providers that share financial and medical responsibility for providing coordinated care in the hopes of limiting unnecessary spending. ACOs that meet quality thresholds may share in the cost savings they achieve for Medicare. ACOs also may agree to a downside risk in exchange for a potentially larger share of savings.

Navigating the program's rules has proven to be a challenge, and many ACOs have decided to withdraw from the program. In September 2014, a CMS study concluded that although ACOs are an important first step toward greater efficiency and quality, their impact on spending may not be as great as initially thought.[16]

Public Reporting and Transparency

The ACA also requires widespread public reporting of hospital and physician quality performance data. Until now, CMS only has reported on whether a physician participated in federal quality reporting programs. However, starting in 2014, CMS will begin to release physician quality performance data to the public, with the goal of releasing performance data on all physicians by 2015.

The pace at which CMS is releasing data to the public has been a major concern of organized medicine given the questionable significance of current measure sets, the subjectivity of patient satisfaction measures, and ongoing concerns about the methodologies used to calculate quality and cost performance. Questions have also been raised about the most appropriate format in which to present this data. Whereas CMS tends to favor consumer-friendly formats, such as star ratings, health care providers have concerns about arbitrary thresholds that result in inappropriate distinctions among professionals whose performance is not statistically different.

In addition to public reporting of quality data, in 2014, CMS released data summarizing utilization and payments for procedures and services provided by physicians under Medicare. Related to this effort, CMS is also in the process of giving private qualified entities unprecedented access to Medicare claims data to pair with private payer data to provide consumers with more complete information about quality and utilization.

ONGOING CHALLENGES AND COMMON THEMES
Inadequate Measures

The nation still has a long way to go with regard to quality measurement. Although CMS continues to move away from claims-based, process-of-care measures, these types of measures still form most of the available PQRS measure set. It also is still not clear to what extent many of these measures lead to better outcomes and are true indictors of higher-quality care. Even among the PQRS measures that neurosurgeons tend to report—such as those that focus on perioperative, stroke, and low back pain care—few are nuanced and actionable enough to be considered meaningful across each of the neurosurgical subspecialties. With so few relevant measures and an increasing reporting burden, neurosurgeons inevitably will be forced to rely on "low-hanging fruit," such as smoking cessation and medication reconciliation measures, that will further distance them from the quality improvement goals of the program.

Physicians are also affected by inadequate hospital-level measures. Although it is the institution and not the individual physician who is held directly accountable for these measures, individual physician actions are nevertheless scrutinized for their contribution to the institution's overall quality of care. Furthermore, hospital-level measures often lack a sufficient level of granularity to accurately evaluate quality and determine the root of a potential problem. For example, all-cause hospital readmissions measures fail to exclude or adjust for readmissions related to trauma, staged procedures, or other situations that are outside the surgeon's and institution's control.

At both the physician and hospital level, patient satisfaction measures are gaining considerable traction. Although well intentioned, their subjective nature and tendency to focus on factors outside a physician's control (like patient wait times) brings into question whether they are appropriate for accountability purposes. Even factors within a physician's control, such as courtesy, can be grossly misrepresented when a patient does not hear what he or she is told, such as to lose weight or quit smoking. Furthermore, when used for accountability purposes, they may put pressure on physicians to ignore what is best for the patient to make the patient happy. The overprescription of pain medications as a result of patient satisfaction surveys is a common example that has recently received attention in Congress, but other examples include ordering a routine MRI for back pain or antibiotics for a viral infection when requested by a patient, even if not clinically indicated.[17]

There is also little evidence of an association between patient satisfaction scores and better clinical outcomes. In fact, a 2012 study found that patients who were more satisfied with their physicians had higher health care costs, were hospitalized more frequently, and had higher death rates compared with less-satisfied patients.[18]

Although quality measurement remains an imperfect science, policymakers are beginning to address some of the most pressing challenges, especially those related to individual physician reporting. In the PQRS, a growing number of measures focus on patient outcomes and rely on more robust clinical data, gathered via registries and EHRs, that capture a more complete picture of quality.

The American Taxpayer Relief Act of 2012, in particular, requires that CMS begin recognizing qualified clinical data registries (QCDR) as a new PQRS reporting mechanism in 2014. For the very first time, QCDRs give physicians the option to qualify for the PQRS by reporting on homegrown, specialty society–developed and collected measures rather than the limited and often inadequate set of existing PQRS measures. The QCDR requirements come with their own set of challenges but offer physicians unprecedented flexibility to chose measures that are most meaningful and relevant to their practice. It also encourages innovation in measurement by shifting the dial toward more meaningful, more informed, and more patient-centered measures guided by the profession.

Flawed Methodologies

Although measures used in federal quality initiatives are adjusted for clinical factors, such as multiple comorbidities or the severity of a patient's illness, they are still not adjusted for sociodemographic factors out of fear that this could set a lower expectation for care provided to these patients and mask critical disparities.[19] However, a recent report commissioned by the Obama Administration criticized current quality measures as fundamentally flawed, noting that current policies may be unfairly penalizing physicians and hospitals that treat large numbers of these patients. Concern about the effect this could have on patient access has been so great around this issue that a bipartisan group of US Senators introduced legislation in 2014 to require that Medicare take the financial status of hospital patients into account when deciding whether to punish a hospital for too many readmissions.

Attribution is equally concerning. The growth in all-encompassing measures intended to encourage better care coordination, such as all-cause readmission, all-cause mortality, and Medicare spending per beneficiary cost measures, has resulted in physicians and hospitals being held accountable for decisions outside their control. The more broadly defined the outcome, the more difficult it is to apportion measured improvement among the many physicians that may see a patient during an episode of care and the many factors that may have contributed to the outcome—some within the control of the health care provider and some that are not. Furthermore, the patient's role in his or her outcome is a factor that is still largely ignored.

There is also currently no alignment between the cost and quality measures used to calculate value-based performance adjustments, which only serves to erode confidence in the accuracy of these value judgments. There is also little alignment of key measures among federal programs and between the public and private sector, further adding to the administratively burdensome and time-consuming process of managing all of these requirements.

Finally, the budget-neutral nature of many of these programs, including the Physician VBM Program, also inevitably creates "losers" who must finance the "winners." Although problematic on its own for its failure to recognize personal improvement, this type of program also results in uncertainty as to how strong a physician's performance actually needs to be each year to qualify for a bonus payment and to support infrastructure investments needed to perform well. This situation is especially concerning for smaller practices and individual practitioners who cannot dedicate the same level of resources as large practices do to reporting compliance.

Insufficient Data and Barriers to Information Exchange

Although newer policies that give health care professionals more control over measure selection are a move in the right direction, meaningful measures simply do not yet exist for many important aspects of health care, including neurosurgery. This includes reliable and widely available measures for things that matter most to patients, such as experience of care and outcomes that reflect how well they can function, work, and engage in life's daily activities. Developing proper measures requires a significant investment in data collection and analysis and time.

The nation also continues to lack reliable and consistent information on which to evaluate cost of care and resource use. As a result, CMS continues to rely on broad cost measures that inappropriately assign accountability to physicians for treatment decisions and services they may not have delivered and often cannot control. As with quality measures, the development of meaningful and accurate cost measures will require investments in a more robust data collection infrastructure.

Clinical data registries hold the key to overcoming these current obstacles, and a recent surge in federal attention to the value of registries is encouraging. Nevertheless, multiple challenges must first be addressed before the true value of clinical data collected from registries can be fully realized. In addition to the significant investment of resources needed to launch and maintain the long-term data collection of a registry, important regulatory challenges must be addressed before specialties can use this data for true quality improvement. For example, regulations originally intended for human research protections are often applied unnecessarily to registries focused solely on quality improvement, which can interfere with serial enrollment and hamper more longitudinal data collection.

Interoperability is also an ongoing challenge for both registries and EHRs and severely limits the potential of health information exchange. The current inability to merge data from different sources limits the effectiveness of any measures developed to date and our ability to develop new and better ones. Despite widespread of adoption of EHRs, it is still common for office-based practices, clinics, hospitals, and emergency departments to face insurmountable barriers when trying to share data.

EHR systems also do not yet fit seamlessly into clinical practice, a problem that is accentuated in specialized fields such as neurosurgery. Other challenges, such as work flows that lack clinical intuition and drop down menus that fail to adequately capture the full range of clinical scenarios, tend to distract and frustrate physicians rather than aid them in providing high-quality care. Poor system design also provokes potentially harmful workarounds by users, such as overriding warnings due to alarm fatigue, checking boxes without verification, and cutting and pasting medical details without actually updating them. Although EHRs hold tremendous promise for higher quality and more efficient care, they can also pose serious patient safety risks if not designed and used properly.

Balancing the Need for Big Data

Transparency mandates and the increasing collection of data via registries and EHRs have given the public unprecedented access to data, but the mechanisms to translate and properly use those data have not been developed at the same speed. This slow development resulted in an information overload that has left physicians, patients, payers, and even policymakers confused rather than more informed. There is also a fear that too much cost sensitivity can compromise care if patients skip or delay needed treatments.

It also is not clear to what extent consumers value and actually use these data to make more informed decisions. A recent study found that although patients selecting a physician for a first-time visit were likely to choose one ranked in the best-performing or average tier, patients who had an ongoing relationship with a physician in a lower-performing tier were no more apt to switch than patients with higher-ranked physicians.[20] Although public access to such data has the potential to revolutionize health care, it must be approached in a thoughtful and deliberate manner to be effective.

The new liability threats that these mandates have potentially created also cannot be ignored. This concern is widespread enough to have provoked multiple legislative vehicles that aim to ensure that these federal quality mandates are not used outside their intended purpose, to create new standards of care for medical liability lawsuits[21] and to create liability protections for those physicians who adhere to evidence-based guidelines developed by physicians.[22]

Cumulative Nature of Penalties

In FY 2014, 2 of 3 hospitals lost money from the combined effects of federal quality and readmissions programs.[9] These cuts come on top of recent reductions in special payments received by hospitals that treat large numbers of low-income people.[9] Combined, the hospital quality programs have the potential to strip away as much as 5.5% of Medicare payments from the worst-performing hospitals starting in FY 2015.[9]

Meanwhile, physicians may be at risk for losing more than 10% of their Medicare Part B payments in the coming years given the cumulative application of penalties associated with the PQRS, VBM, and EHR incentive programs. The impact on reimbursement will likely be even higher given the indirect impact of hospital quality mandates.

Rapid Implementation

One of the most consistent criticisms of CMS is its failure to carefully evaluate the impact of its policies before widespread implementation. Although most of the public, including organized medicine, believe that tracking and even holding health care providers accountable for quality and value is a good thing, the speed and seemingly reckless nature in which this has been carried out has substantially eroded physician trust and engagement in the process. Furthermore, most physicians have not received any formal education or training in quality reporting nor do they have the additional resources or time needed to comply with the increasingly complex requirements of multiple federal quality reporting mandates.

SUMMARY

The practice of medicine has entered an era of unprecedented scrutiny in which regulatory accountability is at an all time high. Although physicians feel this burden on multiple fronts, specialties such as neurosurgery are in the unique position of having to contend with both physician-level mandates and pressure from their institutions to help satisfy facility-level mandates. Up until recently, neurosurgeons have had relative flexibility to choose quality improvement strategies that worked best for their practice, regardless of whether they aligned with federal strategies. However, the increasing mandatory and punitive nature of these federal initiatives has altered the landscape, making it increasingly difficult for even neurosurgeons to absorb the potential financial and reputational impact.

Value-based health care is here to stay. The challenge on the road ahead will be to convince policy makers to tighten the reigns on implementation and to focus less on winners and losers and more on the careful development of a robust data infrastructure that can allow us to more accurately identify gaps in care and answer questions about appropriate treatment in a manner that is meaningful to both physicians and patients. Without a serious reevaluation of these strategies, these programs will, at best, have limited effectiveness and, at worst, lead to critical deteriorations in patient quality, safety, and access to care.

REFERENCES

1. Edney A. U.S. Health system among least efficient before obamacare. New York (NY): Bloomberg LP; 2014. Available at: http://www.bloomberg.com/news/2014-09-18/u-s-health-system-among-least-efficient-before-obamacare.html. Accessed September 29, 2014.
2. Davis K, Stremikis K, Squires D, et al. Mirror, mirror on the wall, 2014 update: how the U.S. health care system compares internationally. New York (NY): The Commonwealth Fund; 2014. Available at: http://www.commonwealthfund.org/publications/fund-reports/2014/jun/mirror-mirror. Accessed September 15, 2014.
3. Schoen C, Osborn R, Squires D, et al. A Survey of Primary Care Doctors in Ten Countries Shows Progress in Use of Health Information Technology, Less in Other Areas. Health Affairs. Accessed December 24, 2014. Available at: http://content.healthaffairs.org/content/31/12/2805.
4. Kohn L, Corrigan J, Donaldson M. To err is human: building a safer health system. Washington, DC: National Academy Press; 1999.
5. Institute of Medicine. Crossing the quality chasm: a new health system for the 21st century. Washington, DC: National Academy Press; 2001.

6. Executive Order of the President. Promoting Quality and Efficient Health Care in Federal Government Administered or Sponsored Health Care Programs. Exec. Order No. 13410, 3 C.F.R. 51089 (2006). August 26, 2006.
7. Rau J. Nearly 1,500 hospitals penalized under medicare program rating quality. Kaiser Health News 2013. Available at: http://www.kaiserhealthnews.org/Stories/2013/November/14/value-based-purchasing-medicare.aspx. Accessed September 20, 2014.
8. Mechanic R. Post acute care- the next frontier for controlling medicare spending. N Engl J Med 2014;370:692–4.
9. Rau J. Medicare fines 2,610 hospitals in third round of readmission penalties. Kaiser News Network 2014. Available at: http://www.kaiserhealthnews.org/Stories/2014/October/02/Medicare-readmissions-penalties-2015.aspx. Accessed October 2, 2014.
10. Refining the Hospital Readmissions Reduction Program. MedPAC Report to Congress. 2013. Available at: http://www.medpac.gov/documents/reports/jun13_ch04_appendix.pdf?sfvrsn=0. Accessed September 29, 2014.
11. 2012 PQRS Experience Report. Centers for Medicare and Medicaid Services. 2012. Available at: http://www.cms.gov/Medicare/Quality-Initiatives-Patient-Assessment-Instruments/PQRS/Downloads/2012-PQRS-and-eRx-Experience-Report.zip. Accessed September 20, 2014.
12. Doctors and hospitals' use of health IT more than doubles since 2012. U.S. Department of Health and Human Services press release. 2013. Available at: http://www.hhs.gov/news/press/2013pres/05/20130522a.html. Accessed September 20, 2014.
13. Centers for Medicare and Medicaid Services. Medicare and Medicaid Incentive Program Data and Program Reports. Available at: http://www.cms.gov/Regulations-and-Guidance/Legislation/EHRIncentivePrograms/DataAndReports.html. Accessed September 20, 2014.
14. Friedberg M, Chen P, Van Busum K, et al. Factors affecting physician professional satisfaction and their implications for patient care, health systems, and health policy. Santa Monica (CA): RAND Corporation; 2013. Available at: http://www.rand.org/pubs/research_reports/RR439.html. Accessed September 20, 2014.
15. Annual Check-Up on Physician Adoption of Health IT (2014). Deloitte. Available at: http://www.deloitte.com/view/en_US/us/Industries/US-federal-government/center-for-health-solutions/dccac173cd978410VgnVCM2000003356f70aRCRD.htm. Accessed September 20, 2014.
16. Pope G, Kautter J, Leung M, et al. Financial and quality impacts of the medicare physician group practice demonstration. Medicare Medicaid Res Rev 2014;4(3). Centers for Medicare and Medicaid Services, Available at: http://www.cms.gov/mmrr/Downloads/MMRR2014_004_03_a01.pdf. Accessed September 20, 2014.
17. Senate Caucus on International Narcotics Control. Letter to Marilyn Tavenner, Administrator, Centers for Medicare and Medicaid Services. 2014. Available at: http://www.grassley.senate.gov/sites/default/files/news/upload/Letter%20to%20CMS%20(Patient%20Surveys)%206-23-14.pdf. Accessed September 20, 2014.
18. Fenton J, Jerant A, Bertakis K, et al. The cost of satisfaction: a national study of patient satisfaction, health care utilization, expenditures, and mortality. Arch Intern Med 2012;172(5):405–11.
19. Pear R. Health law's pay policy is skewed, panel finds. The New York Times 2014. Available at: http://www.nytimes.com/2014/04/28/us/politics/health-laws-pay-policy-is-skewed-panel-finds.html. Accessed September 20, 2014.
20. Alden S. Patients are loyal to their doctors, despite performance scores. Health Behavior News Service 2014. Available at: http://www.cfah.org/hbns/2014/patients-are-loyal-to-their-doctors-despite-performance-scores. Accessed September 29, 2014.
21. H.R. 1473, the "Standard of Care Protection Act".
22. H.R. 4106, the "Saving Lives, Saving Costs Act".

Quality Improvement Tools and Processes

Catherine Y. Lau, MD[a,b,*]

KEYWORDS

- Quality improvement • Quality improvement tools • Quality improvement project management
- Model for Improvement

KEY POINTS

- The Model for Improvement is a popular, easy-to-use method of systematically and successfully implementing a quality improvement project.
- The problem is defined by scoping the current state and describing the existing quality gap. This may be accomplished by performing a literature review, using the 5 Whys tool, flowchart, fishbone diagram, root cause analysis, or failure modes effect analysis.
- The Plan-Do-Study-Act cycle is done successively with small tests of change until process improvement is accomplished; the final set of recommendations can then be implemented on a larger scale throughout the institution and health care system, resulting in greater gains.

INTRODUCTION

Since the publication of the Institute of Medicine (IOM) report *To Err is Human* 15 years ago, there has been substantial interest in improving patient safety and the quality of health care delivered in both medical and surgical fields, with many physicians and health care leaders devoting their careers to effecting positive change.[1–5] With this interest has come the increased adoption of using process improvement tools initially designed in other industries and adapted for use in health care quality and process improvement.[6–8] This article provides a general framework for neurosurgery providers who wish to embark on quality improvement (QI) projects using the Model for Improvement (MFI) and Plan-Do-Study-Act (PDSA) project cycles. Lean and Six Sigma are two other methods to approach QI work, and are not described in this article.

The Model for Improvement and Plan-Do-Study-Act

Because of its ease, logical approach, and emphasis on testing changes using a small-scale and rapid cycle approach, the MFI and the PDSA cycle is a popular framework that has been endorsed by the Institute for Healthcare Improvement as a tool for health care organizations to spearhead and accelerate QI efforts.[9]

The MFI consists of 2 parts (**Fig. 1**):

- Three questions must be addressed:
  - What needs to be accomplished?
  - How can a change be shown to be an improvement?
  - What changes can be made that will result in improvement?
- Use the PDSA cycle to test changes in a real-work setting to ensure that the change results in improvement.

[a] Division of Hospital Medicine, Department of Medicine and Neurological Surgery, University of California, San Francisco, San Francisco, CA, USA; [b] Patient Safety and Quality, Department of Neurological Surgery, 533 Parnassus Avenue, Box 0131, San Francisco, CA 94143, USA
* Patient Safety and Quality, Department of Neurological Surgery, 533 Parnassus Avenue, Box 0131, San Francisco, CA 94143.
E-mail address: clau@ucsf.edu

Neurosurg Clin N Am 26 (2015) 177–187
http://dx.doi.org/10.1016/j.nec.2014.11.016
1042-3680/15/$ – see front matter © 2015 Elsevier Inc. All rights reserved.

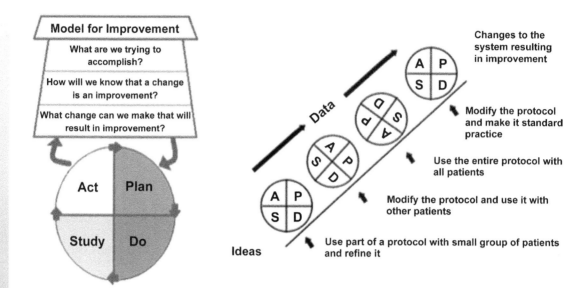

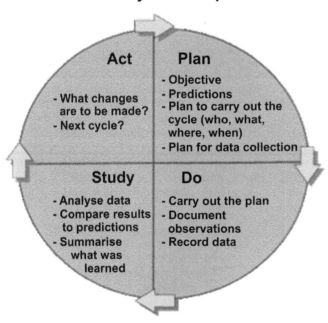

The PDSA Cycle for Improvement

Fig. 1. Engineering change: the MFI and the PDSA project cycle to drive QI. (*Adapted from* Associates in Process Improvement. Available at: www.apiweb.org; and Institute for Healthcare Improvement. Available at: www.ihi.org/resources/Pages/HowToImprove/default.aspx.)

Defining the problem

The main goal of this phase is to address the first question of the MFI: what needs to be accomplished? Project teams must ask themselves what the problem is that they are trying to solve, and whether this is even a problem that is supported by current data. If clinicians suspect that there is a problem but do not have local data to support this or cannot specifically speak to how big the quality gap is, then a needs assessment should be conducted. The goal of the needs assessment is to develop a solid understanding of the current state, highlight how the current state does not meet the quality goal to show the quality gap that needs to be addressed, and explore potential areas for improvement.

Needs assessments can be done in several ways. As an example, consider the reduction of postoperative catheter-associated urinary tract infections (CA-UTI). One method of performing a needs assessment is to conduct a literature search to determine the general prevalence and incidence of the problem, and any evidence-based proven strategies that have been shown to reduce CA-UTI rates.

Another method of performing a needs assessment is to go to where the work is being done by providers. Nursing protocols and workflow for Foley catheter care should be observed and reviewed in addition to surgical provider workflow and order sets for placement and removal of Foley catheters. While performing workflow observations, the QI team may use the following tools to gather and organize their data:

- Five Whys tool
- Flowcharts
- Fishbone diagram
- Failure modes and effects analysis

Five Whys Tool

The 5 Whys tool (**Fig. 2**) is a simple technique for determining the root cause of a problem. It was made popular by the Toyota Production System.[10] Asking "Why?" no fewer than 5 times allows the answers to come from frontline providers who have direct experience with the process being examined. Continue the process of asking "Why?" until the root cause of the problem is identified. This process allows project team members to save time by devoting efforts to the underlying cause of the problem, rather than aimlessly pursuing other strategies that may have no effect on the outcome. The 5 Whys tool is best suited for simple to moderately difficult problems. More complex problems benefit from a more detailed needs assessment and scoping approach, although using the 5 Whys may still yield useful insights.

Flowcharts

A tool that may be used in more complex problems is the flowchart, which is a visual method of listing each separate step of a process in

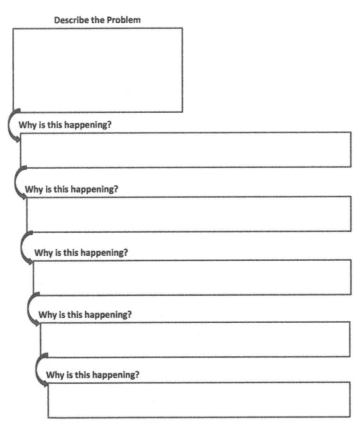

Fig. 2. The 5 Whys tool.

sequential order to help clarify steps in a complex process and allow team members to gain a shared understanding of the process of collecting data, identifying problems, and focusing improvement discussions. **Fig. 3** shows an example of a flowchart describing the discharge process. Flowcharts may also be used to identify steps that do and do not add value to the customer, which is the patient in most health care QI projects. Flowcharts also allow teams to identify delays, unnecessary work, communication failures, and added expense. As a process analysis tool, flowcharts allow QI teams to have a consensus-built tool to drive the design of new process improvements.

Fishbone Diagram

The fishbone diagram (**Fig. 4**), or cause-and-effect diagram, is another graphical process analysis tool that allows teams to understand that there are many causes that contribute to an effect, displays the relationship of the causes to each other and to the end effect, and identifies areas for improvement. The fishbone diagram is one method of graphically displaying the results of a root cause analysis (RCA), which is described in greater detail later in this article.

Failure Modes and Effects Analysis

A failure modes and effects analysis (FMEA) is a systematic, proactive method for evaluating a process to identify:

- Where the process may fail
- How the process may fail
- The relative impacts of the different failure points
- The higher-risk failure components of the process that are most in need of change to redesign the process and prevent harm

A multidisciplinary team selects a high-risk process to evaluate and begins by listing the steps in the process, similar to a flowchart. For each step in the process, the team lists the failure modes (things that can go wrong with the process) and failure causes. The team then assigns numeric values for each failure mode based on the likelihood of occurrence, likelihood of detection (with lower likelihood of detection rated as being higher risk for causing harm), and severity. Based on these numeric values, a risk priority number (RPN) is then assigned for each failure mode. Failure modes that have the highest RPN are then chosen for improvement efforts. Thus, an FMEA may be performed to better understand crucial

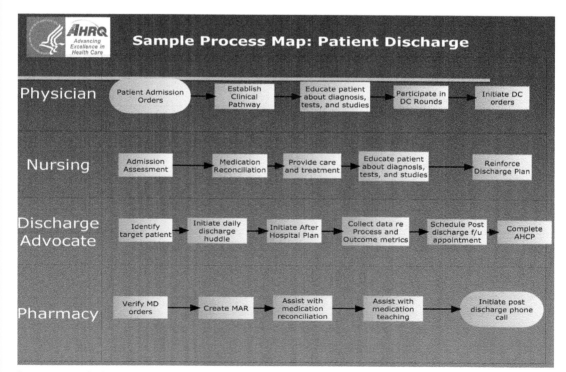

Fig. 3. Patient discharge flowchart. DC, discharge. (*From* Slide 8: Project RED: Module 3: The re-designed discharge process: patient admission and care and treatment education: Slide 8. Rockville (MD): Agency for Healthcare Research and Quality; 2011. Available at: http://www.ahrq.gov/professionals/systems/hospital/red/module3/slide8.html.)

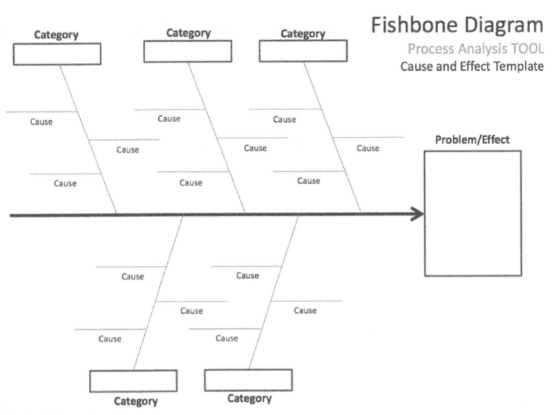

Fig. 4. Fishbone diagram.

processes that must be improved to avoid adverse events or errors (**Table 1**).

Root Cause Analysis

Similar to an FMEA, an RCA is a systematic process involving a multidisciplinary team to determine the root cause or causes of an adverse event or near miss.[11] However, unlike an FMEA, which is a proactive method of looking at a high-risk process, an RCA is a reactive process that is performed after an event has occurred. Similar to the 5 Whys tool, RCA teams often ask "Why" 5 times to reach the root cause of the event. The focus of an RCA is on flawed systems issues and processes rather than placing blame on individual health care providers. The RCA team then designs and implements risk reduction strategies, evaluates the changes, and communicates the results of the change back to the stakeholders.

Forming the team
A critical component of the QI process that is often overlooked is assembling the right people to ensure a successful improvement effort. Assembling the team should happen concurrently with defining the problem. Most effective teams consist of an executive sponsor and providers from multiple disciplines with varying levels of training. It is critical to include team members who are familiar with the different parts of the proposed process change. The Institute for Healthcare Improvement (IHI) advocates that effective teams should represent 4 different areas of expertise in the health care organization: clinical leadership or a physician/nurse champion, technical expertise, day-to-day leadership, and an executive sponsor.[8] Careful thought in strategically choosing team members and ensuring that all stakeholders have a voice in the project help with success in implementation, spread, and sustainability of the QI project.

Setting the aims and the objectives
Once the problem has been defined and the project team that engages the key stakeholders in the process has been assembled, the team should come to a consensus about the overall aims and objectives of the project. Well-designed projects often set SMART objectives, or objectives that are:

- S = specific
- M = measurable
- A = achievable
- R = realistic
- T = timely or time sensitive

Table 1
Failure Modes and Effects Analysis (FMEA) example: inpatient pain control

Process	Failure Mode	Failure Causes	Failure Effects	Likelihood of Occurrence (1–10)	Likelihood of Detection (1–10)	Severity (1–10)	Actions to Reduce Failure
Assessment of patient	Inaccurate evaluation	• Lack of articulation • Cultural and language	Poor control	8	5	2	• Standard scale • Cultural training
Analgesic choice and route	Wrong medication selected	• Renal function • Age • Allergies • Interaction	• Wrong dosing • Allergic response	2	5	8	• Decision support tools
Ordering modification	• Wrong dose • Monitoring • Wrong patient	• Deficit in knowledge • Similar patient names	• Overdose or underdose • ADR	—	—	—	—
Order faxed to pharmacy	• Order not received • Delay in processing	• Unaware of order	• Delays	—	—	—	—
Medication prepared	• Wrong drug • Wrong dilution	• Products stored near each other	• ADR	—	—	—	—

Abbreviation: ADR, adverse drug event.

To go back to the example of reducing CA-UTI rates on a neurosurgical inpatient service, a SMART objective for this project might be to reduce neurosurgical inpatient service CA-UTI rates by 10% within 1 year. Rather than referring to SMART objectives, the IHI project guide advocates the use of aim statements, which are essentially the same thing.

A project charter (see Appendix A) should also be drafted at this point to help clarify the project participants, project description and aims, current state description, and initial timeline and budget. In order for QI projects to be done well, it is important to obtain internal departmental or external funding and/or support to allow adequate protected time and personnel to perform the project, analyze the results, and sustain and spread change practices. Other items on the project charter include choosing evaluation metrics and selecting and testing changes. These steps are next in the MFI.

Establishing measures

At this stage, the QI project team needs to answer the second question in the MFI: how can a change be shown to be an improvement? Donabedian[12] first described a framework for organizing quality metrics into 3 categories several decades ago. This framework of structural, process, and outcomes measures (**Fig. 5**) allows the QI team to use their knowledge of the organization they are trying to change to propose changes that provide good structure, which increases the likelihood of good processes, which in turn increases the likelihood of a good outcome.

Most QI initiatives typically choose process measures as a measurement strategy because most QI projects are designed to change processes, or what is done. For the CA-UTI reduction project, a process measure to follow could include checking whether patients had their Foley catheters discontinued within 24 to 48 hours after surgery.

It is imperative to include at least 1 outcome measure in each project to show any change in patient outcomes rather than just changes in the health care delivery process. This outcome may be harder to measure because some outcomes are not common or are difficult to measure over time. In addition, outcomes measures may be confounded by interventions other than the QI project team's proposed interventions. For the CA-UTI reduction project, the outcome measure would be the neurosurgical service's CA-UTI rate.

In addition, it is prudent for QI project teams to consider balancing metrics, or a method of measuring unintended consequences of the proposed change. For the CA-UTI reduction project, one unintended potential consequence of being stricter with postoperative Foley catheter removal may be increased sacral wounds or decubitus ulcers caused by a decreased ability to keep this area clean and free from moisture. Thus, sacral hospital-acquired pressure ulcers may be the balancing metric for this project.

Once the process, outcomes, and balancing metrics are chosen, a more rigorous baseline data collection process can begin. Decisions to made regarding data collection are:

- From what sources will baseline data be obtained and can this process be automated moving forward?
- How much baseline data should be obtained?
  - Be mindful that obtaining baseline data should not require months of time-intensive work. The goal is to yield enough data to start the QI improvement process.

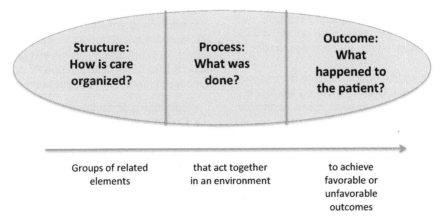

| Structure: How is care organized? | Process: What was done? | Outcome: What happened to the patient? |

| Groups of related elements | that act together in an environment | to achieve favorable or unfavorable outcomes |

Fig. 5. Donabedian's[12] framework of structure, process, and outcomes measures. (*Adapted from* Donabedian A. The quality of care: how can it be assessed? JAMA 1988;260:1745–6.)

- How often will data be analyzed moving forward? Weekly? Monthly? Quarterly?
- Who will complete this work?
- How will these results be distributed to project stakeholders?
  - QI dashboards or scorecards are a popular method of providing data feedback to project stakeholders. The goal of creating a quality dashboard or scorecard is to better understand provider and institutional performance by standardizing metrics, data sources, and reporting frequency. This method allows targeted interventions, increases transparency, establishes accountability, and helps build a culture of safety. Remember that a QI dashboard or scorecard is only as good as the integrity of the data sources and metrics that it contains. Furthermore, dashboards generally provide a top-level view of overall performance. Drill-downs using previously described methods are often needed to fully understand the performance and cause of quality lesions.

Selecting changes

The next step is to compile as many ideas as possible that address the quality gap. This is the third step of the MFI, in which the QI team asks themselves what changes can be made that will result in improvement. These change ideas may come from evidence-based best-practice guidelines, team brainstorming sessions, or work done by other departments both within and outside the organization.

In order to pare the potential number of change ideas into a succinct list of those that are most likely to be successful, the QI project team should ensure that the change idea candidates are able to address the 4 quality improvement pillars that have been shown to support change efforts[7]:

- Education: show providers and frontline staff why this matters and how to do things correctly, more efficiently, with less likelihood of error.
- Data audit and feedback: provide team-based and, if possible, individual-based feedback.
- Systems change: design new workflow, personnel, or electronic medical record changes to directly support the change efforts.
- Culture change: show providers and frontline staff that the QI project can be done successfully and share team success stories. Create short-term wins by thanking providers, providing achievable goals, and having team celebrations when goals are reached.

Testing changes

After performing the above-mentioned carefully thought-out planning process, the QI project team is ready to test the changes. Because not all change results in improvement but improvement results from a change, it is important not to rely too heavily on 1 change idea. To mitigate this risk, the fundamental principle of the PDSA cycle is to rapidly test small-scale tests of change by planning (which has already been done); doing a small-scale pilot; studying the results of the pilot using predetermined process, outcomes, and balancing metrics; and acting on the results of the pilot to then begin the next planning cycle to test the next or revised change based on what was previously learned (see **Fig. 1**).

Before the QI project is complete, there are often several PDSA cycles that are performed to decide which of the original proposed changes lead to the desired improvement outcome. It is common for several combinations of the initial proposed changes to eventually be combined to have the desired effect on the quality measurement and outcome.

Implementing, spreading, and sustaining changes

Once several PDSA cycles have been completed, a finalized protocol and proven set of recommendations can be made to result in standard work and system-wide changes to improve health care outcomes. Changing human behavior is difficult even on a small scale and more so on a broad, organizational level, and a great number of books and articles have been written to provide strategies to make change less hard and more attainable.[13–18] In order to increase the chances for success, the issues of implementation, spread, and sustainability must be addressed early during project design rather than being addressed in a reactive, ad-hoc manner.

In addition to ensuring that the QI project team addresses the 4 QI pillars, management science expert John Kotter[19] from Harvard Business School lists 8 sequential steps of change that a successful leader and project team addresses:

- Establish a sense of urgency
- Create a guiding coalition
- Develop a clear shared vision
- Communicate the vision for buy-in
- Empower people to act on the vision for broad-based action
- Create short-term wins
- Never let up by consolidating and building on gains
- Incorporate changes into institutional culture

Table 2
Key differences between QI projects and RCTs

	QI Projects	RCTs
Goal	Improve clinical practice	Generate new knowledge
Methods	• Identify best practices • Tests observable • Bias present • Just enough data • Dynamic hypothesis • Sequential tests • Ongoing tracking and follow-up • PDSA	• Establish new practice • Tests blinded • No bias • All possible data • Fixed hypothesis • One large test • Data collection ends with study • Plan-Do-Study-Publish
End result	Change in performance, then publication	Publication, then change in clinical practice

By addressing these steps, project leaders can help improve the chances for success of their QI project.

KEY DIFFERENCES BETWEEN QUALITY IMPROVEMENT PROJECTS/RESEARCH AND HEALTH CARE SCIENCE RESEARCH

There are several notable differences between QI projects and the gold standard of health care clinical science research, the randomized control trial (RCT). Although the goal of RCTs is to generate new clinical knowledge, the goal of QI projects is to improve clinical practice to make it safer, less prone to error, more efficient, and of higher value. Because of these differing goals, the methods taken in QI projects and RCTs also are divergent. **Table 2** lists these differences.

SUMMARY/DISCUSSIONS

The MFI is a popular, easy-to-use method of systematically and successfully managing a QI project. Defining the problem is done by scoping the current state and describing the existing quality gap by performing a literature review and using the 5 Whys tool, flowchart, fishbone diagram, RCA, or failure modes effect analysis. The project team is then formed, representing key stakeholders, and the aim statement or SMART objective is determined. Measures are then chosen, baseline data are obtained, and changes to the

process are proposed and selected. A change is then tested, and results are collected and analyzed with the goal of guiding the next test of change. The PDSA is done successively with small tests of change until process improvement is accomplished. The final set of recommendations can then be implemented on a larger scale throughout the institution and health care system, resulting in greater gains.

REFERENCES

1. Kohn LT, Corrigan J, Donaldson MS. To err is human: building a safer health system. Washington, DC: National Academy Press; 2000.
2. Institute of Medicine. Crossing the quality chasm: a new health system for the 21st century. Washington, DC: National Academy Press; 2001.
3. Chassin MR, Galvin RW. The urgent need to improve health care quality: Institute of Medicine National Roundtable on Health Care Quality. JAMA 1998;280:1000–5.
4. Berwick DM, Calkins DR, McCannon CJ, et al. The 100,000 Lives campaign: setting a goal and a deadline for improving health care quality. JAMA 2006;295:324–7.
5. James JT. A new, evidence-based estimate of patient harms associated with hospital care. J Patient Saf 2013;9:122–8.
6. Nelson EC, Batalden PB, Ryder JC, editors. The clinical improvement action guide. Oakbrook Terrace (IL): Joint Commission on Accreditation of Healthcare; 1998.
7. Langley GJ, Moen RD, Nolan KM, et al. The improvement guide: a practical approach to enhancing organizational performance. San Francisco (CA): Jossey-Bass Publishers; 2009.
8. Agency for Healthcare Research and Quality Website: human factors engineering. Accessed September 8, 2014. Available at: psnet.ahrq.gov/primer.aspx?primerID=20.
9. Institute for Healthcare Improvement Resources website. Accessed September 8, 2014. Available at: www.ihi.org/resources/Pages/HowtoImprove/default.aspx.
10. Ohno T. Toyota production system: beyond large-scale production. Portland (OR): Productivity; 1988.
11. Agency for Healthcare Research and Quality Website: root cause analysis. Accessed September 8, 2014. Available at: psnet.ahrq.gov/primer.aspx?primerID=10.
12. Donabedian A. The quality of care: how can it be assessed? JAMA 1988;260:1743–8.
13. Kotter J. Leading change. Cambridge (MA): Harvard Business Press Books; 1996.
14. Goleman D. Leadership that gets results. Cambridge (MA): Harvard Business Review; 2000. Reprint R00204.
15. Kotter J. Accelerate: building strategic agility for a faster-moving world. Cambridge (MA): Harvard Business Press Books; 2014.

16. Bodenheimer T. The science of spread: how innovations in care become the norm. Oakland (CA): California Healthcare Foundation; 2007.
17. Massoud MR, Nielsen GA, Nolan K, et al. A framework for spread: from local improvements to system-wide change: Institute for Healthcare Improvement innovation series white paper. Cambridge (MA): IHI; 2006. Available at: www.ihi.org/IHI/Results/WhitePapers/AFrameworkforSpreadWhitePaper.htm.
18. Berwick DM. Disseminating Innovations in Health Care. JAMA 2003;289:1969–75.
19. Accessed September 8, 2014. Available at: www.kotterinternational.com/our-principles/changesteps.

APPENDIX A: PROJECT CHARTER TEMPLATE

Project Name:		Date:

PROJECT PARTICIPANTS

Executive Sponsor:	Project Champion/Leader:	Project Manager:
Stakeholders: Those that will be affected positively and negatively by the change. Often a stakeholder buy-in or commitment to change is necessary for project implementation.	**Core Team Members:** Those who will undertake all tasks necessary to design, build and implement the final solution.	**Ad Hoc Team Members:** Those who will provide additional resources, direction and support.

PROJECT DESCRIPTION

Executive Summary:

Business Case: captures the reasoning for initiating a project or task to convince a decision maker to take action. Include what problem or situation triggered the initiative and what benefit, value or return is expected.

Problem Statement: provides a clear description of an issue facing an individual or group. It generally includes the scope and magnitude of the problem.

Project Objective / Aims (SMART objective, should be measurable):

Current State Description / High Level Process Map

Current State Problems: lists the issues identified with the current state and how they contribute to the overall problem.

Deliverables (different than objectives):

Tangible things that will be created to support the project. They may include process maps, survey instruments, and/or educational materials.
STRUCTURE (new personnel, processes in EMR, that must be built)

Evaluation (metrics to evaluate project progress)

OUTCOMES: (patient level benefits – e.g., cost, mortality, LOS)

PROCESSES: (changes in the steps of care delivery that are necessary to achieve those outcomes)

Initial Initiatives / Small tests of change

Timeline

Schedule (target date):
Start Date:
End Date:
Budget, if applicable (amount):

NEXT STEPS AND ACTION ITEMS

Cost-Effectiveness Research in Neurosurgery

Corinna C. Zygourakis, MD[a],*, James G. Kahn, MD, MPH[b]

KEYWORDS

• Cost-effectiveness • Cost-utility • QALY • Neurosurgery • Spine surgery

KEY POINTS

• A cost-effectiveness analysis (CEA) reports the added cost per added quality-adjusted life year (QALY) by moving from less to more expensive interventions; the focus is on differences in cost and effectiveness among options, so the result is called the incremental cost-effectiveness ratio (ICER).
• With the exception of spine surgery, there is a relative paucity of cost-effectiveness studies in the field of neurosurgery; and many of these use inconsistent cost metrics, variable outcome measures, and data sets that are poorly matched to the analysis.
• It is of utmost important for this field to establish and adhere to guidelines for cost and CEA methodology and reporting so that results can be appropriately compared among neurosurgery cost-effectiveness studies and with interventions in other medical fields.

INTRODUCTION

Cost and value (defined as the quality or outcomes of care compared with cost) are increasingly important components of health care. Despite a wealth of CEAs in many areas of medicine, there has been little research addressing the cost of neurosurgical procedures until recently. This is particularly problematic because this specialty represents one of the most expensive areas in medicine. According to the Centers for Disease Control and Prevention, there were approximately 1.2 million neurosurgical procedures performed in the United States in 2010.[1] The cost of lumbar laminectomies alone exceeded $2 billion, and spinal fusions cost $12.8 billion nationwide in 2011.[2]

This article first discusses the general principles of CEAs, then reviews the cost-related research that has been done to date in the neurosurgical subspecialties, primarily spine and also trauma, functional, vascular, pediatric, and tumor neurosurgery. Finally, the need for standardization of cost and cost-effectiveness metrics within neurosurgery is highlighted and an easy-to-use set of metrics to guide future research in neurosurgical cost-effectiveness is defined.

PRINCIPLES OF COST-EFFECTIVENESS ANALYSES

A CEA is a type of economic analysis that compares the costs and health outcomes of 2 or more courses of action.[3] CEAs are often expressed in terms of a ratio of cost per health gain. The most commonly used health outcomes measure in the United States and Europe is QALYs. A QALY reflects both the quantity and quality of the years gained by a medical intervention, and is equal to time (years) × quality (ie, utility). Health utility is on a scale from 0 to 1, with 0 indicating death and 1 representing perfect health. Direct methods to estimate health state utility include time tradeoff, standard gamble, and visual analog scale. Indirect methods include the Health Utility Index,[4]

a Department of Neurological Surgery, University of California, San Francisco, 505 Parnassus Avenue, Room 779M, San Francisco, CA 94143, USA; b Philip R. Lee Institute for Health Policy Studies, Global Health Economics Consortium, University of California, San Francisco, 3333 California St., Suite 265, Box 0936, San Francisco, CA 94118, USA
* Corresponding author.
E-mail address: zygourakisc@neurosurg.ucsf.edu

Neurosurg Clin N Am 26 (2015) 189–196
http://dx.doi.org/10.1016/j.nec.2014.11.008
1042-3680/15/$ – see front matter © 2015 Elsevier Inc. All rights reserved.

EuroQoL–5 Dimension (EQ-5D),[5] and Short Form–6 Dimension (SF-6D).[6] A single year spent in perfect health yields 1 QALY, and effective medical interventions increase QALYs. To compare 2 interventions (eg, treatments A and B), an ICER, which equals (cost of B – cost of A)/(QALYS with B – QALYs with A), is calculated. The use of ICERs enables the cost of achieving a certain benefit to be compared with similar ratios calculated for other health interventions, providing a broader context in which to make judgments about the value for money of a particular health intervention.[3] In the United States, ICERs less than $150,000 are typically considered cost effective, because this represents 2 times the gross domestic product per capita.[7]

A cost-utility analysis is a specific type of CEA that uses health utilities expressed as QALYs (described previously). CEAs can also include other health outcomes, such as cost per death averted or added year of life. A cost-benefit analysis, distinct from a CEA, assigns a monetary value to health outcomes, usually based on a population's "willingness to pay" for those outcomes. Thus, it calculates the net monetary cost or savings of an intervention. It is used less frequently than CEAs in medicine.[3]

A rigorous CEA must specify its cost methods. Costs include both direct costs (eg, resources consumed by the surgical procedure, such as surgical implants and hospital stay, and the costs of future medical care) and time costs (eg, due to loss of productivity from the morbidity of a surgical procedure). In the literature, hospital-allowed charges (ie, what the hospital is paid by the insurance company) are often used as a proxy for direct cost. Importantly, crude (billed) hospital charges can bear little resemblance to economic cost[8]; and use of hospital charges as a proxy for cost may lead researchers to draw unwarranted conclusions.[9] The best measure of cost is actual resource utilization,[9] which can be difficult to calculate but is available via some hospital cost-accounting systems. Many articles in the literature are forced to use insurance payments, specifically the Centers for Medicare and Medicaid Services reimbursement values for specific diagnosis-related group and current procedural terminology codes, as estimates for cost.[10]

Several additional aspects of CEA methods should also be reported in each study. These include the analytical time period and perspective (eg, that of society or health care payers), the discount rate, the type of sensitivity or uncertainty analysis performed, and the selected cost-effectiveness threshold (if used). All these criteria are reported in the Cost-Effectiveness Analysis Registry,[11] which is a comprehensive database of 4007 cost-utility analyses that have been assessed by reviewers with training in cost-effectiveness and decision analysis. The CEA model structure and input values must be transparent and thoroughly documented and justified, typically with some detail in online supplemental documents.

COST-EFFECTIVENESS ANALYSES IN NEUROSURGERY

A comprehensive PubMed search for "cost-effectiveness" and "neurosurgery" had 691 hits, although only a small subset of these results were true CEAs. A more refined search ("cost-effectiveness" [ti] "cost utility" [ti] neurosurgery) helped narrow the list to 140 articles. A search of the Cost-Effectiveness Analysis Registry (search terms, "neurosurgery" and "spine") revealed fewer than 50 verified cost-utility analyses in the field of neurosurgery up to early 2013, a majority of which are in the subspecialty of spine.[12–25] Admittedly, there has been an increased interest in this area recently, with a significant rise in the number of neurosurgery cost-effectiveness studies published over the past 2 years. A majority of purported cost-effectiveness neurosurgery studies, however, do not adhere to the CEA methodology described previously. Many of these are actually cost comparison (ie, descriptive comparisons of cost differences) rather than cost-effectiveness studies. They also have several limitations, including inconsistent use of cost methods (direct vs indirect costs, charges vs payments), variable outcome measures, and potentially noncomparable data sets (ranging from large national databases, such as the Nationwide Inpatient Sample database, to small, single-institution series).

SPINE: THE LEADER IN NEUROSURGERY COST-EFFECTIVENESS

Driven largely by the high costs of their procedures and insurance companies' demands for justification of their interventions, spine surgeons were among the first neurosurgeons to enter the cost-effectiveness field. One of the earliest studies, published in 2008, showed the cost-effectiveness of lumbar laminectomy, compared with nonoperative treatment, for lumbar disc herniation at 2 years (ICER $69,403).[26] Using the same Spine Patient Outcomes Research Trial data, this research group also found that lumbar laminectomy was a cost-effective treatment option compared with nonoperative treatment for spinal stenosis with and without degenerative spondylolisthesis at 2 years (ICER <$150,000).[27] These findings were supported by a study in 2010 showing that lumbar laminectomy was more effective than nonsurgical care or X-STOP Interspinous Process Decompression System for treatment of symptomatic lumbar spinal stenosis (ICER = $28,256 for laminectomy compared with conservative management at 4-year follow-up).[28] More recently, several studies have looked at the cost-effectiveness of decompression alone versus instrumented fusion for grade I L4/5 spondylolisthesis ($56,610/QALY for decompression alone vs >$100,000/QALY gained for decompression with various types of fusion),[29] the cost/QALY gained for transforaminal lumbar interbody fusion (TLIF) for grade I degenerative spondylolisthesis (2-year cost of $42,854 per QALY gained),[30] and the cost-effectiveness of revision surgery for same-level recurrent lumbar stenosis and adjacent-segment disease (2-year cost of $80,594 per QALY gained).[31–33] Much of this work comes from the same research group (led by Matthew McGirt, MD, formerly of Vanderbilt University) performing analysis on a small set of patients at a single institution.[30–33]

Similar to this body of work on degenerative lumbar disease, several groups have investigated the cost-effectiveness of different surgical treatment options for cervical spine disease,[34,35] metastatic spine tumors,[36,37] and adult spinal deformity.[38] Researchers have also examined the cost-effectiveness of specific spinal implants, such as bone morphogenic protein ($136,207/QALY gained),[39] femoral head allografts,[40] and polyetheretheketone anterior cervical cages (>$100,000/QALY gained),[41] as well as the cost-effectiveness of certain intraoperative techniques like neurophysiological monitoring[42] and O-arm confirmation of lumbar pedicle screw placement.[43] With the increasing popularity of minimally invasive spine (MIS) surgery, many recent spine CEAs have focused on determining the cost-effectiveness of newer minimally invasive techniques, such as the minimally invasive TLIF or tubular discectomy, compared with the traditional open approaches.[21,44–48] Results for MIS surgery have been mixed, with some studies suggesting that minimally invasive approaches are cost effective[45,46,48] but others showing equivalent cost-effectiveness for minimally invasive and open approaches.[21]

Despite the growing number of studies on spinal surgery cost-effectiveness, there are many limitations of this work. First, many of these studies are simply cost descriptions[34,49–51] rather than true CEAs, as discussed previously. These studies use widely different measures of cost, from hospital-based charges to Medicare reimbursement rates, which can substantially influence the results of a cost-effectiveness study,[14] and are discussed in further detail later. Finally, most of these are retrospective single-institution studies. To make systems-level treatment recommendations, more robust CEAs from prospective multicenter studies are needed, such as the currently underway Verbiest trial in the Netherlands comparing operative with nonoperative treatment of neurogenic claudication due to lumbar stenosis[52] and the Netherlands Cervical Kinematics double-blind randomized multicenter study comparing the cost-effectiveness of anterior cervical discectomy with and without interbody fusion and arthroplasty.[53]

COST-EFFECTIVENESS ANALYSES IN OTHER AREAS OF NEUROSURGERY: MOVING BEYOND SPINE

Despite the growing literature focused on cost-effectiveness in spinal surgery, there are only a handful of articles addressing cost issues in other neurosurgical subspecialties. In the authors' comprehensive literature review, 7 articles were identified addressing cost-effectiveness in neurosurgical trauma.[15,54–59] Three studies addressed the cost-effectiveness of decompressive hemicraniectomy for severe traumatic brain injury (TBI): 1 from the United States[54] and another from Europe[55] reported that decompressive hemicraniectomy was a cost-effective treatment option for patients with severe TBI (even if they were >80 years old [eg, €17,900/QALY gained]), but a study from western Australia concluded that surgery was not a cost-effective option for patients with severe TBI when the predicted risk of an unfavorable outcome was greater than 80% ($682,000/QALY).[56] Another study found that surgical decompressive hemicraniectomy was more cost-effective than a barbiturate coma for refractory intracranial hypertension (ICER = $9,565).[57] Finally, 2 studies examined the cost-effectiveness of radiographic imaging for traumatic minor head injury in adults[15] and in children.[58]

In the realm of functional neurosurgery, 3 recent studies[60–62] examined the cost-effectiveness of microvascular decompression for trigeminal neuralgia compared with radiosurgery and percutaneous rhizotomy ($4,931/QALY for surgery vs $7,768/QALY for radiosurgery and $602/QALY for percutaneous rhizotomy).[60,61] None of these studies compared microvascular decompression with medical therapy, which is an important target for future work. A recent study from Hong Kong looked at the ICER of deep brain stimulation versus medical therapy for Parkinson disease (ICER = $123,110 at 1 year and $62,846 at

2 years).[63] This analysis did not calculate cost-effectiveness over patient expected lifetime, however. Two international studies[64,65] also showed cost-effectiveness of surgical treatment of epilepsy compared with continued medical therapy (ICER = $25,020 to $69,451 Canadian dollars),[64,65] which promises to be an exciting area of cost-effectiveness research for the functional neurosurgeon.

Only 3 published works have applied cost-effectiveness techniques to pediatric neurosurgery, with 1 group performing a cost comparison analysis for endoscopic-assisted craniectomy versus open cranial vault remodeling for sagittal synostosis,[66] another looking at the cost-effectiveness of endoscopic third ventriculostomy versus shunt for hydrocephalus,[67] and another looking at the costs and benefits of neurosurgical intervention for infants with hydrocephalus in sub-Saharan Africa ($59 to $126/disability-adjusted life year averted).[68] The cost-effectiveness literature in vascular neurosurgery is similarly sparse[12,24,69–72]; and studies comparing the cost of surgical clipping versus endovascular treatment of ruptured aneurysms provide contradictory results.[73–76]

NEUROSURGICAL ONCOLOGY COST-EFFECTIVENESS ANALYSES

As in trauma, functional, pediatric, and vascular neurosurgery, there is a paucity of literature addressing the cost of neurosurgical oncology (ie, brain tumor treatment),[77–85] and a majority of these articles are from outside the United States.[20,86–95] The authors' research group, therefore, has focused efforts on performing the first rigorous CEAs with decision-tree analyses for the management of benign brain tumors, including vestibular schwannomas, prolactinomas (prolactin-secreting pituitary tumors), and meningiomas. Their vestibular schwannoma CEA using direct hospital cost data found that surgery is a cost-effective alternative to radiation when patients are diagnosed with a vestibular schwannoma at less than 45 years old (ICER <$150,000). For vestibular schwannoma patients greater than or equal to 45 years old, radiation is the most cost-effective treatment option.[96] In a prolactinoma CEA analysis, despite higher up-front surgical costs, surgery was the less expensive treatment option over a patient's expected lifespan ($428 per 1% reduction in serum prolactin level for surgery vs $921 for bromocriptine and $1621 for cabergoline) because medically treated patients must often remain on either bromocriptine or cabergoline indefinitely. In the authors' CEA model, surgery is a cost-effective alternative to cabergoline and bromocriptine at all ages of diagnosis less than 80 years old.[97]

DISCUSSION

This article provides a brief summary of the basic principles of CEAs as well as a review of the cost-related research in all subspecialties of neurosurgery, including spine, trauma, functional, pediatrics, vascular, and tumor neurosurgery. The limitations of much of the neurosurgery cost-effectiveness work that has been performed to date are emphasized. Many of the studies discussed in this article are not true CEAs but rather cost studies. Even the studies that are CEAs often use different cost metrics, variable outcome measures, and unreliable data sets, making it difficult to draw definitive conclusions from them. A particularly nice study showed how the choice of cost method (hospital-based cost analysis using charges multiplied by cost-to-charge ratios vs Medicare reimbursements) substantially influenced the final results of a cervical spine surgery CEA.[14] Medicare reimbursements may underestimate real cost whereas hospital charges can grossly overestimate true costs.

It is, therefore, of utmost important for this field to establish guidelines for cost and CEA methods and reporting so that results between studies can be appropriately compared. The authors propose that every neurosurgery cost-effectiveness article be held to the basic standards of CEA analysis used by the Cost-Effectiveness Analysis Registry.[11] More specifically, every neurosurgery cost-utility analysis should have correctly calculated QALYs and ICERs and should explicitly report the analytical time period and analytical perspective (eg, from the societal or health care payer perspective), the currency used, the discount rate, the type of sensitivity or uncertainty analysis performed, and the selected cost-effectiveness threshold (if used). In addition, model design and input values should be sufficiently described to permit replication and comparison with other analyses that might use a different structure or input values.

Finally, to make systems-level treatment recommendations, greater generalizability is needed, building the CEAs on prospective multicenter studies, a few examples of which are already under way in Europe.[52,53] In the United States, the authors hope that such studies will become possible with further developments of the new national clinical databases, such as the National Neurosurgery Quality and Outcomes Database.[98]

REFERENCES

1. Center for Disease. Available at: http://www.cdc.gov/nchs/data/nhds/4procedures/2010pro4_number procedureage.pdf. Accessed September 27, 2014.
2. Center for Disease. Available at: http://www.cdc.gov/nchs/data/hus/hus13.pdf - 116. Accessed September 27, 2014.
3. World Health Organization. Introduction to Drug Utilization Research. 2003. Available at: http://apps.who.int/medicinedocs/en/d/Js4876e/. Accessed September 27, 2014.
4. Horsman J, Furlong W, Feeny D, et al. The health utilities index (HUI): concepts, measurement properties and applications. Health Qual Life Outcomes 2003;1:54.
5. Rabin R, de Charro F. EQ-5D: a measure of health status from the EuroQol Group. Ann Med 2001;33:337–43.
6. Brazier J, Roberts J, Deverill M. The estimation of a preference-based measure of health from the SF-36. J Health Econ 2002;21:271–92.
7. Cost-effectiveness thresholds. World Health Organization. Available at: http://www.who.int/choice/costs/CER_thresholds/en/. Accessed September 27, 2014.
8. Brill S. Bitter pill: why medical bills are killing us. Time Magazine 2013. 16–55.
9. Finkler S. The distinction between cost and charges. Ann Intern Med 1982;96:102–9.
10. Tumeh JW, Moore SG, Shapiro R, et al. Practical approach for using Medicare data to estimate costs for cost-effectiveness analysis. Expert Rev Pharmacoecon Outcomes Res 2005;5:153–62.
11. Cost-effectiveness Analysis Registry. Available at: http://www.cearegistry.org. Accessed September 9, 2014.
12. Jethwa PR, Punia V, Patel TD, et al. Cost-effectiveness of digital subtraction angiography in the setting of computed tomographic angiography negative subarachnoid hemorrhage. Neurosurgery 2013;72:511–9 [discussion: 519].
13. Parker SL, McGirt MJ. Determination of the minimum improvement in pain, disability, and health state associated with cost-effectiveness: introduction of the concept of minimum cost-effective difference. Neurosurgery 2012;71:1149–55.
14. Whitmore RG, Schwartz JS, Simmons S, et al. Performing a cost analysis in spine outcomes research: comparing ventral and dorsal approaches for cervical spondylotic myelopathy. Neurosurgery 2012;70:860–7 [discussion: 867].
15. Smits M, Dippel DW, Nederkoorn PJ, et al. Minor head injury: CT-based strategies for management–a cost-effectiveness analysis. Radiology 2010;254:532–40.
16. Malmivaara K, Hernesniemi J, Salmenpera R, et al. Survival and outcome of neurosurgical patients requiring ventilatory support after intensive care unit stay. Neurosurgery 2009;65:530–7 [discussion: 537–8].
17. Papatheofanis FJ, Williams E, Chang SD. Cost-utility analysis of the cyberknife system for metastatic spinal tumors. Neurosurgery 2009;64:A73–83.
18. North RB, Kidd D, Shipley J, et al. Spinal cord stimulation versus reoperation for failed back surgery syndrome: a cost effectiveness and cost utility analysis based on a randomized, controlled trial. Neurosurgery 2007;61:361–8 [discussion: 368–9].
19. Stein SC, Burnett MG, Zager EL, et al. Completion angiography for surgically treated cerebral aneurysms: an economic analysis. Neurosurgery 2007; 61:1162–7 [discussion: 1167–9].
20. Cho DY, Tsao M, Lee WY, et al. Socioeconomic costs of open surgery and gamma knife radiosurgery for benign cranial base tumors. Neurosurgery 2006; 58:866–73 [discussion: 866–73].
21. van den Akker ME, Arts MP, van den Hout WB, et al. Tubular diskectomy vs conventional microdiskectomy for the treatment of lumbar disk-related sciatica: cost utility analysis alongside a double-blind randomized controlled trial. Neurosurgery 2011;69:829–35 [discussion: 835–6].
22. Rasanen P, Ohman J, Sintonen H, et al. Cost-utility analysis of routine neurosurgical spinal surgery. J Neurosurg Spine 2006;5:204–9.
23. King JT Jr, Sperling MR, Justice AC, et al. A cost-effectiveness analysis of anterior temporal lobectomy for intractable temporal lobe epilepsy. J Neurosurg 1997;87:20–8.
24. Nussbaum ES, Heros RC, Erickson DL. Cost-effectiveness of carotid endarterectomy. Neurosurgery 1996;38:237–44.
25. Pickard JD, Bailey S, Sanderson H, et al. Steps towards cost-benefit analysis of regional neurosurgical care. BMJ 1990;301:629–35.
26. Tosteson AN, Skinner JS, Tosteson TD, et al. The cost effectiveness of surgical versus nonoperative treatment for lumbar disc herniation over two years: evidence from the Spine Patient Outcomes Research Trial (SPORT). Spine 2008;33:2108–15.
27. Tosteson AN, Lurie JD, Tosteson TD, et al, SPORT Investigators. Surgical treatment of spinal stenosis with and without degenerative spondylolisthesis: cost-effectiveness after 2 years. Ann Intern Med 2008;149:845–53.
28. Burnett MG, Stein SC, Bartels RH. Cost-effectiveness of current treatment strategies for lumbar spinal stenosis: nonsurgical care, laminectomy, and X-STOP. J Neurosurg Spine 2010;13:39–46.
29. Alvin MD, Lubelski D, Abdullah KG, et al. Cost-utility analysis of instrumented fusion versus decompression alone for grade i l4-5 spondylolisthesis at 1-year follow-up: a pilot study. J Spinal Disord Tech 2014. [Epub ahead of print].

30. Adogwa O, Parker SL, Davis BJ, et al. Cost-effectiveness of transforaminal lumbar interbody fusion for Grade I degenerative spondylolisthesis. J Neurosurg Spine 2011;15:138–43.

31. Adogwa O, Owens R, Karikari I, et al. Revision lumbar surgery in elderly patients with symptomatic pseudarthrosis, adjacent-segment disease, or same-level recurrent stenosis. Part 2. A cost-effectiveness analysis: clinical article. J Neurosurg Spine 2013;18:147–53.

32. Adogwa O, Parker SL, Shau DN, et al. Cost per quality-adjusted life year gained of revision neural decompression and instrumented fusion for same-level recurrent lumbar stenosis: defining the value of surgical intervention. J Neurosurg Spine 2012;16:135–40.

33. Adogwa O, Parker SL, Shau DN, et al. Cost per quality-adjusted life year gained of laminectomy and extension of instrumented fusion for adjacent-segment disease: defining the value of surgical intervention. J Neurosurg Spine 2012;16:141–6.

34. Tumialan LM, Ponton RP, Gluf WM. Management of unilateral cervical radiculopathy in the military: the cost effectiveness of posterior cervical foraminotomy compared with anterior cervical discectomy and fusion. Neurosurg Focus 2010;28:E17.

35. Alvin MD, Lubelski D, Abdullah KG, et al. Cost-utility analysis of anterior cervical discectomy and fusion with plating (ACDFP) versus posterior cervical foraminotomy (PCF) for patients with single-level cervical radiculopathy at 1-year follow-up. J Spinal Disord Tech 2014. [Epub ahead of print].

36. Fehlings MG, Nater A, Holmer H. Cost-effectiveness of surgery in the management of metastatic epidural spinal cord compression (MESCC): a systematic review. Spine 2014;39(22 Suppl 1):S99–105.

37. Furlan JC, Chan KK, Sandoval GA, et al. The combined use of surgery and radiotherapy to treat patients with epidural cord compression due to metastatic disease: a cost-utility analysis. Neuro Oncol 2012;14:631–40.

38. Terran J, McHugh BJ, Fischer CR, et al. Surgical treatment for adult spinal deformity: projected cost effectiveness at 5-year follow-up. Ochsner J 2014;14:14–22.

39. Alvin MD, Derakhshan A, Lubelski D, et al. Cost-utility analysis of one and two-level dorsal lumbar fusions with and without recombinant human bone morphogenic protein-2 at 1-year follow-up. J Spinal Disord Tech 2014. [Epub ahead of print].

40. Brown DA, Mallory GW, Higgins DM, et al. A cost-effective method for femoral head allograft procurement for spinal arthrodesis: an alternative to commercially available allograft. Spine 2014;39:E902–6.

41. Virk SS, Elder JB, Sandhu HS, et al. The cost effectiveness of polyetheretheketone (PEEK) cages for anterior cervical discectomy and fusion. J Spinal Disord Tech 2014. [Epub ahead of print].

42. Ney JP, van der Goes DN, Watanabe JH. Cost-benefit analysis: intraoperative neurophysiological monitoring in spinal surgeries. J Clin Neurophysiol 2013;30:280–6.

43. Sanborn MR, Thawani JP, Whitmore RG, et al. Cost-effectiveness of confirmatory techniques for the placement of lumbar pedicle screws. Neurosurg Focus 2012;33:E12.

44. Al-Khouja LT, Baron EM, Johnson JP, et al. Cost-effectiveness analysis in minimally invasive spine surgery. Neurosurg Focus 2014;36:E4.

45. Sulaiman WA, Singh M. Minimally invasive versus open transforaminal lumbar interbody fusion for degenerative spondylolisthesis grades 1-2: patient-reported clinical outcomes and cost-utility analysis. Ochsner J 2014;14:32–7.

46. Parker SL, Mendenhall SK, Shau DN, et al. Minimally invasive versus open transforaminal lumbar interbody fusion for degenerative spondylolisthesis: comparative effectiveness and cost-utility analysis. World Neurosurg 2014;82:230–8.

47. Parker SL, Adogwa O, Davis BJ, et al. Cost-utility analysis of minimally invasive versus open multilevel hemilaminectomy for lumbar stenosis. J Spinal Disord Tech 2013;26:42–7.

48. Parker SL, Adogwa O, Bydon A, et al. Cost-effectiveness of minimally invasive versus open transforaminal lumbar interbody fusion for degenerative spondylolisthesis associated low-back and leg pain over two years. World Neurosurg 2012;78:178–84.

49. McCarthy IM, Hostin RA, Ames CP, et al, International Spine Study Group. Total hospital costs of surgical treatment for adult spinal deformity: an extended follow-up study. Spine J 2014;14:2326–33.

50. Parker SL, Adogwa O, Witham TF, et al. Post-operative infection after minimally invasive versus open transforaminal lumbar interbody fusion (TLIF): literature review and cost analysis. Minim Invasive Neurosurg 2011;54:33–7.

51. Ray WZ, Ravindra VM, Jost GF, et al. Cost effectiveness of subaxial fusion–lateral mass screws versus transarticular facet screws. Neurosurg Focus 2012;33:E14.

52. Overdevest GM, Luijsterburg PA, Brand R, et al. Design of the Verbiest trial: cost-effectiveness of surgery versus prolonged conservative treatment in patients with lumbar stenosis. BMC Musculoskelet Disord 2011;12:57.

53. Arts MP, Brand R, van den Akker E, et al. The Netherlands Cervical Kinematics (NECK) trial. Cost-effectiveness of anterior cervical discectomy with or without interbody fusion and arthroplasty in the treatment of cervical disc herniation; a double-blind randomised multicenter study. BMC Musculoskelet Disord 2010;11:122.

54. Whitmore RG, Thawani JP, Grady MS, et al. Is aggressive treatment of traumatic brain injury cost-effective? J Neurosurg 2012;116:1106–13.

55. Malmivaara K, Kivisaari R, Hernesniemi J, et al. Cost-effectiveness of decompressive craniectomy in traumatic brain injuries. Eur J Neurol 2011;18: 656–62.

56. Ho KM, Honeybul S, Lind CR, et al. Cost-effectiveness of decompressive craniectomy as a lifesaving rescue procedure for patients with severe traumatic brain injury. J Trauma 2011;71:1637–44 [discussion: 1644].

57. Alali AS, Naimark DM, Wilson JR, et al. Economic evaluation of decompressive craniectomy versus barbiturate coma for refractory intracranial hypertension following traumatic brain injury. Crit Care Med 2014;42:2235–43.

58. Holmes MW, Goodacre S, Stevenson MD, et al. The cost-effectiveness of diagnostic management strategies for children with minor head injury. Arch Dis Child 2013;98:939–44.

59. Hofmeijer J, van der Worp HB, Kappelle LJ, et al. Cost-effectiveness of surgical decompression for space-occupying hemispheric infarction. Stroke 2013;44: 2923–5.

60. Sivakanthan S, Van Gompel JJ, Alikhani P, et al. Surgical management of trigeminal neuralgia: use and cost-effectiveness from an analysis of the Medicare claims database. Neurosurgery 2014;75:220–6.

61. Fransen P. Cost-effectiveness in the surgical treatments for trigeminal neuralgia. Acta Neurol Belg 2012;112:245–7.

62. Pollock BE, Ecker RD. A prospective cost-effectiveness study of trigeminal neuralgia surgery. Clin J Pain 2005;21:317–22.

63. Zhu XL, Chan DT, Lau CK, et al. Cost-effectiveness of subthalmic nucleus deep brain stimulation for treatment of advanced Parkinson's disease in Hong Kong: a prospective study. World Neurosurg 2014. [Epub ahead of print].

64. Bowen JM, Snead OC, Chandra K, et al. Epilepsy care in ontario: an economic analysis of increasing access to epilepsy surgery. Ont Health Technol Assess Ser 2012;12:1–41.

65. Widjaja E, Li B, Schinkel CD, et al. Cost-effectiveness of pediatric epilepsy surgery compared to medical treatment in children with intractable epilepsy. Epilepsy Res 2011;94:61–8.

66. Vogel TW, Woo AS, Kane AA, et al. A comparison of costs associated with endoscope-assisted craniectomy versus open cranial vault repair for infants with sagittal synostosis. J Neurosurg Pediatr 2014;13: 324–31.

67. Garton HJ, Kestle JR, Cochrane DD, et al. A cost-effectiveness analysis of endoscopic third ventriculostomy. Neurosurgery 2002;51:69–77 [discussion: 77–8].

68. Warf BC, Alkire BC, Bhai S, et al. Costs and benefits of neurosurgical intervention for infant hydrocephalus in sub-Saharan Africa. J Neurosurg Pediatr 2011;8:509–21.

69. Jabbarli R, Shah M, Taschner C, et al. Clinical utility and cost-effectiveness of CT-angiography in the diagnosis of nontraumatic subarachnoid hemorrhage. Neuroradiology 2014;56(10):817–24.

70. Malmivaara K, Juvela S, Hernesniemi J, et al. Health-related quality of life and cost-effectiveness of treatment in subarachnoid haemorrhage. Eur J Neurol 2012;19:1455–61.

71. Koffijberg H, Buskens E, Rinkel GJ. Aneurysm occlusion in elderly patients with aneurysmal subarachnoid haemorrhage: a cost-utility analysis. J Neurol Neurosurg Psychiatry 2011;82:718–27.

72. Greving JP, Rinkel GJ, Buskens E, et al. Cost-effectiveness of preventive treatment of intracranial aneurysms: new data and uncertainties. Neurology 2009;73:258–65.

73. Hoh BL, Chi YY, Lawson MF, et al. Length of stay and total hospital charges of clipping versus coiling for ruptured and unruptured adult cerebral aneurysms in the Nationwide Inpatient Sample database 2002 to 2006. Stroke 2010;41:337–42.

74. Zubair Tahir M, Enam SA, Pervez Ali R, et al. Cost-effectiveness of clipping vs coiling of intracranial aneurysms after subarachnoid hemorrhage in a developing country–a prospective study. Surg Neurol 2009;72:355–60 [discussion: 360–1].

75. Maud A, Lakshminarayan K, Suri MF, et al. Cost-effectiveness analysis of endovascular versus neurosurgical treatment for ruptured intracranial aneurysms in the United States. J Neurosurg 2009;110:880–6.

76. King JT Jr, Glick HA, Mason TJ, et al. Elective surgery for asymptomatic, unruptured, intracranial aneurysms: a cost-effectiveness analysis. J Neurosurg 1995;83:403–12.

77. Mukherjee D, Patil CG, Todnem N, et al. Racial disparities in Medicaid patients after brain tumor surgery. J Clin Neurosci 2013;20:57–61.

78. Sonig A, Khan IS, Wadhwa R, et al. The impact of comorbidities, regional trends, and hospital factors on discharge dispositions and hospital costs after acoustic neuroma microsurgery: a United States nationwide inpatient data sample study (2005-2009). Neurosurg Focus 2012;33:E3.

79. Marko NF, LaSota E, Hamrahian AH, et al. Comparative effectiveness review of treatment options for pituitary microadenomas in acromegaly. J Neurosurg 2012;117:522–38.

80. Makary M, Chiocca EA, Erminy N, et al. Clinical and economic outcomes of low-field intraoperative MRI-guided tumor resection neurosurgery. J Magn Reson Imaging 2011;34:1022–30.

81. Long DM, Gordon T, Bowman H, et al. Outcome and cost of craniotomy performed to

treat tumors in regional academic referral centers. Neurosurgery 2003;52:1056–63 [discussion: 1056–63].

82. Mehta M, Noyes W, Craig B, et al. A cost-effectiveness and cost-utility analysis of radiosurgery vs. resection for single-brain metastases. Int J Radiat Oncol Biol Phys 1997;39:445–54.

83. Banerjee R, Moriarty JP, Foote RL, et al. Comparison of the surgical and follow-up costs associated with microsurgical resection and stereotactic radiosurgery for vestibular schwannoma. J Neurosurg 2008;108:1220–4.

84. Rutigliano MJ, Lunsford LD, Kondziolka D, et al. The cost effectiveness of stereotactic radiosurgery versus surgical resection in the treatment of solitary metastatic brain tumors. Neurosurgery 1995;37: 445–53 [discussion: 453–5].

85. Lester SC, Taksler GB, Kuremsky JG, et al. Clinical and economic outcomes of patients with brain metastases based on symptoms: an argument for routine brain screening of those treated with upfront radiosurgery. Cancer 2014;120:433–41.

86. Martino J, Gomez E, Bilbao JL, et al. Cost-utility of maximal safe resection of WHO grade II gliomas within eloquent areas. Acta Neurochir 2013;155: 41–50.

87. Vuong DA, Rades D, van Eck AT, et al. Comparing the cost-effectiveness of two brain metastasis treatment modalities from a payer's perspective: stereotactic radiosurgery versus surgical resection. Clin Neurol Neurosurg 2013;115:276–84.

88. Undabeitia J, Liu BG, Catalan G, et al. Clinical and economic analysis of hospital acquired infections in patients diagnosed with brain tumor in a tertiary hospital. Neurocirugia 2011;22:535–41.

89. Vuong DA, Rades D, Le AN, et al. The cost-effectiveness of stereotactic radiosurgery versus surgical resection in the treatment of brain metastasis in Vietnam from the perspective of patients and families. World Neurosurg 2012;77:321–8.

90. Tan SS, van Putten E, Nijdam WM, et al. A microcosting study of microsurgery, LINAC radiosurgery, and gamma knife radiosurgery in meningioma patients. J Neurooncol 2011;101:237–45.

91. Lee WY, Cho DY, Lee HC, et al. Outcomes and cost-effectiveness of gamma knife radiosurgery and whole brain radiotherapy for multiple metastatic brain tumors. J Clin Neurosci 2009;16:630–4.

92. Wellis G, Nagel R, Vollmar C, et al. Direct costs of microsurgical management of radiosurgically amenable intracranial pathology in Germany: an analysis of meningiomas, acoustic neuromas, metastases and arteriovenous malformations of less than 3 cm in diameter. Acta Neurochir 2003;145:249–55.

93. Mendez I, Jacobs P, MacDougall A, et al. Treatment costs for glioblastoma multiforme in Nova Scotia. Can J Neurol Sci 2001;28:61–5.

94. van Roijen L, Nijs HG, Avezaat CJ, et al. Costs and effects of microsurgery versus radiosurgery in treating acoustic neuroma. Acta Neurochir 1997;139: 942–8.

95. Zhen JR, Yu Q, Zhang YH, et al. Cost-effectiveness analysis of two therapeutic methods for prolactinoma. Zhonghua Fu Chan Ke Za Zhi 2008;43:257–61 [in Chinese].

96. Zygourakis C, Oh T, Sun M, et al. Surgery is costeffective treatment for young patients with vestibular schwannomas: decision tree modeling of surgery, radiation, and observation. Neurosurg Focus 2014; 37(5):E8. [Epub ahead of print].

97. Zygourakis C, Imber B, Han S, et al. Surgery is more cost-effective than medical therapy for treatment of prolactinomas. Submitted.

98. The National Neurosurgery Quality and Outcomes Database. Available at: http://www.neuropoint.org/NPA%20N2QOD.html. Accessed September 27, 2014.

Economics, Innovation, and Quality Improvement in Neurosurgery

Christopher D. Witiw, MD[a], Vinitra Nathan[a],
Mark Bernstein, MD, MHSc, FRCSC[a,b],*

KEYWORDS

- Economics • Quality improvement • Innovation • Neurosurgery • Cost effectiveness • Cost utility
- Willingness to pay

KEY POINTS

- Innovation to improve patient care is a cornerstone of neurologic surgery; these improvements often are measured in quality outcome metrics while economic metrics are frequently held to lesser consideration.
- As the strain of limited health care resources grows, assessment of the cost incurred to improve quality has become increasingly more important; the means of assessing innovations in terms of economic measures are reviewed, and the considerations for willingness-to-pay thresholds are discussed.
- Innovations within neurosurgery are presented in a framework structured on quality and economic metrics; this provides a conceptual means for neurosurgeons and policy makers to assess current innovations and to highlight areas in which further investigation and cost assessment are needed.

INTRODUCTION

The highly specialized and complex nature of neurologic surgery is inherently associated with slim margins for error and the ever-present potential of life-altering adverse events. This has driven innovation within the field since the early days of Harvey Cushing,[1] and an implicit obligation to provide or incorporate new ideas, technologies, or surgical techniques has remained a cornerstone of the specialty. In the modern era of evidence-based medicine, these improvements in quality are measured in clinical outcome metrics such as length of survival, disease-free survival, and quality of life. Conversely, the inclusion of innovations that specifically optimize efficiency and focus on economic measures is less ingrained in the traditions and training of neurosurgeons.

Austerity measures in the face of the recent global economic downturn, beginning in the first decade of the 21st century, have been implicated in a decline in access and quality of patient care.[2] Although it seems that government investment in health care services is back on the increase, an aging population and increasing life expectancies will continue to drive health care expenditures to higher levels. In 2005, aggregate health care expenditures were US $5572 per capita—of these, $1615 per capita was surgical specific. Aggregate health care expenditures are predicted to increase to $8832 per capita by 2025 with $2561 per capita being surgical specific. Put in other terms, aggregate health care expenditures will comprise one-fourth of the US economy in 2025 and surgical-specific expenditures will comprise one-fourteenth. The predicted growth

[a] Division of Neurosurgery, Toronto Western Hospital, University of Toronto, 399 Bathurst Street, Toronto, Ontario M5T 2S8, Canada; [b] Joint Centre for Bioethics, University of Toronto, 155 College Street, Suite 754, Toronto, Ontario M5T 1P8, Canada
* Corresponding author. Toronto Western Hospital, 399 Bathurst Street, 4WW-448, Toronto, Ontario M5T 2S8, Canada.
E-mail address: Mark.Bernstein@uhn.ca

Neurosurg Clin N Am 26 (2015) 197–205
http://dx.doi.org/10.1016/j.nec.2014.11.003

between 2005 and 2025 is nearly 60%.[3] Innovations that reduce the costs and improve the efficiency of patient care are needed to obviate impending critical stresses on the health care system. Investigations that combine endpoints for quality and economic metrics are essential to evaluate these new innovations. However, studies of this nature are the exception rather than the norm in the neurosurgical literature.

The aim of this article is 2-fold. First, the authors present a summary of the current tools for evaluating the gains in quality afforded by innovations in neurosurgery in terms of cost effectiveness and review the factors that determine willingness to pay for quality gains. Second, examples are provided from the specialty organized in a conceptual framework based on quality of care and economic metrics. This framework highlights areas in which innovation has enhanced quality and concomitantly improved costs and calls attention to areas in which further assessment is needed.

ASSESSING QUALITY AND ECONOMICS IN NEUROSURGERY

Increasing costs and government pressures for increasing accountability of health care expenditures have driven a movement toward value-based health care systems in which effectiveness and cost of care must both be taken into consideration. The ultimate goal is to implement innovations that provide maximal improvement in quality at minimal cost. To address this from an evidence-based perspective, numerous means of quantifying and optimizing health-related quality of life (HRQoL) and cost effectiveness have been devised and are used with increasing frequency to assess innovations.

Health-Related Quality Outcomes in Neurosurgery

The value of an individual's HRQoL is determined by incorporating health and functional status along with overall quality of life factors such as socioeconomic status and social support.[4] This defines the multifactorial influence that a disease or treatment has had on an individual. HRQoL is typically quantified through 1 of 2 means: health status instruments or preference-based instruments.

Health status instruments generally take the form of multiple-choice questionnaires that quantify a patient's quality of life based on several domains and provide a summative score representative of their overall HRQoL. Health status instruments such as these are valuable but do not convey important information about a patient's own valuation of their current health state. Preference-based

HRQoL instruments take this into account directly by having a patient assign a value to their current health state or indirectly through statistical inference. By the indirect approach, the individual describes their current health in multiple domains through completion of a questionnaire, and then a predetermined utility function is used to calculate a preference value. Such an instrument, often used within neurosurgery, is the EuroQoL-5D. This instrument is based on the 5 domains of mobility, self-care, usual activities, pain/discomfort, and anxiety/depression.[5] The single value produced by the utility function is generally expressed on a scale of 0 to 1. Zero represents death and 1 represents perfect health. This value can be used as a weighting factor for a year of life in a current health state. If a patient has a state of health with a preference score of 0.5 before an intervention and the preference score increases to 0.7 after an intervention, they have gained 0.2 utility units per year. This weighting factor is the basis of the commonly reported quality-adjusted life year (QALY) and can be used in standardized calculations of the cost of improving quality.[6] This will be discussed further in the next discussion.

Economic Evaluation in Neurosurgery

When assessing the total cost of an innovation, numerous expenditures need to be accounted for such as the direct upfront costs to the health care system, costs of associated complications, third-party payer costs, and lost opportunity costs including time away from work, school, and family. These provide a basis for assessment of the economics of a new innovation, which may be conducted by several techniques.

The most simplistic of these is a cost minimization analysis, whereby the quality outcomes of a new innovation have already been determined to be equivalent to the standard of care. In this case, the costs associated with the new innovation can be directly compared with the costs of the standard of care to determine which is more efficient from an overall perspective. An example of this type of analysis in the literature is a comparison of simple decompression versus anterior subcutaneous transposition for the treatment of ulnar neuropathy. Both treatments were deemed equally effective in a prospective, randomized, controlled trial.[7] The direct and indirect costs of the procedures were then compared in a separate cost minimization analysis, which led to the conclusion that a simple decompression was associated with significantly lower costs than an anterior subcutaneous transposition (€1124 vs €2730, in 2005).[8]

Unfortunately, this simple means of assessment is often not applicable, as quality outcomes are frequently changed by a new innovation. In such case, a cost-effectiveness analysis can be more appropriate, provided the outcomes are expressed in common units. The cost effectiveness is often expressed using an incremental cost-effectiveness ratio (ICER) in which the cost of improvement from the innovation is expressed in terms of 1 unit of outcome improvement.

incorporated into a single general outcome measure: the QALY. This is calculated by determining total life-years gained from an intervention and expressing each year as weighted to the quality of life in that year. The quality weighting is determined from the HRQoL. The results of this cost-utility analysis are expressed as cost per QALY gained.[10] An example of this is a cost-utility analysis of surgical intervention for patients with cervical spondylotic myelopathy in which

$$\text{ICER} = \frac{\text{Cost}_{new} - \text{Cost}_{standard \ practice}}{\text{Quality Outcome}_{new} - \text{Quality Outcome}_{standard \ practice}}$$

An example of this analysis is the cost effectiveness of sacral anterior root stimulation for rehabilitation of bladder dysfunction in spinal cord–injured patients compared with standard medical treatments. In an assessment of the neurosurgical innovation, the investigators expressed the results of their ICER calculations as the cost per additional patient with complete and voluntary micturition.[9] This type of cost-effectiveness analysis is valuable; however, it is restricted by the inability to calculate differences in multidimensional outcomes and a paucity of standard benchmarks for what individuals are willing to pay. Because there is not a standard value for what society or an individual would be willing to pay for the specific outcome of having an additional spinal cord–injured patient achieve complete and voluntary micturition, it is difficult to say if sacral anterior root stimulation should be included in general practice based on the findings of this study.

A utility-based metric allows for the combination of multidimensional outcomes into a single standard index and is the basis of a cost-utility analysis. In this subtype of cost-effectiveness analysis, multidimensional outcomes are

the clinical effectiveness of surgical intervention was expressed relative to the direct medical costs of the intervention.[11] The results of the calculation yielded a finding indicating that the cost of surgical intervention was $32,916 canadian dollar (CAD) per QALY gained. This is a recognizable and standardized means of reporting cost per unit of quality gained and can be assessed in a standardized way, against an individual or society's willingness to pay for that improvement (see later discussion). **Table 1** provides a summary of the aforementioned methods of evaluating economics in neurosurgery.

Willingness-to-Pay Threshold in Current Practice

The willingness to pay is simply the price that an individual is willing to pay to receive 1 unit of improved quality (**Fig. 1**).[12] The question of whether the benefits (which are sometimes marginal) from an innovation are worth the cost to an individual or society as a whole is challenging, and the willingness-to-pay threshold is highly controversial. The perception of what is cost effective is influenced by burden of disease, uncertainty

Table 1
Methods for analyzing health care–related costs

Method	Characteristics	Assumptions	Units
CMA	Direct cost comparison	Equivalent outcomes	Cost difference
CEA	Comparison in terms of cost and effectiveness	No outcome equivalency assumed	Ratio of cost to difference in outcome
CUA	Subtype of CEA in which QALY gained is the outcome measure	No outcome equivalency assumed	Ratio of cost to QALY gained

Abbreviations: CEA, cost-effectiveness analysis; CMA, cost-minimization analysis; CUA, cost-utility analysis.

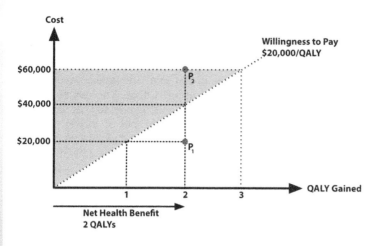

Fig. 1. The relationship between the willingness-to-pay threshold and the incremental cost-effectiveness ratio. In this hypothetical scenario, the willingness-to-pay threshold is set at $20,000 per QALY gained. An innovation that costs $20,000 and has a net benefit of 2 QALYs gained is represented by P_1. This innovation is likely to be accepted, as the ICER is $10,000 per QALY gained and less than the willingness-to-pay threshold. An innovation that costs $60,000 and has the same net benefit of 2 QALYs is represented by P_2. This innovation is unlikely to be accepted with an ICER of $30,000 per QALY gained, which is greater than the willingness-to-pay threshold. (*Adapted from* Claxton K, Briggs A, Buxton MJ, et al. Value based pricing for NHS drugs: an opportunity not to be missed? BMJ 2008;336(7638):252; with permission.)

within the calculations, the net costs, a nation's economic state, standard of living, and many others.[13] For this reason, the willingness-to-pay threshold is better represented as a range rather than a fixed value (**Fig. 2**).[14] In the United Kingdom, the National Institutes for Health and Clinical Excellence is responsible for considering this question and tasked with the decision to implement or reject new innovations. This organization has publicly announced their definition for cost-effective treatments to range from somewhere between $40,000 to $60,000 US per QALY.[15] A reported 3-tiered system suggested an innovation with an ICER of less than $20,000 CAD per QALY gained should be strongly supported, an ICER

between $20,000 and $100,000 CAD per QALY gained should be given moderate support, and those innovations with an ICER that exceeds $100,000 CAD per QALY gained should be given weak support.[16] The World Health Organization (WHO) cites an even more generalizable range of 1 to 3 times a nation's gross domestic product per capita as the willingness to pay for one QALY gained.[17] Taking this into consideration, to make appropriate and fair decisions regarding investment in new health care innovations, it is important that the ICER be established through rigorous study and that those responsible for resource allocation are transparent in their decisions regarding willingness to pay.

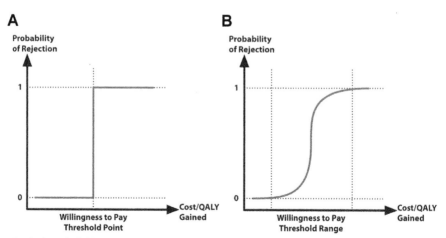

Fig. 2. Hypothetical probability curves represent the likelihood of an innovation being rejected as a function of its calculated incremental cost-effectiveness ratio (cost/QALY gained). (*A*) Probability curve represents the willingness-to-pay threshold as a point. (*B*) Probability curve represents the willingness to pay as a range. (*Adapted from* Devlin N, Parkin D. Does NICE have a cost-effectiveness threshold and what other factors influence its decisions? A binary choice analysis. Health Econ 2004;13(5):438; with permission.)

INNOVATIONS IN NEUROSURGERY FROM AN ECONOMICS AND QUALITY PERSPECTIVE

Innovation in neurosurgery is a key driver for improved patient outcomes. Patient beneficence, through improved quality of care, should remain the primary consideration of the innovator, and novel techniques or technologies should be assessed in an ethical manner.[18] Under ideal circumstances, an innovation that has demonstrable gains in patient outcomes would be incorporated into general practice. However, the increased strain on health care resources has made consideration of the cost of these quality improvements increasingly more important. The preceding section outlines the current approaches to determining the costs of quality improvement, but even in the modern era of evidence-based medicine this analysis is not routinely done.

This section provides examples of innovations organized in a practical framework, structured upon their influence on quality and economic metrics (**Table 2**). Some of these have been appropriately assessed by cost effectiveness or cost-utility studies, but many have not. The aim is not to provide a systematic or comprehensive review of all neurosurgical innovations in terms of quality and economics but to provide a conceptual means for neurosurgeons and policymakers to assess innovations and to highlight areas in which further investigation and cost assessments are needed.

Innovations That Decrease Cost and Improve Quality

The ultimate goal of innovation in neurosurgery is to improve patient care quality and reduce costs. There are several examples within the neurosurgical literature of this. One that has gained recent attention is the administration of intrawound vancomycin powder for posterior spinal surgery. Two cohorts of patients undergoing posterior spinal fusion in the trauma setting were compared: one group received prophylactic intravenous (IV) antibiotics and intrawound vancomycin powder and the control group received IV antibiotics alone. A significantly decreased rate of infection was found in the cohort that received vancomycin powder with no adverse events noted from its

Table 2
Examples of innovations in neurosurgery organized by quality and economic metrics

		Economic Metrics	
		Cheaper	**More Costly**
Quality Metrics	**Improved**	Intrawound vancomycin powder for posterior spinal surgery Godil et al,[19] 2013; Emohare et al,[20] 2014	Intrathecal baclofen infusion for spasticity Sampson et al,[30] 2002
		SCS for failed back surgery syndrome North et al,[21] 2007	Upfront CT angiography for the diagnosis of nontraumatic SAH Jabbarli et al,[31] 2014
		IES for resection of WHO grade II gliomas in eloquent areas Martino et al,[22] 2013	Screening for asymptomatic carotid stenosis Lee et al,[32] 1997
	Undetermined or Controversial	Minimally invasive TLIF for degenerative spondylolisthesis vs open TLIF Parker et al,[23] 2012; Parker et al,[24] 2013	rhBMP for 1 and 2 level dorsal lumbar fusions Alvin et al,[33] 2014
		Spinal anesthesia for lumbar spine surgery Kahveci et al,[25] 2014	Synthetic dural substitute membranes vs autologous tissues for duraplasty Sabatino et al,[34] 2014
		Outpatient cranial and spinal surgery Purzner et al,[26] 2011, McGirt et al,[27] 2014	Intraoperative MRI for neurosurgical treatment of glioblastoma Kubben et al,[35] 2014; Senft et al,[36] 2011

Abbreviations: CT, computed tomography; IES, intraoperative electrical stimulation; MRI, magnetic resonance imaging; rhBMP, recombinant human Bone morphogenic protein; TLIF, transforaminal lumbar interbody fusion; SAH, subarachnoid hemorrhage; SCS, spinal cord stimulation.

use. Cost comparison found a savings of $438,165 per 100 posterior spinal fusion procedures for trauma when vancomycin powder was used for prophylaxis.[19] Similar findings of vancomycin powder use in patients undergoing posterior spinal surgery with or without instrumentation were reported.[20] Charges generated by readmission to treat surgical site infection were $1,232,274 for the group who received IV antibiotic prophylaxis alone, whereas no repeat surgical intervention was needed in the group receiving vancomycin powder in addition to IV antibiotics. The only cost incurred by this group was $1,152, which is the total cost of the vancomycin powder for all patients in the cohort.

Spinal cord stimulation (SCS) for failed back surgery is touted as less expensive and more effective than reoperation. A cost-utility analysis of SCS versus reoperation for failed back surgery syndrome using the data from a randomized, controlled trial found that the mean cost for reoperation was $36,341 and $34,371 for SCS. The mean QALYs gained in the final treatment group that underwent SCS compared with the group that had reoperation were significantly higher, and the cost/QALY calculation favored the SCS group.[21] Such a finding of concomitant quality and economic gain should push policy makers toward more widespread implementation of SCS in appropriately selected patients with failed back surgery syndrome instead of reoperation.

An innovation showing improvement in quality and costs in patients with WHO grade II gliomas in eloquent areas of the brain is the use of intraoperative electrical stimulation (IES).[22] When comparing 2 similar cohorts in which one underwent awake craniotomy with IES-assisted resection and the other resection under general anesthetic, the mean cost per QALY was found to be $12,222 in the IES group and $31,927 in the control group. The IES group was also noted to have a decrease in morbidity and improved preservation of their professional function. This study is highly suggestive of the benefits in terms of quality and costs of awake craniotomy with IES in this patient population and should be given strong consideration for funding despite marginally greater upfront costs.

Innovations That Reduce Cost but Leave Quality Unchanged

The previous section provides some examples of innovations that likely improve patient quality outcomes and reduce costs to the health care system. However, innovations that reduce costs while providing the same level of quality as the standard of care are also highly valuable. An increasing body of evidence is emerging from the minimally invasive spinal surgery literature to suggest that long-term outcomes are equivalent for minimally invasive procedures, whereas upfront costs are reduced. It has been shown that minimally invasive transforaminal lumbar interbody fusion (TLIF) for lumbar spondylolisthesis is associated with significant cost savings from both hospital and societal perspectives when compared with open TLIF. However, there was no significant difference in patient-reported outcomes at 2-year follow-up.[23,24] Spinal anesthetic for lumbar spine surgery instead of general anesthesia is another concept that is gaining more attention. It has been found that spinal anesthesia was clinically as effective as a general anesthetic while being associated with a significant reduction in anesthetic time and postoperative length of stay and can be delivered at nearly one-third of the cost of a general anesthetic.[25] Of note, however, there was a significant reduction in surgeon satisfaction while operating on patients who were under a spinal anesthetic compared with those under a general anesthetic.

Another example of cost-reductive measures is outpatient cranial and spine surgery. In a prospective study of 1003 patients who underwent outpatient brain tumor or spinal surgery at a single institution, there were no negative outcomes attributable to early discharge and an estimated savings of $1,123,200 in inpatient-associated costs alone.[26] Another study found that patients undergoing 1- or 2-level anterior cervical discectomy and fusion on an outpatient basis had a significant reduction in 3-month costs per patient when compared with a similar inpatient cohort ($20,043 vs $27,123) with similar QALYs gained.[27]

These studies are highly suggestive that outpatient cranial and spinal surgery can be effective cost-saving measures and can be implemented without affecting quality of patient care. In fact, an argument could be made that these outpatient procedures may improve patient care quality. There is qualitative evidence in the literature to suggest that patients have a high satisfaction with outpatient cranial surgery, and a reduced length of hospital stay likely lowers the risk of hospital-related complications such a nosocomial infections, thromboembolism, and medical errors.[28,29] However, this remains to be further quantified in a cost-utility study.

Innovations That Improve Quality but Increase Cost

Some of the most difficult decisions in health care resource allocation involve the implementation of innovations that have been found to improve quality of patient care but at increased cost. At the heart of this decision-making process is the previously described willingness-to-pay threshold. To make informed and appropriate decisions, the ICER of these innovations should be determined through rigorous investigation.

A good example of this is intrathecal baclofen infusion for spasticity. Intrathecal infusion of baclofen in patients with severe spasticity is found to improve mobility in bedbound patients and improve in pain symptoms when compared with medical treatment.[30] An investigation into this innovation found an ICER that was in the range of $10,550 to $19,570 per QALY gained, which is under the generally accepted willingness-to-pay threshold in most western societies. Another example of quality improvement that comes at a generally accepted cost is the used of upfront computed tomography (CT) angiography in the diagnosis of nontraumatic subarachnoid hemorrhage (SAH). A study on the cost effectiveness of CT angiography found that upfront CT angiography in patients with nontraumatic SAH raised the diagnostic costs by approximately €81 per patient. When accounting for the determined reduction in radiation exposure and reduced risk of complications related to conventional angiography, which may be avoided by first obtaining a CTA, the costs were €43,406.42 per QALY.[31] This figure falls under the generally accepted willingness-to-pay threshold for an innovation.

The results of these investigations are contrasted by a study of the cost effectiveness of widespread screening for asymptomatic carotid stenosis, which found that the cost effectiveness of the screening relative to no screening was $120,000 per QALY.[32] This value is far greater than generally accepted willingness-to-pay thresholds and explains why widespread screening for carotid stenosis is not done.

Costly Innovations Without Clear Improvement in Outcomes

The final category in our conceptual framework is innovations that do not improve outcomes and elevate costs to the health care system. Studies with such findings are important, as they inform future investigations into similar innovations and guide appropriate monetary allocation within the health care system.

A recent cost-utility analysis of recombinant human bone morphogenetic protein (rhBMP) use for 1- and 2-level dorsal lumbar fusions found that improvements in quality outcomes were similar for both their cohorts (rhBMP and autograft vs autograft alone). However, the cost-utility ratio for the control group was $143,251 per QALY gained compared with $272,414 per QALY gained in the rhBMP cohort.[33] These numbers were only from a single year of follow-up but nonetheless suggest that the use of rhBMP for operative interventions of this type should be considered carefully until the results from long-term studies are available.

A comparison of autologous galea-pericranial duraplasty with commercially available dural substitutes used a prospective cohort of 185 patients undergoing supratentorial elective neurosurgery with a minimum of 12-month follow-up. Ninety-three patients had duraplasty with galea-pericranium and 92 had duraplasty with Tutopatch (Tutogen Medical GmbH).[34] No statistically significant difference in cerebrospinal fluid leaks, postoperative infections, or wound dehiscence was found. The only notable difference between the 2 groups was an increased average cost of €267 per patient for those receiving the synthetic dural substitute. This study suggests that stronger consideration should be given to autologous duraplasty, but this study was limited by its nonrandomized nature and postoperative pain not being included as an outcome measure.

Another costly innovation that has questionable influence on quality metrics is intraoperative MRI (iMRI) for treatment of malignant glioma. A recent interim analysis of a small, randomized, controlled trial comparing iMRI with conventional neuronavigation-guided surgery for suspected supratentorial glioblastomas did not show any advantage with respect to extent of resection, clinical performance, or survival for iMRI.[35] However, this is contrasted by the only other randomized, controlled trial, which found a statistically improved extent of resection in the iMRI group but without endpoints assessing quality of life or length of survival.[36] Given the current evidence, there is no clear quality improvement obtained from the added expense of iMRI, but this is an area in which further investigation is needed.

SUMMARY

Herein we provided a review of the analytical tools available for determining the cost incurred by quality improvement from new innovations in neurosurgery and the influence this has on the willingness to pay for these innovations. This discussion is supplemented with examples from the neurosurgical literature, organized in a conceptual framework, structured around their influence on quality and economic metrics. The aim of this report was not to present a systematic or comprehensive review of all neurosurgical innovations in terms of quality and economics but to include examples of studies that have presented new innovations in a way that allows for more informed decision making regarding appropriate health care resource allocation.

REFERENCES

1. Toledo-Pereyra LH. Innovation according to cushing. J Invest Surg 2008;21(3):97–100.
2. Kentikelenis A, Karanikolos M, Reeves A, et al. Greece's health crisis: from austerity to denialism. Lancet 2014;383(9918):748–53.
3. Munoz E, Munoz W 3rd, Wise L. National and surgical health care expenditures, 2005-2025. Ann Surg 2010; 251(2):195–200.
4. Guyatt GH, Feeny DH, Patrick DL. Measuring health-related quality of life. Ann Intern Med 1993;118(8): 622–9.
5. Rabin R, de Charro F. EQ-5D: a measure of health status from the EuroQol Group. Ann Med 2001; 33(5):337–43.
6. Ament JD, Kim KD. Standardizing cost-utility analysis in neurosurgery. Neurosurg Focus 2012;33(1):E4.
7. Bartels RH, Verhagen WI, van der Wilt GJ, et al. Prospective randomized controlled study comparing simple decompression versus anterior subcutaneous transposition for idiopathic neuropathy of the ulnar nerve at the elbow: part 1. Neurosurgery 2005;56(3):522–30 [discussion: 522–30].
8. Bartels RH, Termeer EH, van der Wilt GJ, et al. Simple decompression or anterior subcutaneous transposition for ulnar neuropathy at the elbow: a cost-minimization analysis–Part 2. Neurosurgery 2005;56(3):531–6 [discussion: 531–6].
9. Bénard A, Verpillot E, Grandoulier AS, et al. Comparative cost-effectiveness analysis of sacral anterior root stimulation for rehabilitation of bladder dysfunction in spinal cord injured patients. Neurosurgery 2013;73(4):600–8 [discussion: 608].
10. Robinson R. Cost-utility analysis. BMJ 1993; 307(6908):859–62.
11. Fehlings MG, Jha NK, Hewson SM, et al. Is surgery for cervical spondylotic myelopathy cost-effective? A cost-utility analysis based on data from the AOSpine North America prospective CSM study. J Neurosurg Spine 2012;17(1 Suppl): 89–93.
12. Claxton K, Briggs A, Buxton MJ, et al. Value based pricing for NHS drugs: an opportunity not to be missed? BMJ 2008;336(7638):251–4.
13. King JT Jr, Tsevat J, Lave JR, et al. Willingness to pay for a quality-adjusted life year: implications for societal health care resource allocation. Med Decis Making 2005;25(6):667–77.
14. Devlin N, Parkin D. Does NICE have a cost-effectiveness threshold and what other factors influence its decisions? A binary choice analysis. Health Econ 2004;13(5):437–52.
15. McCabe C, Claxton K, Culyer AJ. The NICE cost-effectiveness threshold: what it is and what that means. Pharmacoeconomics 2008;26(9):733–44.
16. Laupacis A, Feeny D, Detsky AS, et al. How attractive does a new technology have to be to warrant adoption and utilization? Tentative guidelines for using clinical and economic evaluations. CMAJ 1992;146(4):473–81.
17. Zhao FL, Yue M, Yang H, et al. Willingness to pay per quality-adjusted life year: is one threshold enough for decision-making?: results from a study in patients with chronic prostatitis. Med Care 2011; 49(3):267–72.
18. Bernstein M, Bampoe J. Surgical innovation or surgical evolution: an ethical and practical guide to handling novel neurosurgical procedures. J Neurosurg 2004; 100(1):2–7.
19. Godil SS, Parker SL, O'Neill KR, et al. Comparative effectiveness and cost-benefit analysis of local application of vancomycin powder in posterior spinal fusion for spine trauma: clinical article. J Neurosurg Spine 2013;19(3):331–5.
20. Emohare O, Ledonio CG, Hill BW, et al. Cost savings analysis of intrawound vancomycin powder in posterior spinal surgery. Spine J 2014. http://dx.doi.org/10.1016/j.spinee.2014.03.011. pii:S1529–9430(14)00252-6.
21. North RB, Kidd D, Shipley J, et al. Spinal cord stimulation versus reoperation for failed back surgery syndrome: a cost effectiveness and cost utility analysis based on a randomized, controlled trial. Neurosurgery 2007;61(2):361–8 [discussion: 368–9].
22. Martino J, Gomez E, Bilbao JL, et al. Cost-utility of maximal safe resection of WHO grade II gliomas within eloquent areas. Acta Neurochir (Wien) 2013; 155(1):41–50.
23. Parker SL, Adogwa O, Bydon A, et al. Cost-effectiveness of minimally invasive versus open transforaminal lumbar interbody fusion for degenerative spondylolisthesis associated low-back and leg pain over two years. World Neurosurg 2012;78(1–2):178–84.
24. Parker SL, Mendenhall SK, Shau DN, et al. Minimally invasive versus open transforaminal lumbar interbody fusion for degenerative spondylolisthesis: comparative effectiveness and cost-utility analysis. World Neurosurg 2013. http://dx.doi.org/10.1016/j.wneu.2013.01.041. pii:S1878–8750(13)00102-2.
25. Kahveci K, Doger C, Ornek D, et al. Perioperative outcome and cost-effectiveness of spinal versus general anesthesia for lumbar spine surgery. Neurol Neurochir Pol 2014;48(3):167–73.

26. Purzner T, Purzner J, Massicotte EM, et al. Outpatient brain tumor surgery and spinal decompression: a prospective study of 1003 patients. Neurosurgery 2011;69(1):119–26 [discussion: 126–7].

27. McGirt MJ, Godil SS, Adamson TE, et al. Samuel hassenbusch young neurosurgeon award 139 anterior cervical diskectomy and fusion in the ambulatory care setting: defining its value across the acute and post-acute care episode. Neurosurgery 2014; 61(Suppl 1):205.

28. Khu KJ, Doglietto F, Radovanovic I, et al. Patients' perceptions of awake and outpatient craniotomy for brain tumor: a qualitative study. J Neurosurg 2010;112(5):1056–60.

29. Boulton M, Bernstein M. Outpatient brain tumor surgery: innovation in surgical neurooncology. J Neurosurg 2008;108(4):649–54.

30. Sampson FC, Hayward A, Evans G, et al. Functional benefits and cost/benefit analysis of continuous intrathecal baclofen infusion for the management of severe spasticity. J Neurosurg 2002;96(6):1052–7.

31. Jabbarli R, Shah M, Taschner C, et al. Clinical utility and cost-effectiveness of CT-angiography in the diagnosis of nontraumatic subarachnoid hemorrhage. Neuroradiology 2014;56:817–24.

32. Lee TT, Solomon NA, Heidenreich PA, et al. Cost-effectiveness of screening for carotid stenosis in asymptomatic persons. Ann Intern Med 1997;126(5):337–46.

33. Alvin MD, Derakhshan A, Lubelski D, et al. Cost-utility analysis of one and two-level dorsal lumbar fusions with and without recombinant human bone morphogenic protein-2 at 1-year follow-up. J Spinal Disord Tech 2014. [Epub ahead of print].

34. Sabatino G, Della Pepa GM, Bianchi F, et al. Autologous dural substitutes: a prospective study. Clin Neurol Neurosurg 2014;116:20–3.

35. Kubben PL, Scholtes F, Schijns OE, et al. Intraoperative magnetic resonance imaging versus standard neuronavigation for the neurosurgical treatment of glioblastoma: a randomized controlled trial. Surg Neurol Int 2014;5:70.

36. Senft C, Bink A, Franz K, et al. Intraoperative MRI guidance and extent of resection in glioma surgery: a randomised, controlled trial. Lancet Oncol 2011; 12(11):997–1003.

Volume-Outcome Relationships in Neurosurgery

Jason M. Davies, MD, PhD[a], Alp Ozpinar, BS[b],
Michael T. Lawton, MD[a],*

KEYWORDS

- Neurosurgery - Volume - Outcomes - Surgery

KEY POINTS

- For a variety of neurosurgical conditions, increasing surgeon and hospital volumes correlate with improved outcomes, such as mortality, complication rates, length of stay, hospital charges, and discharge disposition.
- Neurosurgeons can improve patient outcomes at the population level by changing practice and referral patterns to regionalize care for select conditions at high-volume specialty treatment centers.
- Individual practitioners should be aware of where they fall on the volume spectrum and understand the implications of their practice and referral habits on their patients.

INTRODUCTION

Evidence is mounting that patient morbidity and mortality rates decrease when high-volume physicians and centers perform certain medical or surgical procedures (**Tables 1** and **2**). These volume-outcome relationships (VORs) have been demonstrated for common procedures, such as hip and knee replacements, and more complex procedures, such as pancreaticoduodenectomy and abdominal aortic aneurysm repair. Data such as these have been used to support changes in the delivery of care, with centralization of patients and procedures at specialized centers in efforts to increase volumes and thereby improve overall patient outcomes.

During the past decade, neurosurgeons have begun to study the impact of surgeon and institutional volume on a variety of outcomes across the neurosurgical subspecialties. Positive relationships have been shown between higher volume and improved length of stay, mortality, complications, charges, and discharge dispositions. This article summarizes current evidence for VORs in neurosurgery to examine the basis for centralization of neurosurgical services. For each subspecialty (tumor, vascular, spine, pediatrics, functional, and neurotrauma), the literature for relevant studies is reviewed, the pertinent VORs that have been studied to date are summarized, and the implications of these data are discussed.

INTRACRANIAL TUMOR

Surgery for tumor treatment is among the most highly studied of the neurosurgical specialties. Multiple studies of patients with intracranial tumors have shown improved outcomes at higher-volume centers. Some look across the spectrum of tumors, whereas others concentrate the analyses on specific subsets of tumors.

[a] Department of Neurological Surgery, University of California, San Francisco, 505 Parnassus Avenue, San Francisco, CA 94143, USA; [b] Oregon Health Sciences University, School of Medicine, 3181 SW Sam Jackson Park Rd, Portland, OR 97239, USA
* Corresponding author. Department of Neurological Surgery, University of California, San Francisco, 505 Parnassus Avenue, M780, Box 0112, San Francisco, CA 94143-0112.
E-mail address: lawtonm@neurosurg.ucsf.edu

Neurosurg Clin N Am 26 (2015) 207–218
http://dx.doi.org/10.1016/j.nec.2014.11.015
1042-3680/15/$ – see front matter © 2015 Elsevier Inc. All rights reserved.

neurosurgery.theclinics.com

Table 1
Hospital caseload volume-outcome relationships

Specialty	Subspecialty	Author	Stratification	Volume Threshold	Mortality	Disposition	Length of Stay	Complications
Tumor	All	Long et al,[1] 2003	Dichotomous	>50/y	RR, 0.71; P<.05		6.8 vs 8.8 d; P<.001	
	All	Cowan et al,[2] 2003	Quartile	>29/y		OR, 0.58; 95% CI, 0.35–0.97; P = .04		
	All	Nuno et al,[3] 2012	Quintiles	>139/y	OR, 0.56; 95% CI, 0.37–0.83	OR, 0.71; 95% CI, 0.59–0.91	6.4 vs 8.0 d	
	Supratentorial primaries	Barker et al,[4] 2005 Craniotomy	Quintile	>41/y	OR, 0.75; 95% CI, 0.62–0.90; P = .003	OR, 0.77; 95% CI, 0.70–0.85; P<.001	NS	OR, 1.67; 95% CI, 1.13–2.45; P = .009
		Biopsy	Quintile	>11/y	OR, 0.54; 95% CI, 0.35–0.83; P = .006	OR, 0.67; 95% CI, 0.56–0.80; P<.001		
		Trinh et al,[5]	Quartile/decile	>35/y	OR, 0.76; 95% CI, 0.63–0.90; P<.001	OR, 1.29; 95% CI, 1.21–1.37; P<.01	19% shorter; P<.001	OR, 0.93; 95% CI, 0.97–0.99; P = .040
	Metastasis	Barker,[6] 2004	Quintile	>17/y	OR, 0.79; 95% CI, 0.59–1.03; P = .09	OR, 0.75; 95% CI, 0.65–0.86		
	Transsphenoidal pituitary tumors	Barker et al,[7] 2003	Quartile	>24/y	OR, 0.54; CI, 0.31–0.95; P = .03	OR, 0.74; 95% CI, 059–0.92; P = .007	P = .02	OR, 0.77; 95% CI, 0.61–0.97; P = .03
	Meningioma	Curry et al,[8] 2010	Quartile	>17/y	OR, 0.74; 95% CI, 0.59–0.93	OR, 0.71; 95% CI, 0.62–0.80		
		Ambekar et al,[9] 2013	Quartile	>16/y	OR, 0.5; 95% CI, 0.38–0.66; P<.001	OR, 0.8; 95% CI, 0.74–0.86; P<.001		
	Acoustic neuroma	Barker et al,[10] 2003	Quartile	>36/y	NS	OR, 0.47; 95% CI, 0.37–0.58; P<.001	P = .01	OR, 0.75; CI, 0.64–0.89, P<.001
	Chordoma	Jones et al,[11] 2014	Dichotomous	>40	HR, 0.49; 95% CI, 0.28–0.86; P = .013			

Subcategory	Study, Year	Volume definition	Volume threshold	Outcome 1	Outcome 2	Outcome 3
Clip		Dichotomous	>20	P = .001		P = .0242
Coil				P = .0053		NS
Ruptured	Johnston,[13] 2000	Quartile	>45/y	NS		
Unruptured				NS		
Ruptured	Hattori et al,[14] 2007	Tertile	>50/y	NS		
Unruptured			>50/y	NS		
	Bardach et al,[15] 2002	Quartile	>20/y	OR, 0.57; 95% CI, 0.48–0.67; P<.001	OR, 0.44; 95% CI, 0.36–0.53; P<.001	OR, 1.21; 95% CI, 1.09–1.33; P = .001
	Cross et al,[16] 2003	Quartile	>35/y	OR, 0.71; 95% CI, 0.62–0.83; P<.001		
	Boogaarts et al,[17] 2014	Dichotomous		OR, 0.85; 95% CI, 0.72–0.99; P = .00		
	Solomon et al,[18] 1996	Quartile	>30/y	OR, 0.57; 95% CI, 0.27–0.86; P = .009	NS	
	McNeill et al,[19] 2013	Continuous, per 100 patients per year		RR, 0.76; 95% CI, 0.67–0.87; P = .009	NS	
Carotid stenosis	Cebul et al,[20] 1998	Dichotomous	>62/y	OR, 0.29; 95% CI, 0.12–0.69; P = .006		
	Wennberg et al,[21] 1998	Tertile	>21/y	1.7% vs 2.5%; volume OR not reported; P = .001		
	Cowan et al,[22] 2002	Tertile	>100/y	NS		
Pediatrics — Tumor	Smith et al,[23] 2004	Quartile	>20/y	OR, 0.52; 95% CI, 0.28–0.94; P = .03	OR, 0.52; 95% CI, 0.39–0.71; P<.001	NS
VPS	Smith et al,[24] 2004	Quartile	>121/y	OR, 0.38; 95% CI, 0.18–0.81; P = .01	NS	
Spine	Dasenbrock et al,[25] 2012	Quintile	>394/y	NS	NS	
Trauma	Clement et al,[26] 2013	Quintile	>59/y	OR, 0.59; 95% CI, 0.41–0.87	NS	
Functional — Epilepsy	McClelland et al,[27] 2011	Dichotomous				
	Englot et al,[28] 2012	Tertile	>15/y			RR, 0.93; 95% CI, 0.93–097; P<.001
MVD	Kalkanis et al,[29] 2003	Quartile	>19/y	NS	OR, 0.50; 95% CI, 0.31–0.82; P = .006	OR, 0.59; 95% CI, 0.35–0.98; P = .04
DBS	Eskandar et al,[30] 2003	Quartile	>120/y	OR, 0.14; 95% CI, 0.04–0.49; P = .002	OR, 0.69; 95% CI, 0.50–0.96; P = .007	NS
	Sharma et al,[31] 2013	Quartile	NA	NS	OR, 0.28; 95% CI, 0.14–0.56; P<.001	NS

Table 2
Surgeon caseload volume-outcome relationships

Specialty	Subspecialty	Author	Stratification	Volume Threshold	Mortality	Disposition	Length of Stay	Complications
Tumor	All	Long et al,[1] 2003	Dichotomous	>50/y	OR, 0.42; 95% CI, 0.22–0.84; P = .01			
	All	Cowan et al,[2] 2003	Quartile	>21/y				
	Supratentorial primaries	Barker et al,[4] 2005						
		Craniotomy	Quintile	NA		OR, 0.60; 95% CI, 0.45–0.79; P<.001		
		Biopsy	Quintile	NA		OR, 0.79; 95% CI, 0.70–0.89; P<.001		
		Trinh et al,[5]	Quartile/decile	>12/y	OR, 0.43; 95% CI, 0.32–0.55; P<.001	NS		OR, 0.91; 95% CI, 0.84–0.99; P = .040
	Metastasis	Barker,[6] 2004	Quintile	>7/y		OR, 0.49; 95% CI, 0.30–0.80; P = .004	OR, 0.51; 95% CI, 0.40–0.64	
	Transsphenoidal pituitary tumors	Barker et al,[7] 2003	Quartile	>6/y	NS	OR, 0.62; 95% CI, 0.41–0.94; P = .02	P<.001	OR, 0.76; 95% CI, 0.65–0.89; P = .005
	Meningioma	Curry et al,[8] 2010	Quartile	>5/y	NS		OR, 0.71; 95% CI, 0.62–0.80	
		Ambekar et al,[9] 2013	Quartile	>2/y	OR, 0.43; 95% CI, 0.27–0.69; P<.001		OR, 0.63; 95% CI, 0.56–0.70; P<.001	
	Acoustic neuroma	Barker et al,[10] 2003	Quartile	>33/y	NS	OR, 0.46; 95% CI, 0.31–0.67; P<.001	P = .009	NS
Vascular	Carotid stenosis	Cebul et al,[20] 1998	Dichotomous	>21/y	NS			
		Cowan et al,[22] 2002	Tertile	>29/y	OR, 0.53; 95% CI, 0.40–0.71; P≤.001			
Pediatrics	Tumor	Smith et al,[23] 2004	Quartile	>15/y	NS	OR, 0.70; 95% CI, 0.50–0.98; P = .04	NS	
	VPS	Smith et al,[24] 2004	Quartile	>65/y	OR, 0.30; 95% CI, 0.13–0.69; P = .005			
Spine		Dasenbrock et al,[25] 2012	Quintile	>81/y	NS	NS	–4.4%; 95% CI, –6.1% to –2.7%; P<.001	
Functional	Epilepsy	McClelland et al,[27] 2011	Dichotomous	>2/y	NS	P<.001		
	MVD	Kalkanis et al,[29] 2003	Quartile	>29/y		OR, 0.30; 95% CI, 0.11–0.80; P = .02		OR, 0.32; 95% CI, 0.13–0.77; P = .01
	DBS	Eskandar et al,[30] 2003	Quartile	>20/y	OR, 0.13; 95% CI, 0.03–0.57; P = .01	NS		NS
		Sharma et al,[31] 2013	Quartile	>12/y	NS	NS		NS

Abbreviations: DBS, deep brain stimulation; HR, hazard ratio; MVD, microvascular decompression; NA, not applicable; NS, not significant; OR, odds ratio; RR, relative risk; VPS, ventriculoperitoneal shunt.
Data from Refs.[1,2,4–10,20,22–25,27,29–31]

All Tumors

Long and colleagues[1] analyzed outcomes from 4723 patients who underwent craniotomies for tumor treatment in 33 Maryland hospitals. Hospitals were divided into high-volume (>50 craniotomies per year) and low-volume (≤50 craniotomies per year) centers based on their annual tumor case volume. High-volume centers provided services with improved mortality rates (2.5% vs 4.9%) and fewer hospital days (6.8 vs 8.8 days), although with adjusted costs slightly higher than those at low-volume hospitals ($15,867 vs $14,045; P<.001). Based on the difference in mortality rates, the authors surmised that if all patients in the state had been treated at the high-volume centers, approximately 46 fewer patients would have died, resulting in a 48.6% reduction in mortality and reflecting an additional adjusted cost of $76,395-per-patient saved.

Cowan and colleagues[2] analyzed 7547 patients from the Nationwide Inpatient Sample (NIS) from 1996 to 1997, dividing providers into volume quartiles based on annual case volume. They found that higher-volume providers had superior outcomes after surgical resection of malignant intracranial tumors despite adjustment for case mix. Mortality at hospitals in the highest-volume quartile was 1.8%, compared with 3.8% for the lowest quartile (P<.001). Mortality rates also varied based on surgeon case volume, with mortality rates ranging from 4.1% for the lowest quartile to 1.4% in the highest (P = .003). In multivariate regression, the authors found that at the highest-volume-quartile hospitals, the risk of mortality was reduced by 42% (odds ratio [OR], 0.58; 95% CI, 0.35–0.97; P = .038), and for high-volume surgeons the risk reduction was 58% (OR, 0.42; 95% CI, 0.22–0.84; P = .012).

Nuno and colleagues[3] analyzed 124,171 patients from the NIS who underwent craniotomies for tumor treatment from 2001 to 2007. They found a wide range in annual case-volume, with the highest 2% and lowest 25% of hospitals treating 322 and 12 cases annually, respectively. High-volume centers performed better with respect to length of stay [LOS], mortality, and discharge outcomes. LOS at high-volume centers was significantly shorter (6.4 vs 8.0 days; P<.001). Multivariate analysis demonstrated that patients treated in low-volume centers had an increased mortality risk (OR, 1.8; CI, 1.2–2.7; P = .006) and were more likely to need additional services at discharge (OR, 1.4; CI, 1.1–1.7; P = .01).

Subspecialty Tumor Outcomes

Supratentorial primary brain tumors

Barker and colleagues[4] analyzed outcomes for 38,028 patients undergoing craniotomies for supratentorial primary brain tumors from 1988 to 2000 in the NIS. High-volume centers had lower in-hospital postoperative mortality rates than centers with lighter caseloads in multivariate analyses, both for craniotomies (>41 admissions per year; OR, 0.75 for a 10-fold larger caseload) and for needle biopsies (>11 admissions per year; OR, 0.54). Patients at high-volume centers were also less likely to experience adverse discharge disposition (craniotomies: OR, 0.77; needle biopsy: OR, 0.67). Over the time frame of the study, large centers experienced some growth in case volume, with the percentage of all primary brain tumors operated on in the United States at the 100 highest-caseload hospitals increasing from 30% to 41%.

Trinh and colleagues[5] analyzed outcomes for 62,514 patients undergoing biopsy or resection of supratentorial brain tumor from 2000 to 2009 in the NIS. The authors found that high-volume surgeons had reduced complication rates (P = .04) and lower in-hospital mortality (P<.0001). High-volume hospitals were found to have reduced in-hospital mortality (P = .003), higher routine discharge proportion (P<.0001), and lower complication rates (P = .04). Patients treated by high-volume surgeons were less likely to experience postoperative hematomas, hydrocephalus, or wound complications. Patients treated at high-volume hospitals were less likely to experience mechanical ventilation, pulmonary complications, or infectious complications.

Metastatic brain tumor

Barker[6] studied outcomes for patients who underwent surgery for treatment of metastatic brain tumors. High-volume centers had lower mortality rates (OR, 0.79; 95% CI, 0.59–1.03; P = .09) and were less likely to have an adverse discharge disposition (OR, 0.75; 95% CI, 0.65–0.86; P<.001). They also analyzed surgeon case volume and found that mortality and adverse discharge disposition were both lower among higher-volume providers (mortality: OR, 0.49; 95% CI, 0.30–0.80; P = .004; discharge disposition: OR, 0.51; 95% CI, 0.40–0.64; P<.001). High-volume providers experienced shorter LOS, and hospital charges were significantly lower when high-volume surgeons performed surgery.

Transsphenoidal pituitary tumors

Barker and colleagues[7] analyzed outcomes for 5497 patients who underwent pituitary operations from 1996 to 2000 in the NIS. They found that higher-volume hospitals and surgeons were associated with superior short-term outcomes after transsphenoidal pituitary tumor surgery (hospital: OR, 0.74 for 5-fold larger caseload, P = .007, surgeon: OR, 0.62; P = .02). Mortality rates in general were low, but varied significantly with case volume from 0.9% at lowest-caseload-quartile hospitals to 0.4% at highest-volume-quartile hospitals (P = .03), and were also significantly better for high-volume surgeons (P = .09). LOS was significantly reduced with high-volume hospitals (P = .02) and surgeons (P<.001). The authors additionally analyzed postoperative complications and found them to occur less frequently with higher-volume hospitals (P = .03) and surgeons (P = .005).

Meningioma

Curry and colleagues[8] analyzed inpatient outcomes after craniotomy for meningioma from 1988 to 2000 in the NIS. High-volume providers demonstrated superior rates for mortality and discharge disposition. Multivariate analyses demonstrated that high-volume hospitals had lower mortality (OR, 0.74; 95% CI, 0.59–0.93; P = .01) and lower rates of adverse discharge disposition (OR, 0.71; 95% CI, 0.62–0.80; P<.001). High surgeon case volume was also significantly correlated with less frequent adverse discharge disposition (OR, 0.71; 95% CI, 0.62–0.80; P<.001). Over the course of the period studied, they found that the annual caseload increased concomitant with a decrease in mortality rates, especially at high-volume centers. Mortality rate reductions were largest at high-volume centers, with the highest quintile experiencing a 72% reduction in the relative mortality rate compared with a 6% increase in the relative mortality rate at lowest-volume centers.

Ambekar and colleagues[9] analyzed outcomes for patients who underwent intracranial meningioma surgery from 2001 to 2010 in the NIS. Patients treated at high-case-volume centers and by high-case-volume physicians experienced lower mortality rates (P<.05) and were less likely to have adverse discharge outcomes (P≤.05). Over the study period, a 54% decrease occurred in the number of hospitals performing 1 surgery per year, and the lowest-volume hospitals showed a 2% relative decrease in mortality over that time frame.

Acoustic Neuroma

Barker and colleagues[10] studied outcomes for 2643 patients after craniotomy for resection of acoustic neuroma. Discharge disposition was significantly better when surgery was performed in high-volume hospitals (OR, 0.47 for 5-fold-larger caseload; P<.001) or by higher-volume surgeons (OR, 0.46; P<.001). Patients who had surgery at lowest-volume-quartile hospitals were 4 times more likely to not be discharged directly home, compared with those treated at highest-volume-

quartile hospitals. Additionally, postoperative complications were less likely for those treated at high-volume hospitals and by high-volume surgeons, and length of stay was also shorter at high-volume hospitals (P = .01) and for high-volume surgeons (P = .009). Hospital charges were lower for high-volume hospitals (P = .006) and surgeons (P = .09).

Skull Base Chordoma

Jones and colleagues[11] analyzed outcomes of 394 patients with chordomas of the skull base from 1973 to 2009 in the Surveillance, Epidemiology, and End Results (SEER) database. High-volume centers were those with at least 40 patients treated during the study period. High-volume centers showed improved survival on multivariate analysis (hazard ratio [HR], 0.490, 95% CI, 0.279–0.860; P = .0129). Survival in this study was different from mortality in NIS-type studies, because the SEER database does not just take into account the index inpatient encounter during which treatment was undertaken, but rather includes follow-up over the course of the disease.

VASCULAR
Aneurysmal Disease

Leake and colleagues[12] analyzed trends in which patients with subarachnoid hemorrhage were treated between 2001 and 2008. The authors found that although in 2001 only 31% of the patients who underwent clipping and 0% (0 of 122 patients) of those who underwent coiling did so at high-volume centers, in 2008 the number treated in high-volume centers had substantially increased to 62% and 68% of patients, respectively. Although the number of high-volume centers performing clipping remained constant at 13 to 15 over the study period, the number of low-volume centers significantly declined from 177 in 2001 to 85 in 2008. Centers performing coiling procedures followed a different trend, with high-volume centers increasing from 0 in 2001 to 16 in 2005 and low-volume centers decreasing in number from 62 in 2001 to 54 in 2008.

Johnston[13] analyzed the effect of the presence of endovascular services and hospital volume on aneurysm treatment outcomes in some 2623 unruptured and 9534 ruptured aneurysm cases from 1994 to 1997. In this study, the authors found no relationship between hospital volume and in-hospital mortality. Hattori and colleagues[14] analyzed outcomes for 11,974 patients after cerebral aneurysm clipping at all 369 core neurosurgical training centers certified by the Japan Neurosurgical Society. Hospitals were divided into tiers by case volume in 2003 (<30, 30–50, ≥50). The authors found no significant correlation between hospital case volume and outcome for either ruptured (P = .483) or unruptured aneurysms (P = .562).

Bardach and colleagues[15] analyzed 12,804 patients presenting in California hospitals with subarachnoid hemorrhage from 1990 to 1999. Hospital volume was stratified into quartiles, with the lowest quartile treating from 0 to 8 cases per year, compared with 19 to 70 cases per year in the highest quartile. Higher-volume hospitals had substantially lower rates of in-hospital mortality (lowest: 49% vs 32% highest; P<.001). Higher-volume hospitals demonstrated longer lengths of stay and higher hospital charges in univariate and multivariable models (all P<.001). The authors additionally noted that only 4.8% of those admitted to hospitals in the lowest-volume quartile were transferred to high-volume centers. Cross and colleagues[16] analyzed administrative data from 18 US states for 16,399 hospitalizations for patients presenting with subarachnoid hemorrhage. Patients treated in low-volume hospitals had a significantly higher mortality rate (OR, 1.4; 95% CI, 1.2–1.6).

Boogaarts and colleagues[17] performed a systematic review and meta-analysis of factors impacting outcomes after aneurysmal subarachnoid hemorrhage. The authors included 4 articles, including the above, representing some 36,600 patients. Meta-analysis using a random effects model showed that high-volume hospitals experienced lower in-hospital mortality rates (OR, 0.77; 95% CI, 0.60–0.97; P = .0001). Although definitions of hospital volume differed across studies, the authors were able to perform recalculation with the dichotomized data that was available. Overall, the analysis found that the mortality rate at high-volume centers was lower than for lower-volume hospitals (OR, 0.85; 95% CI, 0.72–0.99; P = .001; I^2 = 87%).

Solomon and colleagues[18] analyzed 15,376 discharges for subarachnoid hemorrhage and 5638 craniotomies for aneurysm. The authors found that high-volume centers, defined as those performing at least 30 craniotomies for aneurysm treatment annually, had significantly lower mortality rates than hospitals that performed fewer than 30 craniotomies for aneurysm treatment annually (8.8% vs 15.5%; P<.0001). This finding was identical for patients with either ruptured and unruptured aneurysms.

McNeill and colleagues[19] found an inverse linear relationship between hospital subarachnoid hemorrhage case volume and 6-month mortality. The authors found that each 100-patient increase in volume correlated with a 24% reduction in mortality (OR, 0.76; 95% CI, 0.67–0.87). This relationship

was noted to apply across the entire range of hospitals examined, from 29 to 367 cases annually.

Carotid Stenosis

Cebul and colleagues[20] analyzed charts for 678 Medicare beneficiaries who underwent carotid endarterectomy (CEA) between 1993 and 1994 and found that 30-day mortality and nonfatal stroke rates varied by hospital volume (P = .004) in univariate analysis. In multivariate analysis, higher-volume hospitals were associated with a 71% risk reduction (OR, 0.29; 95% CI, 0.12–0.69; P = .006).

Wennberg and colleagues[21] analyzed 113,300 Medicare patients undergoing CEA between 1992 and 1993 and compared mortality rates for patients treated at NASCET- and ACAS-participating hospitals and those at nontrial hospitals. High-volume hospitals in both groups demonstrated better mortality rates. However, in multivariate analysis, trial hospitals had a greater apparent risk reduction (OR, 0.85; 95% CI, 0.69–1.00).

Cowan and colleagues[22] analyzed outcomes of 35,821 patients who underwent CEA from 1996 to 1997 in the NIS. The authors found that greater than 50% of the carotid endarterectomies in the United States were performed by high-volume surgeons. These high-volume surgeons had superior mortality rates compared with low-volume surgeons (0.44% vs 1.10%, respectively; P<.001) and lower postoperative stroke rates (1.14% vs 2.03%, respectively; P<.001). Surgeon specialty and hospital volume were not significantly associated with outcomes in this study.

PEDIATRICS

Smith and colleagues[23,24] analyzed VORs for primary pediatric brain tumors and ventriculoperitoneal shunts. In one study, the authors analyzed 4712 admissions for pediatric brain tumor craniotomy from 1988 to 2000.[23] They defined high-volume hospitals as those performing at least 20 craniotomies annually and found that in-hospital mortality and adverse discharge disposition rates were significantly lower at high-volume hospitals and by high-volume surgeons. Shunting procedures displayed similar trends in outcome. In a second study, Smith and colleagues[24] analyzed 5955 admissions for ventriculoperitoneal shunt placement or revision in pediatric patients from 1998 to 2000. Centers were divided into quartiles by volume, with the lowest quartile treating fewer than 28 patients annually, and the highest quartile treating at least 121 annually. The in-hospital mortality rate was 0.8% at lowest-volume centers and 0.3% at highest-volume centers. Surgeon case volume also correlated with outcomes, with low-volume providers who performed fewer than 9 shunts annually showing a mortality rate of 0.8% compared with 0.1% for the highest-volume providers, who each performed at least 65 shunting procedures annually. The study found no significant difference in LOS or hospital charges based on hospital or surgeon volume.

SPINE

A paucity of studies has examined VORs for spinal surgery. Dasenbrock and colleagues[25] examined 48,971 admissions for spine surgery from 2005 to 2008 in the NIS. Mortality rates did not differ significantly among surgeons, but complication rates were significantly associated with volume. Surgeon case volume was divided into quintiles, and very-low-volume surgeons were found to have significantly higher rates of complications compared with very-high-volume surgeons (OR, 1.38; 95% CI, 1.19–1.60; P = .001). However, complication rates were not significantly different between other surgeon volume quintiles. Furthermore, no effect was detected for hospital case volume with respect to either mortality or complications.

TRAUMA

Clement and colleagues[26] analyzed patients with neurotrauma from 2006 in the NIS and showed a volume threshold corresponding to significantly improved mortality. Hospitals treating fewer than 6 neurotrauma cases annually had an in-hospital mortality rate of 14.9%, whereas those treating 6 to 11, 12 to 23, 24 to 59, and 60 or more patients annually had mortality rates of 8.0%, 8.3%, 9.5%, and 10.0%, respectively. The authors found that volume did not correlate with either hospital charges or hospital LOS.

FUNCTIONAL
Epilepsy

McClelland and colleagues[27] analyzed patients admitted for anterior temporal lobectomy for temporal lobe epilepsy from 1988 to 2003 in the NIS. The authors found an overall morbidity rate, including codes for new postoperative morbidity and adverse discharge disposition, of 10.8%. Surgeon volume was not correlated with postoperative morbidity.

Englot and colleagues[28] analyzed hospitalizations for 6652 patients with intractable localized epilepsy who underwent surgical lobectomy or partial lobectomy from 1990 to 2008 in the NIS. The authors found that patients undergoing

surgery at high-volume centers had a lower risk of adverse events than those undergoing resection at middle- or low-volume hospitals (high: 6.1%; middle: 10.2%; low: 12.9%). They found that the most common adverse event was stroke or other neurologic complications, and this occurred significantly more frequently at low-volume (3.9%) versus high-volume (1.3%) centers.

Pain

Kalkanis and colleagues[29] analyzed outcomes from 1590 patients following microvascular decompression for treatment of trigeminal neuralgia, hemifacial spasm, and glossopharyngeal neuralgia. Higher-volume hospitals (P = .006) and surgeons (P = .02) both exhibited superior outcomes at discharge, including fewer complications (hospital: P = .04; surgeon, P = .01), lower adverse discharge disposition (5.1% lowest quartile vs 1.6% highest quartile), and lower hospital charges (P = .007). The authors did not find correlation between volume and mortality or length of stay. Hospital charges were slightly higher at higher-volume hospitals (P = .007).

Deep Brain Stimulation

Eskandar and colleagues[30] analyzed 1761 admissions for surgery for Parkinson disease from 1996 to 2000 in the NIS. High-volume centers demonstrated lower in-hospital mortality rates (P = .002) and fewer adverse discharge dispositions (P = .0070) compared with lower-volume hospitals. The authors additionally found that charges were lower at higher-volume centers (P<.001).

Sharma and colleagues[31] analyzed 2244 admissions for surgical treatment of Parkinson disease from 2006 to 2010 in the NIS. During this time frame, most of the procedures were performed at high-volume centers (64.8%; n = 1453), which demonstrated higher rates of adverse discharge disposition (OR, 3.543; 95% CI, 1.781–7.048; P<.001) and lower hospital charges. In contrast, patients treated by low-volume surgeons and hospitals had significantly higher rates of postoperative complications.

DISCUSSION

Researchers have identified robust VOR across the spectrum of neurosurgical disease. It is noteworthy that relationships observed at the hospital and surgeon levels are not necessarily equivalent. Although some of this may be statistical artifact from smaller numbers of providers than hospitals being identified in the data sets, this observation implies that the improved outcome effect is not altogether from gifted surgeon's hands but rather reflects the impact of the care delivery system as a whole. Care for patients undergoing neurosurgery involves multiple specialties and numerous interventions. Value for the patient is created by various providers and combined efforts over the course of the entire hospital stay. The benefits of one procedure and its respective outcome depend on the effectiveness of interventions throughout the patient care cycle.[32] High-volume centers tend to have not only high-volume surgeons but also well-functioning and experienced supporting teams consisting of neurotrained nurses, neurologists, neuroradiologists, neurointerventionalists, neuropathologists, neuroanesthesiologists, and neurorehabilitation specialists.[33–36]

Limitations

Although the strength of evidence varies across the studies, most is derived from a common source: administrative data sets, such as the annual NIS. The strength of these data sets is their ability to aggregate and analyze cases from across the county over several years, which results in condition-specific cohorts of tens of thousands for even some rare conditions, allowing researchers to overcome institutional biases and to power more insightful statistical measures. However, the granularity of detail for these data is limited. For instance, the NIS is derived from International Classification of Diseases, Ninth Revision (ICD-9) billing codes, which has drawn criticism because of (1) the lack of specificity in procedure and diagnosis codes, (2) the fact that codes are assigned by professional coders instead of physicians, and (3) the scarcity of granular detail regarding the hospital course.

The billing codes are asymmetrically distributed across the spectrum of diseases and procedures, with certain ones being represented in granular detail, whereas others are lumped into catchall categories. The ICD, Tenth Revision (ICD-10) seeks to rectify the lack of specificity with a massive expansion in the numbers of codes. These data are already becoming available in parts of Europe and Asia, where the use of ICD-10 billing codes is ongoing. Other locales, such as the United States, are adopting the new codes more slowly, and therefore it will yet be several years before these data become available to researchers.

Coding by professional coders has raised concern over the accuracy of diagnoses and procedures, in the sense that both a given entity is accurately represented in the billing data and the data are complete, with an accounting of all procedures and diagnoses. Data generated for billing purposes and then used for health services research will never be perfect and likely vary from site to site, with some being more complete and accurate than others.

Billing codes are summative tools to describe a hospital stay to payors, but they capture neither quotidian details, such as sodium values or anatomic details, nor specialty-specific outcomes, such as modified Rankin or Glasgow Outcome Scale scores. The limitations of these data must be understood when assessing the validity of surrogate measures and drawing conclusions. For neurosurgery, these data can be powerfully useful because many of the diseases treated are rare, so that even data from tertiary care centers cannot adequately power statistical analyses. In the absence of more comprehensive national registries, analyses of administrative data sets paired with appropriately rigorous statistical methods should be used to legitimately inform decision makers regarding population-level questions.

Evolving Care Paradigms

VORs have been demonstrated for both common and infrequently performed procedures. For many neurosurgical procedures, the proven relationships between surgical case volume and outcomes take the concept of quality improvement outside the sphere of what a single surgeon, service, or hospital can do, and indicate the need for cooperation at the regional or specialty level, wherein case volume can be sufficiently high to drive significant changes in quality. Some conditions have threshold effects, whereas others demonstrate more dose-dependent improvements in outcomes with higher volumes. Perhaps it is not surprising that good VOR studies do not exist for some of the most common neurosurgical procedures, such as discectomy or laminectomy, because it is the low-volume surgeons and centers that are outliers and the high global volume of these procedures means that vast majority perform above the performance threshold.

If as a specialty neurosurgery chose to be proactive in improving patient outcomes at the population level in this way, it would mean that neurosurgeons might need to adjust practice habits. Regionalization of care would necessitate more robust referral networks wherein certain conditions were only treated at a limited number of centers, and not all centers would necessarily specialize in all areas. Bardach and colleagues[37] performed a cost-utility analysis for regionalization of treatment for subarachnoid hemorrhage and found that transferring patients with subarachnoid hemorrhage from low- to high-volume hospitals would result in gains of 1.60 quality-adjusted life-years (QALY) at a cost of $10,548 dollars/QALY. Although some community and academic neurosurgeons may see a change in the variety of elective case types, the overall result would ultimately be beneficial for both patients and the specialty. In addition to better patient outcomes, concentration of cases would allow specialists to hone their skills, more effectively study and evolve treatment paradigms, and improve exposure for trainees dedicated to a particular subspecialty.

Outside forces consisting of payors, government regulators, and medical boards increasingly exert pressures to decrease costs and improve outcomes. Measuring, reporting, and comparing outcomes for neurosurgical specialists are perhaps the most important steps in understanding and improving outcomes. Neurosurgeons must continue to exert leadership in the development of specialty-specific data sources and measures, and implementing appropriate data-driven policy solutions if they are to retain autonomy and protect patients' access to quality care.

SUMMARY

Across a variety of neurosurgical subspecialties and procedure types, the data show that patients have better outcomes when they are managed by high-volume surgeons and at high-volume centers. These findings support regionalization into specialized neurosurgical treatment centers for certain conditions in the interest of improving the quality of care provided. Although this changing treatment paradigm will benefit from support at the level of organized neurosurgery, individual practitioners should be aware of where they fall on the volume spectrum and understand the implications of their practice and referral habits on their patients.

REFERENCES

1. Long DM, Gordon T, Bowman H, et al. Outcome and cost of craniotomy performed to treat tumors in regional academic referral centers. Neurosurgery 2003;52:1056–63 [discussion: 1063–5]. Available at: http://www.ncbi.nlm.nih.gov/pubmed/12699547. Accessed December 13, 2011.
2. Cowan JA, Dimick JB, Leveque JC, et al. The impact of provider volume on mortality after intracranial tumor resection. Neurosurgery 2003;52:48–53 [discussion: 53–4]. Available at: http://www.ncbi.nlm.nih.gov/pubmed/12493100. Accessed July 30, 2013.
3. Nuno M, Mukherjee D, Carico C, et al. The effect of centralization of caseload for primary brain tumor surgeries: trends from 2001-2007. Acta Neurochir 2012; 154:1343–50. Available at: http://www.hubmed.org/display.cgi?uids=22661296.
4. Barker FG Jr, Curry WT, Carter BS. Surgery for primary supratentorial brain tumors in the United States, 1988 to 2000: the effect of provider caseload and centralization of care. Neuro Oncol 2005. http://dx.doi.org/10.1215/S1152851704000146.
5. Trinh V, Davies JM, Berger MS. Surgery for primary supratentorial brain tumors in the United States, 2000–2009: effect of provider and hospital caseload on complication rates. J Neurosurg 2014;14:1–17.
6. Barker FG. Craniotomy for the resection of metastatic brain tumors in the U.S., 1988-2000: decreasing mortality and the effect of provider caseload. Cancer 2004;100:999–1007. http://dx.doi.org/10.1002/cncr.20058. Available at: http://www.ncbi.nlm.nih.gov/pubmed/14983496. Accessed August 26, 2014.
7. Barker FG, Klibanski A, Swearingen B. Transsphenoidal surgery for pituitary tumors in the United States, 1996-2000: mortality, morbidity, and the effects of hospital and surgeon volume. J Clin Endocrinol Metab 2003;88:4709–19. Available at: http://www.hubmed.org/display.cgi?uids=14557445.
8. Curry WT, Carter BS, Barker FG. Racial, ethnic, and socioeconomic disparities in patient outcomes after craniotomy for tumor in adult patients in the United States, 1988-2004. Neurosurgery 2010;66:427–37. http://dx.doi.org/10.1227/01.NEU.0000365265.10141.8E [discussion: 437–8]. Available at: http://www.ncbi.nlm.nih.gov/pubmed/20124933. Accessed July 30, 2013.
9. Ambekar S, Sharma M, Madhugiri VS, et al. Trends in intracranial meningioma surgery and outcome: a Nationwide Inpatient Sample database analysis from 2001 to 2010. J Neurooncol 2013; 114:299–307. http://dx.doi.org/10.1007/s11060-013-1183-6. Available at: http://www.ncbi.nlm.nih.gov/pubmed/23852621. Accessed August 26, 2014.
10. Barker FG 2nd, Carter BS, Ojemann RG, et al. Surgical excision of acoustic neuroma: patient outcome and provider caseload. Laryngoscope 2003;113:1332–43. http://dx.doi.org/10.1097/00005537-200038000-00013. Available at: http://www.ncbi.nlm.nih.gov/pubmed/12897555. Accessed August 26, 2014.
11. Jones PS, Aghi MK, Muzikansky A, et al. Outcomes and patterns of care in adult skull base chordomas from the Surveillance, Epidemiology, and End Results (SEER) database. J Clin Neurosci 2014;21:1490–6. http://dx.doi.org/10.1016/j.jocn.2014.02.008. Available at: http://www.ncbi.nlm.nih.gov/pubmed/24852903. Accessed August 26, 2014.
12. Leake CB, Brinjikji W, Kallmes DF, et al. Increasing treatment of ruptured cerebral aneurysms at

high-volume centers in the United States. J Neurosurg 2011;115:1179–83. http://dx.doi.org/10.3171/2011.7.JNS11590. Available at: http://www.ncbi.nlm.nih.gov/pubmed/21961924. Accessed August 26, 2014.

13. Johnston SC. Effect of endovascular services and hospital volume on cerebral aneurysm treatment outcomes. Stroke 2000;31:111–7. Available at: http://www.ncbi.nlm.nih.gov/pubmed/10625724. Accessed December 14, 2011.

14. Hattori N, Katayama Y, Abe T. Case volume does not correlate with outcome after cerebral aneurysm clipping: a nationwide study in Japan. Neurol Med Chir (Tokyo) 2007;47:95–100 [discussion: 100–1]. Available at: http://www.ncbi.nlm.nih.gov/pubmed/17384490. Accessed August 26, 2014.

15. Bardach NS, Zhao S, Gress DR, et al. Association between subarachnoid hemorrhage outcomes and number of cases treated at California hospitals. Stroke 2002;33:1851–6. Available at: http://www.ncbi.nlm.nih.gov/pubmed/12105365. Accessed December 14, 2011.

16. Cross DT, Tirschwell DL, Clark MA, et al. Mortality rates after subarachnoid hemorrhage: variations according to hospital case volume in 18 states. J Neurosurg 2003;99:810–7. http://dx.doi.org/10.3171/jns.2003.99.5.0810. Available at: http://www.ncbi.nlm.nih.gov/pubmed/14609158. Accessed August 26, 2011.

17. Boogaarts HD, van Amerongen MJ, de Vries J, et al. Caseload as a factor for outcome in aneurysmal subarachnoid hemorrhage: a systematic review and meta-analysis. J Neurosurg 2014;120:605–11. http://dx.doi.org/10.3171/2013.9.JNS13640. Available at: http://www.ncbi.nlm.nih.gov/pubmed/24093633. Accessed August 19, 2014.

18. Solomon RA, Mayer SA, Tarmey JJ. Relationship between the volume of craniotomies for cerebral aneurysm performed at New York state hospitals and in-hospital mortality. Stroke 1996;27:13–7. Available at: http://www.ncbi.nlm.nih.gov/pubmed/8553389. Accessed August 26, 2014.

19. McNeill L, English SW, Borg N, et al. Effects of institutional caseload of subarachnoid hemorrhage on mortality: a secondary analysis of administrative data. Stroke 2013;44:647–52. http://dx.doi.org/10.1161/STROKEAHA.112.681254. Available at: http://www.ncbi.nlm.nih.gov/pubmed/23362086. Accessed August 26, 2014.

20. Cebul RD, Snow RJ, Pine R, et al. Indications, outcomes, and provider volumes for carotid endarterectomy. JAMA 1998;279:1282–7. Available at: http://www.ncbi.nlm.nih.gov/pubmed/9565009. Accessed December 14, 2011.

21. Wennberg DE, Lucas FL, Birkmeyer JD, et al. Variation in carotid endarterectomy mortality in the Medicare population: trial hospitals, volume, and patient characteristics. JAMA 1998;279:1278–81. Available at: http://www.ncbi.nlm.nih.gov/pubmed/9565008. Accessed December 14, 2011.

22. Cowan JA, Dimick JB, Thompson BG, et al. Surgeon volume as an indicator of outcomes after carotid endarterectomy: an effect independent of specialty practice and hospital volume. J Am Coll Surg 2002;195:814–21. Available at: http://www.ncbi.nlm.nih.gov/pubmed/12495314. Accessed September 28, 2014.

23. Smith ER, Butler WE, Barker FG. Craniotomy for resection of pediatric brain tumors in the United States, 1988 to 2000: effects of provider caseloads and progressive centralization and specialization of care. Neurosurgery 2004;54:553–63 [discussion: 563–5]. Available at: http://www.ncbi.nlm.nih.gov/pubmed/15028128. Accessed July 30, 2013.

24. Smith ER, Butler WE, Barker FG. In-hospital mortality rates after ventriculoperitoneal shunt procedures in the United States, 1998 to 2000: relation to hospital and surgeon volume of care. J Neurosurg 2004;100:90–7. http://dx.doi.org/10.3171/ped.2004.100.2.0090. Available at: http://thejns.org/doi/abs/10.3171/ped.2004.100.2.0090?url_ver=Z39.88-2003&rfr_id=ori:rid:crossref.org&rfr_dat=cr_pub=pubmed. Accessed December 13, 2011.

25. Dasenbrock HH, Clarke MJ, Witham TF, et al. The impact of provider volume on the outcomes after surgery for lumbar spinal stenosis. Neurosurgery 2012;70:1346–53. http://dx.doi.org/10.1227/NEU.0b013e318251791a [discussion: 1353–4]. Available at: http://www.ncbi.nlm.nih.gov/pubmed/22610361. Accessed July 30, 2013.

26. Clement RC, Carr BG, Kallan MJ, et al. Volume-outcome relationship in neurotrauma care. J Neurosurg 2013;118:687–93. http://dx.doi.org/10.3171/2012.10.JNS12682. Available at: http://www.ncbi.nlm.nih.gov/pubmed/23240697. Accessed September 28, 2014.

27. McClelland S, Guo H, Okuyemi KS. Population-based analysis of morbidity and mortality following surgery for intractable temporal lobe epilepsy in the United States. Arch Neurol 2011;68:725–9. http://dx.doi.org/10.1001/archneurol.2011.7. Available at: http://www.ncbi.nlm.nih.gov/pubmed/21320984. Accessed August 20, 2014.

28. Englot DJ, Ouyang D, Garcia PA, et al. Epilepsy surgery trends in the United States, 1990-2008. Neurology 2012;78:1200–6. http://dx.doi.org/10.1212/WNL.0b013e318250d7ea. Available at: http://www.pubmedcentral.nih.gov/articlerender.fcgi?artid=3324320&tool=pmcentrez&rendertype=abstract. Accessed August 26, 2014.

29. Kalkanis SN, Eskandar EN, Carter BS, et al. Microvascular decompression surgery in the United States, 1996 to 2000: mortality rates, morbidity rates, and the effects of hospital and surgeon volumes. Neurosurgery 2003;52:1251–61 [discussion: 1261–2],

Available at: http://www.ncbi.nlm.nih.gov/pubmed/12762870. Accessed August 26, 2014.

30. Eskandar EN, Flaherty A, Cosgrove GR, et al. Surgery for Parkinson disease in the United States, 1996 to 2000: practice patterns, short-term outcomes, and hospital charges in a nationwide sample. J Neurosurg 2003;99:863–71. http://dx.doi.org/10.3171/jns.2003.99.5.0863. Available at: http://www.ncbi.nlm.nih.gov/pubmed/14609166. Accessed August 26, 2014.

31. Sharma M, Ambekar S, Guthikonda B, et al. Regional trends and the impact of various patient and hospital factors on outcomes and costs of hospitalization between academic and nonacademic centers after deep brain stimulation surgery for Parkinson's disease: a United States Nationwide Inpatient Sample analysis from 2006 to 2010. Neurosurg Focus 2013;35:E2. http://dx.doi.org/10.3171/2013.8.FOCUS13295. Available at: http://www.ncbi.nlm.nih.gov/pubmed/24175862. Accessed August 26, 2014.

32. Porter ME. What is value in health care? N Engl J Med 2010;363:2477–81. http://dx.doi.org/10.1056/NEJMp1011024. Available at: http://www.ncbi.nlm.nih.gov/pubmed/21142528. Accessed July 11, 2014.

33. Berman MF, Solomon RA, Mayer SA, et al. Impact of hospital-related factors on outcome after treatment of cerebral aneurysms. Stroke 2003;34:2200–7. http://dx.doi.org/10.1161/01.STR.0000086528.32334.06. Available at: http://www.ncbi.nlm.nih.gov/pubmed/12907814. Accessed September 28, 2014.

34. Cowan JA, Ziewacz J, Dimick JB, et al. Use of endovascular coil embolization and surgical clip occlusion for cerebral artery aneurysms. J Neurosurg 2007;107:530–5. http://dx.doi.org/10.3171/JNS-07/09/0530. Available at: http://www.ncbi.nlm.nih.gov/pubmed/17886551. Accessed September 28, 2014.

35. Hoh BL, Rabinov JD, Pryor JC, et al. In-hospital morbidity and mortality after endovascular treatment of unruptured intracranial aneurysms in the United States, 1996-2000: effect of hospital and physician volume. AJNR Am J Neuroradiol 2003;24:1409–20. Available at: http://www.ncbi.nlm.nih.gov/pubmed/12917139. Accessed June 5, 2013.

36. Kramer AA, Zimmerman JE. The relationship between hospital and intensive care unit length of stay. Crit Care Med 2011;39:1015–22. http://dx.doi.org/10.1097/CCM.0b013e31820eabab. Available at: http://www.ncbi.nlm.nih.gov/pubmed/21336128. Accessed September 15, 2014.

37. Bardach NS, Olson SJ, Elkins JS, et al. Regionalization of treatment for subarachnoid hemorrhage: a cost-utility analysis. Circulation 2004;109:2207–12. http://dx.doi.org/10.1161/01.CIR.0000126433.12527.E6. Available at: http://www.ncbi.nlm.nih.gov/pubmed/15117848. Accessed September 28, 2014.

Neurosurgical Checklists
A Growing Need

Scott L. Zuckerman, MD[a], Kyle M. Fargen, MD, MPH[b], J. Mocco, MD, MS[a],*

KEYWORDS

• Quality improvement • Time-out • Checklist • Patient safety • Neurosurgery

KEY POINTS

• Checklists act as forcing functions, mandating series of evidence-based steps that reduce the potential for error caused by inherent human biases.
• The neurosurgical literature contains 2 different types of checklists: (1) routine checklist to be used in planned interventions and (2) emergent checklist to be used in the unplanned event of a complication.
• Neurosurgical checklists, though in their infancy, are continuing to be developed across all subspecialties.
• Most checklists reported in the neurosurgical literature are single-center studies without external validation.
• After checklist development, successful implementation is a nuanced process, requiring collaboration and commitment from all involved parties.

INTRODUCTION

In 1999, the Institute of Medicine published the seminal article "To Err is Human: Building a Safer Health System,"[1] suggesting that anywhere from 44,000 to 98,000 deaths occurred annually in the United States secondary to avoidable medical errors.[1,2] Earlier reports in the 1980s found that 41% of hospitalized patients were admitted because of iatrogenic disease.[3] Gawande and colleagues[4] postulated that of all hospital admissions nationally in 1992, 3% resulted in adverse events and 50% of these events were preventable. The cost of adverse events is not trivial.[4–8] One state documented that adverse medical events led to a mortality rate of 13.6% and costs more than $800 million in a single year.[2,9] The prevention of these avoidable medical errors has contributed to the evolving interest in quality improvement measures, with heavy emphasis on surgical checklists.

In 2008, The World Health Organization (WHO) created the WHO Surgical Safety Checklist.[10] The 19-item checklist sought to address infection prevention and anesthesia-related complications in surgery. In his 2009 book, *Checklist Manifesto: How to Get Things Right,* Atul Gawande espoused the utility of the checklists in error prevention through systematic corrective measures for generally routine tasks.[11] Gawande's work popularized the notion of intrinsic human fallibility and the inability to provide excellent outcomes with total reliance on individual performance.

Medicine has seen an explosion in checklists aimed at improving patient safety. Where general surgery[12–22] and anesthesiology[23–28] have published extensively on the use of checklists, neurosurgery is now following suit. In a field fraught with life-and-death decisions, where a seemingly minor mishap can lead to unforeseen death, the need for

There were no external sources of financial support for this article.
a Department of Neurological Surgery, Vanderbilt University School of Medicine, 1211 Medical Center Dr, Nashville, TN 37232, USA; b Department of Neurological Surgery, University of Florida, 1149 Newell Dr, Gainesville, FL 32610, USA
* Corresponding author. Department of Neurological Surgery, Vanderbilt University Medical Center, T-4224 Medical Center North, Nashville, TN 37232-2380.
E-mail address: jmocco@yahoo.com

Neurosurg Clin N Am 26 (2015) 219–229
http://dx.doi.org/10.1016/j.nec.2014.11.009
1042-3680/15/$ – see front matter © 2015 Elsevier Inc. All rights reserved.

standardizing perioperative activities is paramount. The authors summarize procedural checklists in neurosurgery, from intensive-care-unit (ICU) procedures to specialty-specific operating room (OR) protocols, in hopes of expanding a growing cornerstone of medical and surgical care.

PREPROCEDURE TIME-OUT

The preprocedural time-out is now a universally performed confirmation of the correct patient and correct operative site and side in virtually every OR in the United States, if not the world. One of the earliest studies of a neurosurgical perioperative checklist was conducted by Lyons[29] whereby one US institution published 8 years of experience with an operative checklist across 6313 operations in 6345 patients. Compliance was extremely high at 99.5%, with no episodes of wrong patient or wrong-site surgery. Oszvald and colleagues[30] conducted a similar advanced perioperative checklist in Germany. The investigators identified 1 wrong-sided emergent burr hole and 1 wrong-sided lumbar approach across 8795 procedures involving 12,390 patients.

Two additional studies modified a general surgical checklist in a neurosurgical population. Da Silva-Freitas and colleagues[31] evaluated the previously mentioned modified WHO surgery safety checklist in 44 neurosurgical operations and identified 51 possible sentinel events in 44 operations. Matsumae and colleagues[32] implemented a similar checklist and used an on-duty safety nurse to ensure all safety practices were being met. Since the widespread adoption of the surgical time-out checklist, specialty- and procedure-specific checklists have gained popularity within neurosurgery (summarized in **Table 1**). The sections that follow discuss such checklists by specialty or procedure.

External Ventricular Drain

External ventricular drain (EVD) insertion is a common procedure performed in the ICU setting whereby a catheter is inserted into the cerebral ventricular system, thereby allowing drainage of cerebrospinal fluid. EVDs are integral to the ICU management of neurosurgical patients, most common in aneurysmal subarachnoid hemorrhage[33] and intracranial pressure (ICP) management.[34,35] Several checklists have been developed aimed at preventing infection, as infection may result in increased ICU length of stay and cost as well as patient morbidity and mortality.[36–38]

Kubilay and colleagues[38] evaluated 2928 ventriculostomies over a 4-year period and documented a reduction in EVD infection rate from 9.2% to 0%

after implementation of a best-practice protocol. The protocol was summarized and distributed in succinct checklist form.[38] The checklist included several tasks, including antibiotic administration, hand washing, hair clipping, wide hair clip space for dressing, spectator use of hats and masks, and tunneling the catheter exit site 5 cm from the scalp incision. The investigators successfully implemented a best-practice model in the form of a checklist at a single institution.[39]

A similar study exclusively in cerebrovascular patients showed an equally encouraging decline in EVD infection rates. In more than 1961 ventriculostomies, Harrop and colleagues[40] showed a precipitous decline in infection rate when 2 different antibiotic-impregnated catheters were used, from 6.7% to 1.0% and 7.6% to 0.9% in 2 study time periods. Their procedural protocol included reducing room traffic, electric clippers for hair shaving, full barrier precautions, and a fully gowned surgical scrub for assistance.

Vascular

The treatment of neurovascular patients is complex. The surgical treatments for cerebrovascular disorders continue to evolve and include open surgery or minimally invasive endovascular techniques. Whether for an aneurysm embolization, open clipping, or emergent thrombectomy, checklists have the potential to improve safety in this high-risk patient population.

Endovascular complications range from benign puncture-site hematomas or transient neurologic deficits to aneurysm rupture, arterial dissection, stroke, and thromboembolism.[41,42] Complications of open clipping occur in approximately 20% of patients, including direct brain injury, cranial nerve injury, postoperative hematoma, and ischemic event.[43] Wong JM, et al[44] reviewed the adverse events of open vascular neurosurgery and concluded a significant proportion of technical adverse events could be reduced by standardized protocols, increased teamwork, and communication.

The current literature contains 2 brands of vascular checklists: routine and emergent. Fargen and colleagues[45] proposed that an endovascular checklist should be completed before any endovascular intervention. Checklist implementation in 60 procedures led to a significant reduction in adverse events as well as improved communication among team members.[45] In emergent situations, Taussky and colleagues[46] postulated a checklist in case of aneurysm perforation during coiling. Similarly, Chen[47] formed 2 checklists in the cases of aneurysmal rupture, with the overall

Table 1
Summary of neurosurgical checklists

Author, Year	Procedure	Main Findings
Kubilay et al,[38] 2013	EVD	EVD infection rate decreased from 9.2% to 0% over 4 y after antibiotic-impregnated catheter and procedure checklist implementation.
Harrop et al,[40] 2010	EVD	EVD infection rate decreased from 6.7% to 1.0% and 7.6% to 0.9% in 2 study periods after antibiotic-impregnated catheter and procedure checklist implementation, exclusively in a vascular patient population.
Fargen et al,[45] 2012	Endovascular	It decreased adverse events in 8 out of 9 event types and improved communication after endovascular procedure checklist implementation.
Chen,[47] 2011	Endovascular	There was successful creation of endovascular checklists for aneurysmal rupture and thromboembolic events.
Taussky et al,[46] 2010	Endovascular	There was successful creation of an endovascular checklist in the event of an aneurysmal rupture.
Kramer et al,[56] 2012	Functional	It implemented a 49-step checklist for deep brain stimulation surgery; the use of the checklist decreased the incidence of major errors more than threefold.
Rahmathulla et al,[58] 2012	Tumor	An intraoperative MRI checklist was successfully implemented in 120 craniotomies for tumor resection with no adverse events.
Ladak & Spinner,[67] 2014	Spine	A correct-level spine checklist was successfully created, whereby a second pause occurs when preoperative and intraoperative imaging correlated, such that all members of the surgical team confirm the marked level.
Ryan et al,[68] 2014	Spine	It decreased the spine infection rate from 5.8% to 2.2% after the procedure checklist was implemented.
Sugrue et al,[70] 2013	Spine	There was a multidisciplinary protocol that evaluates safety and risks for patients undergoing high-risk spine surgery.
Ziewacz et al,[69] 2012	Spine	There was an algorithm for the design, development, and implementation for the multidisciplinary response to intraoperative neuromonitoring alerts in spine surgery.
Hommelstad et al,[71] 2013	VP shunt	It decreased the infection rate from 6.5% to 4.3%, with a reduction of 18.4% to 5.7% in children younger than 1 y, after the procedure checklist was implemented.
Kestle et al,[72] 2011	VP shunt	It decreased the infection rate from 8.8% to 5.7% after infection checklist implementation across 4 centers and 21 surgeons.

Abbreviations: EVD, external ventricular drain; VP, ventriculoperitoneal.
  Data from Refs.[38,40,45–47,56,58,67–72]

goals of hemostasis and ICP management, and in the cases of thromboembolic events, with overall goals of thrombolysis and distal perfusion optimization. Chen[47] divided the checklist into individual OR personnel roles, rather than team responsibilities, suggesting an alternate manner to delegate responsibility. Despite the utility and need of the emergent checklists, none were reportedly used in a live patient scenario.

Functional

At the opposite end of the neurosurgical spectrum, functional neurosurgery is often elective and associated with lower risk, yet requires precise planning and technique. Deep brain stimulation (DBS), various pain interventions, and epilepsy surgery offers the return of quality of life to patients with medically refractory disorders.[48–54] The nature of DBS surgery demands absolute precision with respect to electrode placement; a single skipped surgical step could mean incorrect lead placement and subsequent reoperation.

In 2009, Connolly and colleagues[55] described the first checklist specifically designed for DBS and published their results in 28 patients treated for either Parkinson disease or essential tremor.[56] In this relatively small study, 17 patients underwent

DBS without the use of a 49-step checklist compared with 11 with checklist implementation. The use of a checklist decreased the incidence of major errors more than threefold from 11 to 3. All 5 cases with no error used the checklist.

Tumor

Similar to vascular intervention, the removal of brain tumors is equally high stakes. Operations can be long, combined with other services, and make use of intraoperative MRI (ioMRI). Wong and colleagues[57] reviewed most common adverse events seen in intracranial neoplasm surgery, which widely ranged from 9% to 40%. DVT was most common, seen in 3%–26%. Second was worsened neurologic deficit, ranging from 0% to 20%, seen most commonly in eloquent glioma surgery. The authors concluded that helpful strategies to reduce adverse events included: image guidance, intraoperative functional mapping, intraoperative MRI, and DVT, infection, and seizure prophylaxis.

Although the authors did not find any checklists specific to the tumor operation itself, Rahmathulla and colleagues[58] described an overview of the ioMRI room, safety considerations, and checklist and protocols used in these cases to maintain safety in their "zero tolerance environment." Based on their single-institution experience, they used the WHO surgical safety checklist as well as a detailed MRI screening checklist. Before each case, the surgical team engaged in a presurgical briefing huddle, a process that enhanced communication among OR team members. Their checklist yielded 120 ioMRI craniotomies for tumor resection with no preoperative or intraoperative adverse events.

Spine

The United States currently has the highest rate of spine surgery in the world.[59,60] As the incidence of spine surgery and instrumented fusion increases, so do complication rates. Immediate complications include, durotomy (hole made in the dura), pseudomeningocele, transient neurologic deficit, and permanent neurologic deficit, whereas long-term problems range from pseudoarthrosis or adjacent segment disease to hardware failure.

Wrong-level spinal surgery is an uncommon but unforgivable error.[61] Wrong-level surgery is defined as a surgical procedure performed at the correct site but at the wrong level of the operative field. Without intraoperative radiographs, surgeons initially exposed the wrong level 15% of the time in a prospective study of 100 discectomies.[62] A 2010 study by the same investigators found that wrong-site surgery occurred in an average of 6.8 discectomies, respectively, for every 10,000 procedures performed.[61]

Groff and colleagues[63] surveyed 569 spine surgeons to better understand current practices to avoid wrong-level spine surgery. Surgeons obtained imaging after bony removal 16% of time; 50% of surgeons reported wrong-level lumbar spine surgery at least once; greater than 10% reported wrong-sided lumbar spine surgery at least once. Alarmingly, only 40% of respondents believed the Joint Commission time-out helped reduce these errors. Responses to this article raised interesting questions about wrong-level surgery. For instance, even the most experienced and conscientious surgeons can expose and identify the wrong level in transitional segments and redo operations. Furthermore, respondents argued the considerable difference between wrong-site surgery, such as amputation of the wrong arm, which can be prevented by simply marking and confirming the correct arm preoperatively, and wrong-spinal-level surgery, which can only be prevented through anatomic or radiographic confirmation intraoperatively. The investigators concluded wrong-level spine surgery is clearly more difficult to prevent than other wrong-site surgeries and cannot be treated the same.[64]

In 2001, the North American Spine Society (NASS) developed the Sign, Mark, and X-ray program. This program consists of a checklist seeking to improve patient safety and decrease complications, such as wrong-level surgery, during spine operations.[65,66] However, evidence suggests that the NASS checklist is insufficient to minimize wrong-level surgery and is now more than a decade old. In 2014, Ladak and Spinner[67] reported a protocol developed by spine surgeons whereby preoperative imaging must be available during the procedure and intraoperative imaging is required. The surgeon must then correlate the preoperative and intraoperative studies and a second pause must be conducted intraoperatively, so that all members of the surgical team confirm the marked level on the image before executing the procedure.[67]

One institution published their experience preventing spine infections in a pediatric population.[68] After implantation of a standardized protocol aimed at infection reduction, the infection rate decreased from 5.8% to 2.2% over 267 cases. Their protocol was succinctly summarized and completed before most operations and included the following steps: sign on OR door, antibiotic administration and redosing, chlorhexidine gluconate and ethyl alcohol solution hand scrub (Avagard, 3M, St Paul, MN) bacitracin irrigation, antibiotic-impregnated sutures, and drain placement.

Similar to aneurysmal rupture, checklists have been designed to deal with neuromonitoring changes intraoperatively. Ziewacz and colleagues[69] published their findings of designing, developing, and implementing a checklist for neuromonitoring alerts in patients with myelopathy. They outlined the roles of the surgeon, neurophysiologist, and anesthesiologist. The article excellently describes a cogent plan of action in the event of acute monitoring changes. Even more important, this study discusses how a checklist is made and successfully implemented.

An excellent review about protocols in high-risk spine surgery completely outlined protocol-based care in spine surgery.[70] The article first described an extensive preoperative spine workup, which included a multidisciplinary conference between hospitalists, anesthesia, and nursing, and multiorgan system clearance. A multifaceted postoperative approach was also outlined, with complete guidelines regarding hemodynamics, coagulation, metabolic, and pulmonary care. Although the article did not address operative checklists, it described a safe, complex, and standardized process for safely operating on high-risk patients with spine disease.

Pediatrics

Checklists have been used routinely in ventriculoperitoneal shunt procedures across pediatric neurosurgery, mainly aimed at reducing infection.[71,72] A Norwegian study by Hommelstad and colleagues[71] evaluated the effectiveness of a new shunt protocol by comparing 2 time periods across 901 patients, in whom 1404 shunt procedures were performed. The protocol included patient shower, hair removal, OR team wearing surgical hoods, limiting room traffic, patient normothermia, covering instruments until the procedure starts, changing gloves after handling the shunt, and using nontouch techniques whenever possible. Although the investigators saw an overall infection rate decrease from 6.5% to 4.3%, a significant reduction was seen in children younger than 1 year (18.4%–5.7%). Compliance data were missing in 15.6% of cases, and only 192 procedures (24.6%) had 100% compliance. The investigators noted that emergent cases frequently breached protocol. Moreover, the investigators noted that compliance was difficult when multiple surgeons were involved.

A second study conducted by the Hydrocephalus Clinical Research Network (HCRN) evaluated a standardized protocol at 4 institutions aimed at reducing infection, one of the few multi-institution studies. The protocol was developed by reviewing the current literature and prior institutional experience and applied prospectively in the HCRN network. Twenty-one surgeons performed 1571 procedures between 2007 and 2009. The HCRN infection rate decreased significantly from 8.8% before the protocol to 5.7% while using the protocol. The overall protocol compliance was 74.5% and improved over the course of the observation period. The investigators conclude that the protocol was most important in establishing a common baseline with the HCRN. Moreover, the HCRN recorded a 74.5% rate of 100% compliance of all 11 steps and another 20.2% when 10 out of 11 steps were followed. The most common steps missed were antibiotic administration before incision and patient positioning away from the door. The investigators aimed for a shorter, simpler protocol in future iterations, as these have a higher chance of 100% compliance.

Intensive Care Unit

Although not aimed specifically at surgical intervention or bedside procedure, itemized protocols have been used in the ICU setting to improve the care of neurosurgical patients. One institution published their results after tracking 3 interventions in the neurologic ICU setting: mobility,[73] urinary tract infections,[74] and dysphagia screening.[75] All 3 studies championed nursing-administered protocols for ambulation and physical therapy, urinary catheter removal, and bedside swallow tests and were associated with positive improvements in ICU patient care. Outside of neurosurgery, several procedural checklists exist aimed at preventing catheter-related bloodstream infections in procedural checklist form.[76,77]

POSTOPERATIVE DEBRIEFING

One step of neurosurgical operations that has historically received little attention is the postoperative time-out or *debriefing*. Postoperative debriefing is defined as a process that allows *"individuals to discuss individual and team level performance, identify errors made, and develop a plan to improve their next performance following a procedure or event."*[78] Debriefing allows for the identification of failures, near misses, and successes and has been shown to reduce communication issues, which are the primary cause of human error in the surgical setting.[79] Debriefing may look feasible on paper, but implementation has proved difficult.[80]

In the previously mentioned German study by Oszvald and colleagues,[30] their protocol included a portion devoted to *"before transfer out of the OR"* in every time-out procedure. An incomplete checklist was found in only 3% of patients. Although the investigators did not comment specifically on the postprocedure portion of the checklist, they stated the team time-out principles improved the perioperative workup and focus of the entire team and that the focus is drawn to the procedure, expected difficulties, and special needs in the treatment of individualized patients.[30]

One institution recently reported its experience with a debriefing module.[80] In an observational study of cardiac and neurosurgical cases, it was determined that surgeons performed a postsurgical debriefing in less than a quarter of surgical cases.[81] This lack of debriefing was caused by confusion regarding timing and ownership of debriefing, and it was also perceived to delay closing and interfere with standard surgeon workflow. To combat this challenge, in November 2010, a multidisciplinary Perioperative Debrief Task Force, which consisted of surgeons, an anesthesiologist, human factors experts, nurses, and OR staff, was created to make a succinct yet comprehensive surgical checklist to guide structured postoperative debriefings.

Unlike in the preprocedural time-out, the debriefing cues the surgeon to invite performance feedback from the staff involved in the surgical case. Performance feedback is a brief postcase huddle led by the surgeon that allows surgical team members to voice their assessments of the team's safety performance during the case. Despite several successful meetings, formal checklist implementation was not achieved. Factors that affected the ability to implement the debriefing included surgeon buy-in, department chairman buy-in, and administrative barriers.

Debriefing in neurosurgery is yet to be explored. The debriefing process may become a powerful tool in creating team unity and awareness as well as reducing errors, which in turn leads to a more enjoyable working environment for medical personnel and a safer operative experience for the patients.

IMPLEMENTATION
Why Checklists Are Effective

There has been an increasing focus in published medical literature regarding the science behind decision making and strategies to reduce individual biases with the goal of preventing medical errors.[82–84] A full review of this topic as it pertains to neurosurgery may be found elsewhere.[85] In brief, there is increasing evidence to support a dual process theory of decision making whereby

decisions are generated through a combination of 2 processes: systems 1 (intuitive) and 2 (analytical).[86] System 1 refers to the unconscious, intuitive, rapid, effortless, and potentially biased process through which most of our daily decisions are generated (up to 95% of the decisions we make).[83] This process also uses heuristics, or cognitive shortcuts. System 2, on the other hand, is slow, conscious, analytical, tedious, and mentally fatiguing. As fatigue, workload, or distractions increase, we begin to rely increasingly on system 1 for decisions. Unfortunately, unlike system 2, the intuitive process is subject to several important biases[87] and uses unreliable cognitive shortcuts that may result in cognitive errors. Recognition of these inherent weaknesses in clinical decision making has led experts to develop a series of strategies for debiasing medical decisions with the ultimate goal of reducing potentially preventable medical errors.[83,84]

One of the most stringent means of debiasing decisions is through the use of forcing functions. Forcing functions are strategies that mandate that the clinician follow a step, or series of steps, to eliminate shortcuts and absolve the decision-making process from personal bias. Checklists and protocols are 2 of the most widely used and effective types of forcing functions. When checklists are created with evidence-based and/or validated criteria, these tools force the clinician through a series of steps that are resistant to forgetfulness, fatigue, shortcuts, heuristics, and operator variability or preference. When adopted by a health care team and implemented into the care process, checklists ensure uniformity of evidence-based care.

Implementation

The creation of a surgical checklist is in itself a large undertaking, with consensus across several work systems. Wong and colleagues[88] discussed 5 strategies for reducing adverse events, 2 of them being initiating institutional and national protocols and the implementation of the WHO surgical safety checklist. The investigators mention their experience with a surgical checklist and using a system proposed by Pronovost and colleagues in the ICU setting called the 4 Es: engage, educate, execute, and evaluate.[89]

One can imagine various objections to new checklist implementation; any change brings with it dissenters. Usually it is not a dispute of the evidence, rather a cultural problem.[90] Again referring to Pronovost and colleagues' work, any cultural objections should be strongly met with a reference to the evidence. As long as the evidence is there, most objections result in the deliverance of substandard patient care. In essence, any objectors are asking to indirectly harm patients by not subscribing to the new protocol at hand. Cultural inertia can be an obstacle; but again, a strong grounding in evidence-based measures can overcome this. In addition, surgeon and chairman buy-in has also been found to be important in making sure a checklist or new protocol is received well.[80]

The next step, once the checklist is part of the institutional workflow, is to ensure all staff members speak up when protocol steps are skipped, guidelines not followed, or patient safety jeopardized. This process is much more nuanced, combating ingrained hierarchical constraints.

As anesthesiologist Dr Raghunathan[91] mentions in his checklist and culture article, the world is not flat and the influence of power distance on safety interventions is understudied.[91] Although checklists help minimize power distances, surveys and simulation studies may discover patterns of potentially hidden yet problematic interactions that endanger patients. Popular author Malcolm Gladwell[92] explains the Korean airline culture and that preventable errors may be the result of cultural traditions hindering communication. Raghunathan[91] mentions the Power Distance Index (PDI), first mentioned by the Dutch social psychologist Geert Hofstede,[93] defined as distance and inequality across power imbalance in a pyramidal organizational structure. In a high PDI culture, any mistake is treated as a blame game (ie, *How did you make this error?*) in contrast to a more egalitarian system whereby an adverse event is focused on how to improve (ie, *How did this happen?*).

Translating this to the OR, errors or near-miss reports are likely to be first taken as an accusation of failure rather than an opportunity for improvement. These principles are a basis of the Just Culture model, which is gaining popularity among medical professionals as a way to identify and correct individual and systems-based deficiencies to improve quality of care and prevent future medical errors.

The supreme goal in checklist effectiveness should be creating an OR climate where people are comfortable, staff is free to speak up as necessary, and the landscape is democratized. Norton and colleagues[94] evaluated staff member perception after a surgical safety checklist was implemented at Boston Children's Hospital. The results suggested that the surgical staff supported the checklist use and thought it improved safety. One-third of respondents said they witnessed the checklist prevent an error. Most respondents also said the checklist improved efficiency and reduced delays, in stark contrast to the anecdotal

thought that the checklists delay cases. Staff introductions also improved familiarity and created a comfortable environment.

In a similar study, Lau and colleagues[95] created a perioperative educational safety video targeted to the neurosurgical provider audience. A multidisciplinary team, neurosurgery, anesthesia, nurses, neuromonitoring, and administration, determined the objective and content of the video and created the final product. The video focused on open communication, with special emphasis during the timeout and postsurgical debrief to make all team members feel comfortable and important.

Going Forward

Checklists have been developed and tested in a variety of settings within the realm of medicine. In neurologic surgery, checklists have successfully reduced procedural infections, decreased wrong-site surgery, enhanced communication and prevented medical errors. There is no question that checklists play an important role in preventing unnecessary patient harm during surgical procedures.

Unfortunately, most of the checklists presented in this article have not been used or validated outside of the institution in which they were studied. Widespread acceptance of a published checklist requires that health care systems recognize a deficiency, explore the literature for solutions, identify a checklist that may be beneficial, evaluate potential barriers toward checklist implementation, and finally make a concerted team effort to adopt and implement with buy-in from all parties. Given these roadblocks, it is not surprising, even with an increasing literature supporting their use, that the only universally practiced surgical protocol is the institution-specific surgical time-out. Even worse, the surgical time-out practiced by most US hospitals is highly variable and many stray from the validated criteria within the WHO surgical safety checklist.

The US health care system is currently undergoing a paradigm shift from pay-for-services toward pay-for-performance reimbursement, with a focus on quality measures and patient satisfaction. Although checklists do have limitations, in most settings, these limitations do not outweigh the potential benefits toward improving the quality of care provided through reduction in patient-harm events. In concordance with this paradigm shift, we are likely to see increasing utilization of evidence-based protocols to not only standardize care but also as a means of documenting compliance with regulators and obtaining reimbursement. Checklists will likely play an important role in this process in the foreseeable future. It is important to remember that even the surgical time-out, now universally mandated, once met considerable resistance from clinicians before health systems recognized its importance and required its regular use. Similarly, going forward, we are likely to see waning resistance as the benefits of these checklists become increasingly recognized.

REFERENCES

1. Kohn LT, Corrigan J, Donaldson MS. America, C.o.Q.o.H.C.i, I.o. Medicine. To err is human: building a safer health system. In: Kohn LT, Corrigan JM, Donaldson MS, editors. The National Academies Press; 2000.
2. Brennan TA, Leape LL, Laird NM, et al. Incidence of adverse events and negligence in hospitalized patients. Results of the Harvard Medical Practice Study I. N Engl J Med 1991;324(6):370–6.
3. Trunet P, Le Gall JR, Lhoste F, et al. The role of iatrogenic disease in admissions to intensive care. JAMA 1980;244(23):2617–20.
4. Gawande AA, Thomas EJ, Zinner MJ, et al. The incidence and nature of surgical adverse events in Colorado and Utah in 1992. Surgery 1999;126(1): 66–75.
5. Thomas EJ, Studdert DM, Runciman WB, et al. A comparison of iatrogenic injury studies in Australia and the USA. I: context, methods, casemix, population, patient and hospital characteristics. Int J Qual Health Care 2000;12(5):371–8.
6. Wilson RM, Runciman WB, Gibberd RW, et al. The quality in Australian health care study. Med J Aust 1995;163(9):458–71.
7. Thomas EJ, Studdert DM, Burstin HR, et al. Incidence and types of adverse events and negligent care in Utah and Colorado. Med Care 2000;38(3): 261–71.
8. Thomas EJ, Studdert DM, Newhouse JP, et al. Costs of medical injuries in Utah and Colorado. Inquiry 1999;36(3):255–64.
9. Johnson WG, Brennan TA, Newhouse JP, et al. The economic consequences of medical injuries. Implications for a no-fault insurance plan. JAMA 1992; 267(18):2487–92.
10. Haynes AB, Weiser TG, Berry WR, et al. A surgical safety checklist to reduce morbidity and mortality in a global population. N Engl J Med 2009;360(5): 491–9.
11. Gawande, A. (2010). The checklist manifesto: How to get things right. New York: Metropolitan Books.
12. de Vries EN, Prins HA, Bennink MC, et al. Nature and timing of incidents intercepted by the SURPASS checklist in surgical patients. BMJ Qual Saf 2012; 21(6):503–8.
13. Robb WB, Falk GA, Larkin JO, et al. A 10-step intraoperative surgical checklist (ISC) for laparoscopic cholecystectomy-can it really reduce conversion rates to open cholecystectomy? J Gastrointest Surg 2012;16(7):1318–23.
14. Berrisford RG, Wilson IH, Davidge M, et al. Surgical time out checklist with debriefing and multidisciplinary feedback improves venous thromboembolism prophylaxis in thoracic surgery: a prospective audit. Eur J Cardiothorac Surg 2012;41(6):1326–9.
15. Calland JF, Turrentine FE, Guerlain S, et al. The surgical safety checklist: lessons learned during implementation. Am Surg 2011;77(9):1131–7.
16. Buzink SN, van Lier L, de Hingh IH, et al. Risk-sensitive events during laparoscopic cholecystectomy: the influence of the integrated operating room and a preoperative checklist tool. Surg Endosc 2010; 24(8):1990–5.
17. Peyre SE, Peyre CG, Hagen JA, et al. Reliability of a procedural checklist as a high-stakes measurement of advanced technical skill. Am J Surg 2010;199(1): 110–4.
18. de Vries EN, Dijkstra L, Smorenburg SM, et al. The surgical patient safety system (SURPASS) checklist optimizes timing of antibiotic prophylaxis. Patient Saf Surg 2010;4(1):6.
19. Chua C, Wisniewski T, Ramos A, et al. Multidisciplinary trauma intensive care unit checklist: impact on infection rates. J Trauma Nurs 2010; 17(3):163–6.
20. Peyre SE, Peyre CG, Hagen JA, et al. Laparoscopic Nissen fundoplication assessment: task analysis as a model for the development of a procedural checklist. Surg Endosc 2009;23(6):1227–32.
21. de Vries EN, Hollmann MW, Smorenburg SM, et al. Development and validation of the surgical patient safety system (SURPASS) checklist. Qual Saf Health Care 2009;18(2):121–6.
22. DuBose JJ, Inaba K, Shiflett A, et al. Measurable outcomes of quality improvement in the trauma intensive care unit: the impact of a daily quality rounding checklist. J Trauma 2008;64(1):22–7 [discussion: 27–9].
23. Nilsson L, Lindberget O, Gupta A, et al. Implementing a pre-operative checklist to increase patient safety: a 1-year follow-up of personnel attitudes. Acta Anaesthesiol Scand 2010;54(2):176–82.
24. Byrnes MC, Schuerer DJ, Schallom ME, et al. Implementation of a mandatory checklist of protocols and objectives improves compliance with a wide range of evidence-based intensive care unit practices. Crit Care Med 2009;37(10):2775–81.
25. Lingard L, Regehr G, Orser B, et al. Evaluation of a preoperative checklist and team briefing among surgeons, nurses, and anesthesiologists to reduce failures in communication. Arch Surg 2008;143(1):12–7 [discussion: 18].

26. Lingard L, Whyte S, Espin S, et al. Towards safer interprofessional communication: constructing a model of "utility" from preoperative team briefings. J Interprof Care 2006;20(5):471–83.

27. Hart EM, Owen H. Errors and omissions in anesthesia: a pilot study using a pilot's checklist. Anesth Analg 2005;101(1):246–50 [Table of contents].

28. Ziewacz JE, Arriaga AF, Bader AM, et al. Crisis checklists for the operating room: development and pilot testing. J Am Coll Surg 2011;213(2):212–7.e10.

29. Lyons MK. Eight-year experience with a neurosurgical checklist. Am J Med Qual 2010;25(4):285–8.

30. Oszvald Á, Vatter H, Byhahn C, et al. "Team time-out" and surgical safety-experiences in 12,390 neurosurgical patients. Neurosurg Focus 2012;33(5):E6.

31. Da Silva-Freitas R, Martin-Laez R, Madrazo-Leal CB, et al. Establishment of a modified surgical safety checklist for the neurosurgical patient: initial experience in 400 cases. Neurocirugia (Astur) 2012;23(2):60–9 [in Spanish].

32. Matsumae M, Nakajima Y, Morikawa E, et al. Improving patient safety in the intra-operative MRI suite using an on-duty safety nurse, safety manual and checklist. Acta Neurochir Suppl 2011;109:219–22.

33. Gigante P, Hwang BY, Appelboom G, et al. External ventricular drainage following aneurysmal subarachnoid haemorrhage. Br J Neurosurg 2010;24(6):625–32.

34. Dey M, Jaffe J, Stadnik A, et al. External ventricular drainage for intraventricular hemorrhage. Curr Neurol Neurosci Rep 2012;12(1):24–33.

35. Li LM, Timofeev I, Czosnyka M, et al. Review article: the surgical approach to the management of increased intracranial pressure after traumatic brain injury. Anesth Analg 2010;111(3):736–48.

36. Sonabend AM, Korenfeld Y, Crisman C, et al. Prevention of ventriculostomy-related infections with prophylactic antibiotics and antibiotic-coated external ventricular drains: a systematic review. Neurosurgery 2011;68(4):996–1005.

37. Zingale A, Ippolito S, Pappalardo P, et al. Infections and re-infections in long-term external ventricular drainage. A variation upon a theme. J Neurosurg Sci 1999;43(2):125–32 [discussion: 133].

38. Kubilay Z, Amini S, Fauerbach LL, et al. Decreasing ventricular infections through the use of a ventriculostomy placement bundle: experience at a single institution. J Neurosurg 2013;118(3):514–20.

39. Rahman M, Whiting JH, Fauerbach LL, et al. Reducing ventriculostomy-related infections to near zero: the eliminating ventriculostomy infection study. Jt Comm J Qual Patient Saf 2012;38(10):459–64.

40. Harrop JS, Sharan AD, Ratliff J, et al. Impact of a standardized protocol and antibiotic-impregnated catheters on ventriculostomy infection rates in cerebrovascular patients. Neurosurgery 2010;67(1):187–91 [discussion: 191].

41. Lawson MF, Velat GJ, Fargen KM, et al. Interventional neurovascular disease: avoidance and management of complications and review of the current literature. J Neurosurg Sci 2011;55(3):233–42.

42. Dawkins AA, Evans AL, Wattam J, et al. Complications of cerebral angiography: a prospective analysis of 2,924 consecutive procedures. Neuroradiology 2007;49(9):753–9.

43. Bulters DO, Santarius T, Chia HL, et al. Causes of neurological deficits following clipping of 200 consecutive ruptured aneurysms in patients with good-grade aneurysmal subarachnoid haemorrhage. Acta Neurochir (Wien) 2011;153(2):295–303.

44. Wong JM, Ziewacz JE, Ho AL, et al. Patterns in neurosurgical adverse events: open cerebrovascular neurosurgery. Neurosurg Focus 2012;33(5):E15.

45. Fargen KM, Velat GJ, Lawson MF, et al. Enhanced staff communication and reduced near-miss errors with a neurointerventional procedural checklist. J Neurointerv Surg 2012;5(5):497–500.

46. Taussky P, Lanzino G, Cloft H, et al. A checklist in the event of aneurysm perforation during coiling. AJNR Am J Neuroradiol 2010;31(7):E59.

47. Chen M. A checklist for cerebral aneurysm embolization complications. J Neurointerv Surg 2013;5(1):20–7.

48. Halpern C, Hurtig H, Jaggi J, et al. Deep brain stimulation in neurologic disorders. Parkinsonism Relat Disord 2007;13(1):1–16.

49. Kern DS, Kumar R. Deep brain stimulation. Neurologist 2007;13(5):237–52.

50. Yu H, Neimat JS. The treatment of movement disorders by deep brain stimulation. Neurotherapeutics 2008;5(1):26–36.

51. Pereira EA, Green AL, Stacey RJ, et al. Refractory epilepsy and deep brain stimulation. J Clin Neurosci 2012;19(1):27–33.

52. Josephson CB, Dykeman J, Fiest KM, et al. Systematic review and meta-analysis of standard vs selective temporal lobe epilepsy surgery. Neurology 2013;80(18):1669–76.

53. Georgiadis I, Kapsalaki EZ, Fountas KN. Temporal lobe resective surgery for medically intractable epilepsy: a review of complications and side effects. Epilepsy Res Treat 2013;2013:752195.

54. Pereira EA, Green AL, Aziz TZ. Deep brain stimulation for pain. Handb Clin Neurol 2013;116:277–94.

55. Connolly PJ, Kilpatrick M, Jaggi JL, et al. Feasibility of an operational standardized checklist for movement disorder surgery. A pilot study. Stereotact Funct Neurosurg 2009;87(2):94–100.

56. Kramer DR, Halpern CH, Connolly PJ, et al. Error reduction with routine checklist use during deep brain stimulation surgery. Stereotact Funct Neurosurg 2012;90(4):255–9.

57. Wong JM, Panchmatia JR, Ziewacz JE, et al. Patterns in neurosurgical adverse events: intracranial neoplasm surgery. Neurosurg Focus 2012;33(5): E16.

58. Rahmathulla G, Recinos PF, Traul DE, et al. Surgical briefings, checklists, and the creation of an environment of safety in the neurosurgical intraoperative magnetic resonance imaging suite. Neurosurg Focus 2012;33(5):E12.

59. Deyo RA, Gray DT, Kreuter W, et al. United States trends in lumbar fusion surgery for degenerative conditions. Spine (Phila Pa 1976) 2005;30(12): 1441–5 [discussion: 1446–7].

60. Deyo RA, Mirza SK. Trends and variations in the use of spine surgery. Clin Orthop Relat Res 2006;443: 139–46.

61. Devine J, Chutkan N, Norvell DC, et al. Avoiding wrong site surgery: a systematic review. Spine (Phila Pa 1976) 2010;35(9 Suppl):S28–36.

62. Ammerman JM, Ammerman MD, Dambrosia J, et al. A prospective evaluation of the role for intraoperative x-ray in lumbar discectomy. Predictors of incorrect level exposure. Surg Neurol 2006;66(5):470–3 [discussion: 473–4].

63. Groff MW, Heller JE, Potts EA, et al. A survey-based study of wrong-level lumbar spine surgery: the scope of the problem and current practices in place to help avoid these errors. World Neurosurg 2013; 79(3–4):585–92.

64. Francis T, Benzel E. Wrong level spine surgery: a perspective. World Neurosurg 2013;79(3–4):451–2.

65. Society, NAS Sign, Mark & X-ray (SMaX): prevent wrong-site surgery. 2001. Available at: http://www.spine.org/Pages/PracticePolicy/ClinicalCare/SMAX/Default.aspx. Accessed August 10, 2014.

66. JCAHO. Universal protocol for preventing wrong site, wrong procedure, wrong person surgery. 2003. Available at: http://www.jointcommission.org/facts_about_the_universal_protocol/. Accessed August 10, 2014.

67. Ladak A, Spinner RJ. Redefining "wrong site surgery" and refining the surgical pause and checklist: taking surgical safety to another level. World Neurosurg 2014;81(5–6):e33–5.

68. Ryan SL, Sen A, Staggers K, et al. A standardized protocol to reduce pediatric spine surgery infection: a quality improvement initiative. J Neurosurg Pediatr 2014;14(3):259–65.

69. Ziewacz JE, Berven SH, Mummaneni VP, et al. The design, development, and implementation of a checklist for intraoperative neuromonitoring changes. Neurosurg Focus 2012;33(5):E11.

70. Sugrue PA, Halpin RJ, Koski TR. Treatment algorithms and protocol practice in high-risk spine surgery. Neurosurg Clin N Am 2013;24(2):219–30.

71. Hommelstad J, Madsø A, Eide PK. Significant reduction of shunt infection rate in children below 1 year of age after implementation of a perioperative protocol. Acta Neurochir (Wien) 2013;155(3): 523–31.

72. Kestle JR, Riva-Cambrin J, Wellons JC, et al. A standardized protocol to reduce cerebrospinal fluid shunt infection: the hydrocephalus clinical research network quality improvement initiative. J Neurosurg Pediatr 2011;8(1):22–9.

73. Titsworth WL, Hester J, Correia T, et al. The effect of increased mobility on morbidity in the neurointensive care unit. J Neurosurg 2012;116(6):1379–88.

74. Titsworth WL, Hester J, Correia T, et al. Reduction of catheter-associated urinary tract infections among patients in a neurological intensive care unit: a single institution's success. J Neurosurg 2012;116(4): 911–20.

75. Titsworth WL, Abram J, Fullerton A, et al. Prospective quality initiative to maximize dysphagia screening reduces hospital-acquired pneumonia prevalence in patients with stroke. Stroke 2013; 44(11):3154–60.

76. Simpson CD, Hawes J, James AG, et al. Use of bundled interventions, including a checklist to promote compliance with aseptic technique, to reduce catheter-related bloodstream infections in the intensive care unit. Paediatr Child Health 2014;19(4): e20–3.

77. Exline MC, Ali NA, Zikri N, et al. Beyond the bundle - journey of a tertiary care medical intensive care unit to zero central line-associated bloodstream infections. Crit Care 2013;17(2):R41.

78. Salas E, Klein C, King H, et al. Debriefing medical teams: 12 evidence-based best practices and tips. Jt Comm J Qual Patient Saf 2008;34(9): 518–27.

79. Wolf FA, Way LW, Stewart L. The efficacy of medical team training: improved team performance and decreased operating room delays: a detailed analysis of 4863 cases. Ann Surg 2010;252(3):477–83 [discussion: 483–5].

80. Zuckerman SL, France DJ, Green C, et al. Surgical debriefing: a reliable roadmap to completing the patient safety cycle. Neurosurg Focus 2012;33(5):E4.

81. France DJ, Leming-Lee S, Jackson T, et al. An observational analysis of surgical team compliance with perioperative safety practices after crew resource management training. Am J Surg 2008; 195(4):546–53.

82. Croskerry P. The importance of cognitive errors in diagnosis and strategies to minimize them. Acad Med 2003;78(8):775–80.

83. Croskerry P, Singhal G, Mamede S. Cognitive debiasing 1: origins of bias and theory of debiasing. BMJ Qual Saf 2013;22(Suppl 2):ii58–64.

84. Croskerry P, Singhal G, Mamede S. Cognitive debiasing 2: impediments to and strategies for change. BMJ Qual Saf 2013;22(Suppl 2):ii65–72.

85. Fargen KM, Friedman WA. The science of medical decision making: neurosurgery, errors, and personal cognitive strategies for improving quality of care. World Neurosurg 2014;82(1–2):e21–9.

86. Pelaccia T, Tardif J, Triby E, et al. An analysis of clinical reasoning through a recent and comprehensive approach: the dual-process theory. Med Educ Online 2011;16:1–9.

87. Elstein AS. Heuristics and biases: selected errors in clinical reasoning. Acad Med 1999;74(7):791–4.

88. Wong JM, Bader AM, Laws ER, et al. Patterns in neurosurgical adverse events and proposed strategies for reduction. Neurosurg Focus 2012;33(5):E1.

89. Pronovost PJ, Berenholtz SM, Goeschel CA, et al. Creating high reliability in health care organizations. Health Serv Res 2006;41(4):1599–617.

90. Pronovost P. Interventions to decrease catheter-related bloodstream infections in the ICU: the keystone intensive care unit project. Am J Infect Control 2008;36(10):S171.e1–5.

91. Raghunathan K. Checklists, safety, my culture and me. BMJ Qual Saf 2012;21(7):617–20.

92. Gladwell M. Outliers: the story of success. New York: Little Brown and Company; 2008.

93. Hofstede G. Culture's consequences, comparing values, behaviors, institutions, and organizations across nations. Thousand Oaks (CA): Sage Publications; 2001.

94. Norton EK, Singer SJ, Sparks W, et al. Operating room clinicians' attitudes and perceptions of a pediatric surgical safety checklist at 1 institution. J Patient Saf 2014. [Epub ahead of print].

95. Lau CY, Greysen SR, Mistry RI, et al. Creating a culture of safety within operative neurosurgery: the design and implementation of a perioperative safety video. Neurosurg Focus 2012;33(5):E3.

Quality Improvement in Neurological Surgery Graduate Medical Education

Scott L. Parker, MD[a], Matthew J. McGirt, MD[b],
Anthony L. Asher, MD[b], Nathan R. Selden, MD, PhD[c],*

KEYWORDS

- Quality improvement • Resident education • Milestones

KEY POINTS

- Graduate medical education is now subject to the same imperatives for clinical outcomes measurement, continuous quality improvement, and value-based care as all American health care providers.
- Effective fundamental reform requires the engagement of a new generation of practitioners, through systematic training as lifelong learners.
- This article outlines one vision for a national didactic and hands-on outcomes and quality improvement curriculum for US neurological surgery training, which is explicitly coordinated with recent curricular initiatives of the Society of al Surgeons and educational outcomes assessment initiatives of the Accreditation Council for Graduate Medical Education Next Accreditation System.

INTRODUCTION

There are 3 principal rationales for incorporating quality improvement (QI) and patient safety into resident education. First and foremost, patients rightfully expect physicians to provide safe, effective, efficient, equitable, patient-centered, and high-value care. Second, regulatory agencies such as the Accreditation Council for Graduate Medical Education (ACGME) now mandate that residency programs integrate safety and QI training into curricula in order to maintain accreditation status. In addition, modern residents are interested and self-motivated to learn and acquire tools that will enable them to provide high-quality, cost-effective care that will be necessary to their future success in the practice of post–health care reform medicine. Unlike any previous era of health care, profiling the quality and clinical outcomes of individual practitioners is increasingly common. Empowering the next generation of neurosurgeons to engage in a quality-driven consumer market with public and open access to data is vital to the continued health of this specialty.

In 1998, the ACGME developed an initiative, the Outcomes Project, to evolve residency training away from process-based accreditation, toward measuring educational and patient care outcomes.[1] More recently, the ACGME's Next Accreditation System mandates that training programs explicitly link resident-physician education to improved patient care outcomes.[2] This system includes a series of essential developmental milestones that residents must achieve before successfully graduating from an accredited training program. The neurological surgery milestones have been published, and include explicit QI attributes among the

Disclosures: See last page of article.
[a] Department of Neurological Surgery, Vanderbilt University Medical Center, 1161 21st Avenue South, T4224 MCN, Nashville, TN 37232, USA; [b] Carolina Neurosurgery and Spine Associates, 225 Baldwin Avenue, Charlotte, NC 28205, USA; [c] Department of Neurological Surgery, Oregon Health & Science University, 3303 Southwest Bond Avenue, CH8N, Portland, OR 97239, USA
* Corresponding author.
E-mail address: seldenn@ohsu.edu

neurosurgery.theclinics.com

practice-based learning and improvement (PBLI) requirements for residency training.[3]

The ACGME has more recently launched the Clinical Learning Environmental Review (CLER) program as a key part of its 2011 Common Program Requirements.[4,5] CLER incorporates increased emphasis on 6 focus areas, including assessment of patient safety and QI. To date, there has been no formal, standardized curriculum for neurosurgical resident education in QI. This article proposes a potential plan for the implementation of a national program for QI in modern neurosurgical resident education.

THE DEMAND FOR EDUCATING PRINCIPLES OF QUALITY IMPROVEMENT

The Institute of Medicine (IOM) defines health care quality as "The degree to which healthcare services for individuals and populations increase the likelihood of desired health outcomes."[6] According to the IOM, quality care is safe, timely, efficient, patient centered, equitable, and effective. Multiple stakeholders in medicine, including government agencies, private insurers, employer groups, media, and patients increasingly demand that individual physicians and groups objectively account for the effectiveness, quality, and value of their care. Furthermore, Medicare and Medicaid will soon require all US health care professionals to produce data related to health care quality and safety.[7] Through the American Recovery and Reinvestment Act of 2009, the federal government recently allocated several billion dollars for studies that compare the relative outcomes, effectiveness, and appropriateness of medical and surgical interventions.[8]

As a result of such health care reform initiatives, there is now increased emphasis on and scrutiny of the relative quality and value (cost-effectiveness) of care provided by individual physicians. In such an environment, physicians must be well versed in the principles of quality, cost, and value to analyze, improve, and defend the value of their services and of their individual quality outcomes compared with relevant standards. A comprehensive QI curriculum for neurological surgery residents would empower neurosurgeons to proactively influence the validity and relevance of the quality measurements that will inevitably affect their own eventual practices, as well as empower lifelong, practice-based learning.

Lifelong learning, including the so-called science of practice, is defined by 3 key features: (1) the habitual and systematic collection of data inseparable from clinical activity, (2) the analysis of practice data to generate new knowledge, and (3) the application of that knowledge to processes of change in health care.[9] If introduced and engrained early in clinicians' medical education as common practice, these 3 essential activities can become cultural norms and practice habits, and can bend the learning curve to ultimately allow a higher personal ceiling of safe and effective patient care (**Fig. 1**).

EDUCATIONAL PRINCIPLES OF QUALITY IMPROVEMENT

Systematic methods of data collection for process and outcomes measures of clinical care (quality measurement); observational and comparative analyses of patient and disease covariates, procedures, and outcomes (quality analysis); and subsequent implementation of learned knowledge into clinical practice (QI) represent 3 pillars of educational opportunity for neurosurgical QI. The basic principles of each of these components are described here.

Quality Measurement

In the current health care evidence paradigm, neurosurgeons must define effectiveness via outcome metrics that all health care stakeholders deem relevant. No longer will evidence of technical feasibility, radiographic metrics, non–patient-centered outcomes, or isolated safety measures suffice to prove treatment value. Rather than merely presenting the provider's perspective, valid outcome measurements must convey the impact of interventions on the patient's health status. They should measure aspects of health and general well-being that are meaningful to the patient and, ideally, should incorporate multiple domains of the patient's general health and quality-of-life status, disease-specific health, and societal productivity.

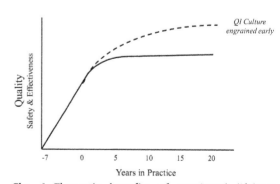

Effect of QI / Practice Based Learning

QI Culture engrained early

Quality Safety & Effectiveness

Years in Practice

Fig. 1. Theoretic benefits of continued lifelong learning for clinicians using their own practice data and experience in a systematic approach to QI.

Patient-reported outcomes are multidimensional constructs that measure patients' perspectives regarding their symptoms, physical function, general health, and quality of life.[10] Several attributes determine how useful an instrument is for measuring outcomes in a particular condition, including reliability, validity, responsiveness, acceptability, feasibility, and ceiling/floor effects (Table 1).[11] A combination of patient-reported outcome measures should be used to provide valid and accurate measurement of the benefit experienced as a result of neurosurgical care. As an example, in lumbar surgery, the N^2QOD (National Neurosurgery Quality and Outcomes Database) registry measures back-specific pain-related functional disability (oswestry disability index [ODI]), generic health status (EQ-5D in quality adjusted life years), and return to work/occupational capacity. These three instruments measure unique aspects of patient benefit. Furthermore, each instrument comprises multiple health domains in its summary score. For EQ-5D, the patient's mobility, self-care, usual activities, pain/discomfort, and anxiety/depression contribute. Hence, it is important to combine appropriate instruments based on performance and reliability (eg, validation) as well as content (distinct aspect of health benefit) when deciding how to measure effectiveness of care during practice-based learning or QI initiatives. Neurosurgeons treat a wide variety of diseases. The ideal outcome measures will therefore vary among cerebrovascular, neuro-oncologic, and spinal disease. As a result, reliance on a wide variety of disease-specific and general health outcome instruments is necessary to quantify the effectiveness of the spectrum of treatments neurosurgeons offer.

Safety of care is equally important in the determination of health care quality. In constructing measures of safety, clinical standards have traditionally considered 30 days as the standard time frame for postoperative morbidity. In the present reform environment, most stakeholders consider the 90-day global (billing) period as most relevant, as it is for measures of safety, morbidity, or unplanned consequences of surgical care such as hospital readmission or reoperation. Neurosurgical providers must be familiar with these common measures used to profile their care (reoperation, readmission, prolonged length of stay, hospital-billed major morbidity codes, and so forth). For meaningful QI, distinguishing major from minor morbidity and procedure-related from non–procedure-related morbidity is crucial to guide meaningful safety measurement and QI.

In addition to the use of appropriate outcomes measures, effective and valid data collection processes are equally important. Which cases are measured; how data are gathered; what the data source is; how the data are stored; and the feasibility, efficiency, and bias associated with quality data collection are fundamentals that, when done improperly, introduce bias and confounding that can significantly reduce the validity of any QI

Table 1
Basic concepts used to determine how good an outcomes instrument is for a particular disease

Concept	Definition
Reliability	• Represents the consistency in producing reproducible results • Variation is measurement error; the less the error, the more reliable the instrument
Validity	• Extent to which an instrument accurately measures what it is supposed to measure
Responsiveness	• The sensitivity of an instrument to detect small but clinically important changes
Acceptability	• Refers to how acceptable a particular instrument is to patients (or respondents) • Determined by mode of administration, administration time, response rate, and percentage of missing data
Feasibility	• Refers to the ease of administration and processing of the questionnaire (response burden) • Self-administered and shorter questionnaires are more feasible than interviewer-administered and longer questionnaires
Ceiling/floor effects	• High ceiling and floor effects highlight the inability of a questionnaire to discriminate severely disabled and mildly disabled patients, respectively • Ceiling effect means that the scores are extremely skewed on the high end; thus, there is no differentiation of these respondents and for improvement in group change (ie, inability to measure change because of a shortcoming of the scale). The inverse is true for floor effect

analysis. The details of observational research methodology are beyond the scope of this article, but are important to include in any neurosurgery QI educational curriculum.

Quality Analysis

In any observational research design, an association between intervention and outcome can only be assessed after ensuring that confounding variables do not result in the observed differences. Whether it is via multivariate risk adjustment or matching 2 cohorts of patients based on baseline characteristics, a multitude of clinically relevant covariate risk factors should be assessed. If there are significant dissimilarities in the patients or disease characteristics between 2 treatment groups, reliable conclusions are not possible. For example, it is not possible to determine whether intraoperative topical antibiotics reduce infection rate if appropriate use of perioperative systemic antibiotics and common risk factors for infection (obesity, diabetes, revision surgery, use of perioperative radiation therapy) are not simultaneously measured at the patient level.

Data derived from administrative (billing) databases that are inaccurately coded or do not collect these clinical risk factors are not risk adjusted, are often arbitrary in their definitions, and can produce information that is either unhelpful or misleading. Without appreciating and understanding bias and confounding variables through the collection of covariates, observations are susceptible to greater random noise than true signal. Effective measurement and analysis of patient-centered, clinically relevant, and risk-adjusted neurosurgical outcomes may allow assessment of independent associations of treatments and patient variables with outcomes. A basic understanding of the concept of quality analysis allows a like-with-like comparison within a surgeon's practice when comparing 2 treatment approaches to a single disease state, determining which is most effective for individual surgeons, at individual hospitals, and for the specific patients they treat in everyday practice. In order to achieve meaningful QI through practice changes, appropriate methods, measures, and analysis are required. Hence, neurosurgical graduate medical education (GME) QI training should include didactic information regarding each of these pillars of evidence-driven QI practice changes.

Quality Improvement

The IOM defines 5 basic tenets for health professionals to meaningfully engage in QI work: (1) continually measure quality of care by examining outcomes; (2) assess current practices compared with relevant better practices, thereby identifying opportunities for improvement; (3) design and test interventions to change the process of care; (4) identify errors and hazards in care and subsequently implement basic safety design principles; and (5) act as effective members of interdisciplinary teams and improve the quality of their own performance through self-assessment and ongoing change.[12] As such, a basic understanding of the concept of QI allows the implementation of safer, more effective, and/or less costly treatments for the patients treated in everyday practice. For QI education, only practicing QI-based changes with measurement and analysis projects allows neurosurgeons in training to build experience and efficiency in applying evidence-based practice changes at both the individual surgeon and neurosurgery service line levels.

INCORPORATING QUALITY IMPROVEMENT EDUCATION INTO NEUROSURGICAL RESIDENT EDUCATION

Health care improvement is not passive but is a participant-driven implementation of specific knowledge and skills.[13] As such, QI cannot be learned solely by passively sitting in a lecture, attending a meeting, or visiting a Web site. Nevertheless, educational materials such as didactic sessions and Web site–based guided learning can play an important role in preparing the learner. QI is an active process, and learning about improvement must be action based. There are a multitude of examples from other medical specialties on integrating a QI curriculum into resident education.[14–21] Most of this experience supports a combination of didactic and project-based work.

In response to the ACGME milestones inclusion of QI projects among the residency goals necessary for graduation, the American Medical Association (AMA) has created the Resident and Fellow Quality Improvement Forum and Project Database.[22] This members-only forum and database is designed to support residents and fellows in creating their own QI initiatives. The forum contains a QI introductory module designed to teach residents: (1) what QI is and why it is important; (2) how to find a good QI initiative; and (3) how to construct a personal QI project. The database consists of QI projects previously submitted by residents and fellows and serves as a central location for sharing of projects and ideas, with a goal of inspiring others to create their own QI initiatives. This AMA infrastructure serves as an excellent example of the creation of a Web-hosted national QI curriculum for a large group of medical trainees. In neurological surgery, a similar infrastructure could include a central databank of completed neurosurgical QI projects over time, along with the core QI didactic curriculum, accessible to all residents in order to encourage a larger collective learning network.

The ultimate goal of a comprehensive QI curriculum should be to encourage the next generation of neurosurgeons to practice continuously and reflexively within the framework of QI. In order to accomplish this, neurosurgical residents should learn QI habits early in training and engrain QI principles as part of their daily practice during residency. Standardized Web-based and easy-to-integrate quality modules can serve this purpose during residency (eg, the federally supported REDCap [Research Electronic Data Capture] registry database).[23]

As residents progress through training, perform more surgical cases, and accrue greater amounts of clinical experience, they can collect more comprehensive data, which can then be subjected to more sophisticated analysis. By the time residents reach their final clinical year, they should have performed several hundred operations in their preidentified quality areas of interest (eg, spine, cerebrovascular system). Increasingly meaningful analyses and reports can be provided to their residency directors at a junior, mid, or senior resident level, based on patients they have had a role in treating (**Table 2**).

An important principle of QI is that the data points relevant to maximizing the quality of real-time practice are identical to those that are useful for practice-based learning. Ideal clinical documentation contains all the same relevant data needed for quality analysis and improvement. As such, residents should be taught the habit of generating, handling, and analyzing their own outcomes data. Introduction of a Web-based registry database module customized by each resident could minimize the practical burden associated with such data collection and empower the data collection enterprise (at the individual, training program, and institutional levels). Only by handling their own data can residents become familiar with confounding variables and bias, allowing them to navigate and discredit the enormous amount of nonvalid quality data and profiling that is generated by payors and outside stakeholders in clinical practice. Just as with surgical skills, practice makes perfect. This process is not a burden when clinicians become familiar with the Web-based or electronic medical record tools that allow easy and standardized clinical data capture.

An integrated QI curriculum should have specific goals and achievement milestones at each level of residency training. At a junior resident level (postgraduate year [PGY] 1–2), these goals should include demonstration of analytical skills regarding each individual's own patient population. At this

Level of Resident	Educational Goals
Table 2 **Building blocks of a QI curriculum**	

Junior resident	• Measure variation in patient demographics, comorbidities, and surgical treatments for common neurosurgical disorders
	• Become familiar with common outcome metrics used in neurosurgical patient populations
	  ○ Process measures
	  ○ Safety measures
	  ○ Longitudinal patient-reported outcomes measures
	• Generate basic reports on variation in patient, disease, and treatment approaches (descriptive statistics)

Midlevel resident	• Record perioperative safety and quality outcomes • Identify associations between safety and patient, disease, or treatment variables • Generate basic reports and understand data on safety and quality (univariate statistics of comparison or association) • Perform root cause analysis on preventable adverse event
Senior resident	• Record and longitudinally track patient-reported outcomes on a select number and subset of patients • Understand effectiveness of treatment options • Engage in a QI project using process measures, safety measures, and effectiveness measures • Submit local residency director approved QI project summary/results to national neurosurgery resident QI databank for national resident shared learning

stage, appreciating variation in patient demographics, comorbidities, disorder variants, and surgical treatments for common neurosurgical disorders is fundamental to future observations of associations between these patient and disease characteristics and surgical outcomes. In addition, residents should perform a root-cause analysis of an adverse event to provide an early understanding of how health services delivery can affect safety.

At a midresident level (PGY 3–4), goals should include data collection and valid analysis of adverse events (minor complication, major complication, global period readmission, and reoperation). Residents should be able to generate basic reports and interpret safety data, including the association of preoperative patient characteristics or other covariates with postoperative complications and morbidity.

In addition, at a senior resident level (PGY 5–7), goals should include the accrual of long-term follow-up data from longitudinal data collection on a subset of patients whom the resident was involved in treating. By enrolling 5 patients per month into a longitudinal follow-up module, residents should be able to conclude training with data on meaningful outcomes (effectiveness of care) on more than 100 patients. These data, possibly analyzed in the context of data from their coresidents (both institutionally and nationally), could be used to begin performing comparative effectiveness analyses at the individual resident, individual program, or collaborative national levels (see **Table 2**).

As part of the curriculum, all residents should access a standardized Web-based didactic curriculum and both contribute to and learn from a continuously growing QI project repository (of shared resident QI experience). Using this strategy, trainees may develop basic and then working knowledge of QI processes, which they can then apply and practice independently. In addition, a comprehensive QI training curriculum should include a completed formal QI project before graduation (**Fig. 2**).

The infrastructure necessary to support such a QI curriculum at more than 100 neurological surgery residency programs nationally is substantial, but may incorporate various public domain components that are also highly scalable, making such a project highly feasible. For example, the malleable Web-based data entry and storage platform, REDCap, offers the possibility of low-cost data entry and basic analysis to fulfill many of the curricular goals discussed earlier (particularly in a learning environment that does not require data validation or auditing).[23] Academic department leadership, through the Society of Neurological Surgeons (SNS), in collaboration with the Congress of Neurological Surgeons (CNS) and American Association of Neurological Surgeons (AANS), is consolidating the educational function of various platforms for hosting online education and testing in neurological surgery residency to

**GME Education of Quality Measurement, Analysis, and Application
for Neurosurgery Quality Improvement & Practice-Based Learning**

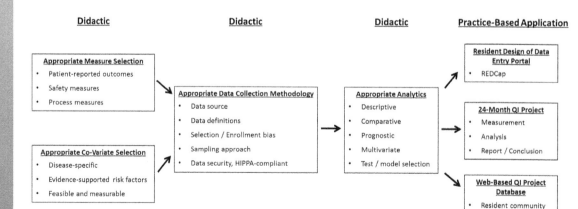

Fig. 2. GME neurosurgery QI should include a balance of didactic and experience-based application. A learned understanding of measure selection, QI project design, and analysis can be applied throughout a 7-year residency experience, culminating with a 24-month QI project within the subspecialty area of the resident's focus.

create a neurosurgical learning portal. This educational venue will be capable of hosting the envisioned didactic QI module with trivial marginal cost. In addition, the curriculum also requires creation of a simple Web-hosted resident QI forum for project sharing and didactic lecture referencing. Together, these components can give neurosurgery residents the tools to measure, record, and critically assess the quality of care in which they are involved.

A QUALITY IMPROVEMENT CURRICULUM AND NEUROSURGERY MILESTONES

For the first time in American GME, a system is in place to systematically define and track agreed-on educational outcomes, or milestones. The ACGME defined a set of comprehensive pedagogical principles, but delegated the choice of individual milestones to educational leaders from each recognized specialty.[24] Individual milestones are organized according to technical and general competencies: medical knowledge and patient care (technical); professionalism, interpersonal skills and communication, PBLI and systems-based practice (SBP) (general).

The milestones are also organized according to a progression of the developmental competency level of individual trainees: level 1, consistent with the development of an incoming postgraduate trainee; level 4, that of a graduating final clinical year resident; and level 5, that of a postresidency fellow or young faculty member. In many cases, groups of milestones are organized progressively across developmental levels, such that related knowledge and skills are benchmarked across training to track increasing skill and independent competence in a particular domain of clinical practice.

The Milestones Group for Neurological Surgery explicitly prioritized the creation of groups of milestones measuring the developmental progression of trainees for QI and safety skills (Selden NR, personal communication, 2014). The SBP milestone sets for neurosurgery include developmental progressions covering hand-offs and checklists, root cause analysis, and error management. The milestone sets for PBLI include developmental progressions covering lifelong learning, data from practice, and evidence-based medicine, as well as clinical registries, hypothesis testing, and research.

The SNS, comprising residency program directors and academic unit leaders, has simultaneously developed the outline of a national knowledge curriculum for neurological surgery: the neurosurgical matrix. Neurosurgical educational societies, including the SNS, CNS, and AANS, are currently working to collate and, if necessary, create didactic and interactive material to fulfill the knowledge areas and skills identified in the matrix curriculum. The proposal outlined here is capable of meeting the QI and outcomes curricular mandates of the SNS neurosurgical matrix.

SUMMARY

The current generation of neurosurgical trainees will soon enter a value-based and quality profiled practice environment. It is the responsibility of this profession, delegated to training programs and neurosurgical societies, to empower these future neurosurgeons to confidently navigate the new challenges. More importantly, they will have the knowledge, skills, and tools for lifelong practice-based learning to maximize the quality of care delivered throughout their careers. In addition, they will be prepared to emulate the tradition of neurological surgery to produce paradigmatic leaders, such as Cushing and Dandy, of advances in American GME.

DISCLOSURES

Dr A.L. Asher is the Director and Dr M.J. McGirt the Vice Director of the National Neurosurgery Quality and Outcomes Database (N²QOD). Drs A.L. Asher and N.R. Selden are Directors of the NeuroPoint Alliance (a nonprofit corporation that owns N²QOD). Dr A.L. Asher is a director of the AANS, Director of the American Board of Neurological Surgery, Chairman of the American Medical Association National Quality Registry Network Research and Privacy Task Force, and a member of the National Quality Forum Surgery Working Group. Dr N.R. Selden is President-elect of the CNS, Chair of the ACGME Milestones Group for Neurological Surgery, and Chair of the Committee on Resident Education of the Society of Neurological Surgeons. None of the authors have personal intellectual property or ownership stakes in any of the projects, curricula, or educational products described here.

REFERENCES

1. Swing SR. The ACGME outcome project: retrospective and prospective. Med Teach 2007;29(7): 648–54.
2. Nasca TJ, Philibert I, Brigham T, et al. The next GME accreditation system–rationale and benefits. N Engl J Med 2012;366(11):1051–6.
3. Selden NR, Abosch A, Byrne RW, et al. Neurological surgery milestones. J Grad Med Educ 2013; 5(1 Suppl 1):24–35.

4. Weiss KB, Wagner R, Bagian JP, et al. Advances in the ACGME Clinical Learning Environment Review (CLER) program. J Grad Med Educ 2013;5(4):718–21.

5. Weiss KB, Wagner R, Nasca TJ. Development, testing, and implementation of the ACGME Clinical Learning Environment Review (CLER) Program. J Grad Med Educ 2012;4(3):396–8.

6. Lohr KN, Schroeder SA. A strategy for quality assurance in Medicare. N Engl J Med 1990;322(10):707–12.

7. Thorpe JH, Weiser C. Medicare quality measurement and reporting programs. 2011. Available at: http://healthreformgps.org/resources/medicare-quality-measurement-and-reporting-programs/. Accessed August 1, 2014.

8. Aston G. Comparative effectiveness. Federal government's push for more data to benefit supply chain. Mater Manag Health Care 2010;19(4):22–5.

9. Asher AL, McCormick PC, Kondziolka D. Introduction: the science of practice: addressing the challenges of modern health care. Neurosurg Focus 2013;34(1):Introduction.

10. Acquadro C, Berzon R, Dubois D, et al. Incorporating the patient's perspective into drug development and communication: an ad hoc task force report of the Patient-Reported Outcomes (PRO) Harmonization Group meeting at the Food and Drug Administration, February 16, 2001. Value Health 2003;6(5):522–31.

11. Lurie J. A review of generic health status measures in patients with low back pain. Spine 2000;25(24):3125–9.

12. Institute of Medicine. Health professions education: a bridge to quality. Washington, DC: National Academies Press; 2003.

13. Armstrong G, Headrick L, Madigosky W, et al. Designing education to improve care. Jt Comm J Qual Patient Saf 2012;38(1):5–14.

14. Zafar MA, Diers T, Schauer DP, et al. Connecting resident education to patient outcomes: the evolution of a quality improvement curriculum in an internal medicine residency. Acad Med 2014;89:1341–7.

15. Maski KP, Loddenkemper T, An S, et al. Development and implementation of a quality improvement curriculum for child neurology residents: lessons learned. Pediatr Neurol 2014;50(5):452–7.

16. Ogrinc G, Ercolano E, Cohen ES, et al. Educational system factors that engage resident physicians in an integrated quality improvement curriculum at a VA hospital: a realist evaluation. Acad Med 2014;89:1380–5.

17. Vinci LM, Oyler J, Johnson JK, et al. Effect of a quality improvement curriculum on resident knowledge and skills in improvement. Qual Saf Health Care 2010;19(4):351–4.

18. Tudiver F, Click IA, Ward P, et al. Evaluation of a quality improvement curriculum for family medicine residents. Fam Med 2013;45(1):19–25.

19. Sepulveda D, Varaklis K. Implementing a multifaceted quality-improvement curriculum in an obstetrics-gynecology resident continuity-clinic setting: a 4-year experience. J Grad Med Educ 2012;4(2):237–41.

20. Patow CA, Karpovich K, Riesenberg LA, et al. Residents' engagement in quality improvement: a systematic review of the literature. Acad Med 2009;84(12):1757–64.

21. Tomolo AM, Lawrence RH, Aron DC. A case study of translating ACGME practice-based learning and improvement requirements into reality: systems quality improvement projects as the key component to a comprehensive curriculum. Postgrad Med J 2009;85(1008):530–7.

22. American Medical Association. Available at: http://www.ama-assn.org/ama/pub/about-ama/our-people/member-groups-sections/resident-fellow-section/rfs-resources/rfs-qi-landing.page?. Accessed August 1, 2014.

23. Harris PA, Taylor R, Thielke R, et al. Research electronic data capture (REDCap)–a metadata-driven methodology and workflow process for providing translational research informatics support. J Biomed Inform 2009;42(2):377–81.

24. Swing SR, Beeson MS, Carraccio C, et al. Educational milestone development in the first 7 specialties to enter the next accreditation system. J Grad Med Educ 2013;5(1):98–106.

Technology and Simulation to Improve Patient Safety

George M. Ghobrial, MD[a], Youssef J. Hamade, MD[b],
Bernard R. Bendok, MD[b], James S. Harrop, MD[a],*

KEYWORDS

- Simulation • Neurosurgery • Surgical simulator • Resident education • Neurosurgical simulator

KEY POINTS

- Neurosurgical education is increasingly looking to integrate surgical procedural based simulators as a tool for operative training and interim evaluation of skills.
- Repetitive surgical training helps the resident develop a mental rehearsal of steps. Simulation allows for that mental rehearsal to begin prior to the first operative experience. This process is particularly beneficial with infrequently encountered pathologies and procedures.
- Using simulation as an interim evaluation tool requires a validated and reliable scoring system, which poses a unique challenge in grading technical skills.

INTRODUCTION TO SIMULATION IN NEUROSURGICAL EDUCATION

Improving the quality and efficiency of surgical education, reducing technical errors in the operating suite, and ultimately improving patient safety and outcomes are common goals in all surgical specialties.[1] Modern medical education at the turn of the 20th century emphasized graduated levels of responsibility through successive years of training.[2] Modern-day simulation tools represent an effort to enhance the training experience because of the limitations of a government-mandated 80-hour work week, and have the goal of providing a well-balanced resident education in a society with a decreasing level of tolerance for medical errors.[2,3]

Early simulator use in medical training has been focused on the rehearsal of clinical scenarios, such as those required in advanced cardiac life support resuscitation training.[4] The use of simulators has expanded rapidly after positive reports correlating technical simulator proficiency with increasing measures of technical expertise in the operating suite.[5] One prospective randomized trial evaluating the use of simulation training among physicians performing laparoscopic inguinal hernia repair found significantly shorter operative times, decreased complication rates, and shorter patient hospital stays compared with those who had no prior simulation training.[6]

ORGANIZED PRESURGICAL TRAINING MODELS

In a recent survey of US neurosurgery program directors, 72% believed that simulation would improve patient outcome, and nearly half of the respondents believed that residents should achieve an agreed upon standard of simulation proficiency before receiving intraoperative training.[7] One formal implementation of simulator training could be in the form of annual objective assessments of resident operative skills. At minimum, because

a Department of Neurological Surgery, Thomas Jefferson University Hospital, Philadelphia, PA, USA;
b Department of Neurological Surgery, Northwestern University Feinberg School of Medicine, Chicago, IL, USA
* Corresponding author.
E-mail address: James.harrop@jefferson.edu

Neurosurg Clin N Am 26 (2015) 239–243
http://dx.doi.org/10.1016/j.nec.2014.11.002
1042-3680/15/$ – see front matter © 2015 Elsevier Inc. All rights reserved.

a direct effect of work-hour restriction is a decrease in operative time for residents, practice runs using a simulator would help them develop a mental "script-based rehearsal" to optimize their time spent in the operating suite.[8]

SIMULATION IN NEUROSURGERY

Simulators can be divided into physical simulators, haptic/computerized simulators, and cadaveric dissection.[3] Cadaveric simulation was the first educational tool to provide anatomic education with preserved 3-dimensional relationships. As a result, this modality has currently provided the most education. Improvements in computer and engineering technology have enabled the recent growth of computerized simulators. Eventually, computer graphics technology and passive 3-dimensional optics became affordable for implementation in neurosimulation. Lastly, techniques of 3-dimensional fabrication have allowed for realistic physical simulators to be developed at a cost affordable for training institutions.

INITIAL USE OF SIMULATION IN NEUROSURGERY RESIDENCY

Surgical "boot camps" for postgraduate first-year residents have been adopted and implemented in the past several years across a variety of surgical specialties, including cardiothoracic surgery,[9] orthopedics,[10] otorhinolaryngology,[11] and neurosurgery.[12] Surveys conducted in neurosurgery found a high level of satisfaction with and knowledge retention of the skills that were emphasized at the neurosurgical boot camp.[12] Appropriate simulators used at postgraduate year one training events have included central line placement, ventriculostomy catheter placement, and trauma craniotomy models.[12]

EXPANSION OF TRAINING ASPECTS ADDRESSED BY SIMULATORS

With the rapid expansion in available simulators, interest in incorporating these into formal training has been increasing. In the past year alone, results of several efforts have been published, with haptic feedback devices demonstrating the various aspects of microsurgical technique that can been taught outside of the operating room, ranging from tumor handling, to volumetric resection, to anatomic accuracy (**Table 1**). These technologies are ideal for techniques such as endovascular treatment of vascular pathologies,[5] craniotomies,[13,14] and endoscopic approaches.[15] In spinal surgery, new simulations are being introduced, such as the durotomy repair,[16] posterior

cervical laminoforaminotomy,[17] and anterior cervical discectomy models.[18] These models have been a welcome addition to prior established simulators for percutaneous pedicle screw fixation.[19] Arguably these skills should be practiced before entry into the operating room, because textbook knowledge alone is insufficient.

CHALLENGES TO DESIGNING A FORMAL CURRICULUM USING SIMULATION IN RESIDENCY EDUCATION

The initial introduction of simulators has already been successfully incorporated into residencies and national meetings, such as the Congress of Neurological Surgeons.[20] In an attempt to fully incorporate neurosurgical simulators into resident education, an educational curriculum and evaluation tool is needed. Several challenges exist to grading surgical skills not encountered with typical testing of knowledge. The first challenge is identifying a participant's knowledge of all skills,[16] so that when repeated examination of the same participant occurs, a frame of reference is established. The second challenge is choosing the right objective structured assessment tool (OSAT) to quantitatively measure a resident's interim performance. All OSATS must be consistent across all examiners and would need to be demonstrated in future study through validation, and interobserver and intraobserver reliability studies.

PROPOSAL FOR VALIDATION OF NEUROSURGICAL SIMULATION SKILLS

One proposed pathway to a more reliable and consistent grading scheme is a video-based OSAT scoring system, rather than a traditional text-based scoring system that purely describes certain techniques on a 10-point scoring scheme.

With this technique, participants can videotape their examinations while following scripted instructions either independently or with a faculty instructor. This system would allow for formal grading by an examiner. One way to validate this method would be to have multiple examiners review and grade a submitted video, using the video-based OSAT to confirm interobserver reliability. Interobserver reliability is believed to be the most important component of implementing an interim grading scheme that limits bias from having different examiners grading annual performance.

THE DUROTOMY REPAIR SIMULATOR AS A MODEL RESIDENCY TRAINING TOOL

Unintended repair of durotomies can be frustrating, adding significant morbidity to a spine

Table 1
Selected simulation efforts using haptic feedback/software in 2014

Author, Year	Title	Journal	Purpose	Design	Metric
Patel et al,[22] 2014	Neurosurgical tactile discrimination training with haptic-based virtual reality simulation	Neurol Res	To determine whether computer simulation w/haptic feedback devices improved handling with surgical instruments	Group that received computer training with haptic simulation demonstrated superior handling compared with group with no prior training	Ability to correctly identify brain lesions in a black box using instrumented tactile response
Hooten et al,[23] 2014	Mixed reality ventriculostomy simulation: experience in neurosurgical residency	Neurosurgery	To assess whether simulation can improve ventriculostomy placement	Physical simulator measuring accuracy	Comparison with controls, distance to foramen of Munro
Azarnoush et al,[24] 2014	Neurosurgical virtual reality simulation metrics to assess psychomotor skills during brain tumor resection	Int J Comput Assist Radiol Surg	Software/haptic feedback to develop tumor handling	Use of NeuroTouch software	Tier 1: volumetric resection (%), normal brain resected (%) Tier 2: tip path, operating room time, pedal activation Tier 3: sum of applied forces (estimating force of manipulation)

Data from Refs.[22–24]

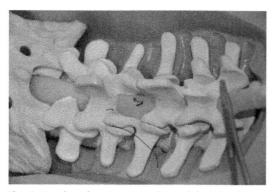

Fig. 1. Lumbar durotomy repair model. A Sawbones model of the lumbar spine is seen with the spinal canal filled with a latex tube distended by a set hydrostatic pressure. Residents are instructed to make a set durotomy (1 cm) and are evaluated by their technique and timeliness under instruction. These simulators are simple, and therefore can be used in a self-directed manner. (Sawbones, Vashon Island, WA.)

procedure. Dural closure of an unintended durotomy often occurs in a technically difficult location, such as the lateral recesses of the lumbar spinal canal. Because these occur at an infrequent rate of 1% to 13%,[21] residents receive little case practice. Furthermore, at the time of dural repair, it would be ideal for residents to have had prior experience with this procedure because of the innate difficulties of closure. In a durotomy repair model,[16] residents can practice dural closure with a variety of suture materials and sizes. Although at its current stage this model does not simulate the difficulties of obscured vision from epidural bleeding or the risk of nerve root injury from suturing, it provides valuable time for the resident to practice watertight dural closure and knot placement (**Fig. 1**). Residents take a multiple-choice pretest and undergo a didactic skills session before closure. Each closure is graded on timeliness, the presence of a watertight closure, and the consistency of suturing in terms of distance between bites and even apposition of the edges of the durotomy. The current steps in improving the value of this tool in interim education is to provide a video-based OSAT wherein the resident can review a video of ideal techniques and emulate that in independent self-guided study and testing.

SUMMARY/DISCUSSION

Modern residency education is looking forward to the number of newly developing simulators becoming available. Incorporation of these simulators is just the first step. Full integration into residency requires a scientific OSAT and a method of independent testing and grading. One proposed method is through a video-based assessment of simulator performance. These simulators represent one key attempt at maximizing the efficiency of resident education in the era of limited duty hours.

REFERENCES

1. Harrop J. Introduction to neurosurgical simulation. Neurosurgery 2013;73(Suppl 1):8.
2. Singh H, Kalani M, Acosta-Torres S, et al. History of simulation in medicine: from Resusci Annie to the Ann Myers Medical Center. Neurosurgery 2013; 73(Suppl 1):9–14.
3. Gasco J, Holbrook TJ, Patel A, et al. Neurosurgery simulation in residency training: feasibility, cost, and educational benefit. Neurosurgery 2013; 73(Suppl 1):39–45.
4. Perkins GD. Simulation in resuscitation training. Resuscitation 2007;73(2):202–11.
5. El Ahmadieh TY, Aoun SG, El Tecle NE, et al. A didactic and hands-on module enhances resident microsurgical knowledge and technical skill. Neurosurgery 2013;73(Suppl 1):51–6.
6. Zendejas B, Cook DA, Bingener J, et al. Simulation-based mastery learning improves patient outcomes in laparoscopic inguinal hernia repair: a randomized controlled trial. Ann Surg 2011;254(3):502–9 [discussion: 509–11].
7. Ganju A, Aoun SG, Daou MR, et al. The role of simulation in neurosurgical education: a survey of 99 United States neurosurgery program directors. World Neurosurg 2013;80(5):e1–8.
8. Marcus H, Vakharia V, Kirkman MA, et al. Practice makes perfect? The role of simulation-based deliberate practice and script-based mental rehearsal in the acquisition and maintenance of operative neurosurgical skills. Neurosurgery 2013;72(Suppl 1):124–30.
9. Macfie RC, Webel AD, Nesbitt JC, et al. "Boot camp" simulator training in open hilar dissection in early cardiothoracic surgical residency. Ann Thorac Surg 2014;97(1):161–6.
10. Sonnadara RR, Garbedian S, Safir O, et al. Orthopaedic Boot Camp II: examining the retention rates of an intensive surgical skills course. Surgery 2012;151(6):803–7.
11. Malloy KM, Malekzadeh S, Deutsch ES. Simulation-based otorhinolaryngology emergencies boot camp: part 1: curriculum design and airway skills. Laryngoscope 2014;124(7):1562–5.
12. Selden NR, Anderson VC, McCartney S, et al. Society of Neurological Surgeons boot camp courses: knowledge retention and relevance of hands-on learning after 6 months of postgraduate year 1 training. J Neurosurg 2013;119(3):796–802.

13. Lobel DA, Elder JB, Schirmer CM, et al. A novel craniotomy simulator provides a validated method to enhance education in the management of traumatic brain injury. Neurosurgery 2013;73(Suppl 1): 57–65.

14. Jabbour P, Chalouhi N. Simulation-based neurosurgical training for the presigmoid approach with a physical model. Neurosurgery 2013;73(Suppl 1): 81–4.

15. Neubauer A, Wolfsberger S. Virtual endoscopy in neurosurgery: a review. Neurosurgery 2013; 72(Suppl 1):97–106.

16. Ghobrial GM, Anderson PA, Chitale R, et al. Simulated spinal cerebrospinal fluid leak repair: an educational model with didactic and technical components. Neurosurgery 2013;73(Suppl 1):111–5.

17. Harrop J, Rezai AR, Hoh DJ, et al. Neurosurgical training with a novel cervical spine simulator: posterior foraminotomy and laminectomy. Neurosurgery 2013;73(Suppl 1):94–9.

18. Ray WZ, Ganju A, Harrop JS, et al. Developing an anterior cervical diskectomy and fusion simulator for neurosurgical resident training. Neurosurgery 2013;73(Suppl 1):100–6.

19. Luciano CJ, Banerjee PP, Sorenson JM, et al. Percutaneous spinal fixation simulation with virtual reality and haptics. Neurosurgery 2013;72(Suppl 1):89–96.

20. Harrop J, Lobel DA, Bendok B, et al. Developing a neurosurgical simulation-based educational curriculum: an overview. Neurosurgery 2013;73(Suppl 1):25–9.

21. Williams BJ, Sansur CA, Smith JS, et al. Incidence of unintended durotomy in spine surgery based on 108,478 cases. Neurosurgery 2011;68(1):117–23 [discussion: 123–4].

22. Patel A, Koshy N, Ortega-Barnett J, et al. Neurosurgical tactile discrimination training with haptic-based virtual reality simulation. Neurol Res 2014. http://dx.doi.org/10.1179/1743132814Y0000000405.

23. Hooten KG, Lister JR, Lombard G, et al. Mixed reality ventriculostomy simulation: experience in neurosurgical residency. Neurosurgery 2014 December; 10 Suppl 4:576–81.

24. Azarnoush H, Alzhrani G, Winkler-Schwartz A, et al. Neurosurgical virtual reality simulation metrics to assess psychomotor skills during brain tumor resection. Int J Comput Assist Radiol Surg 2014. [Epub ahead of print].

Electronic Medical Records and Quality Improvement

Jonathan T. Carter, MD

KEYWORDS

- Electronic health records • Electronic medical records • Quality improvement • Meaningful use

KEY POINTS

- Recent legislation has incentivized American hospitals and providers to rapidly adopt electronic medical records (EMRs) and demonstrate meaningful use of them. This implementation will drive quality improvement for the next 5 to 10 years.
- EMRs allow numerous surgical quality initiatives to be implemented efficiently: examples are the Joint Commission's Surgical Care Improvement Program (SCIP), surgical timeout, and care hand-offs. Such quality initiatives are otherwise difficult or impossible to realize with paper processes.
- Successful implementation of EMRs requires considerable time and money. Patients can be harmed when EMRs are poorly implemented.

INTRODUCTION

Widespread adoption of electronic medical records (EMRs) in the United States is transforming the practice of medicine from a paper-based cottage industry into an integrated health care delivery system. For the purposes of this article, an EMR is defined as a systematic collection of digital health information that theoretically can be shared across different health settings and is designed to accurately capture the state of the patient (or population) at all times. Most physicians and institutions view widespread use of EMRs to be inevitable. But the transformation has not been painless. Many have questioned whether the substantial investment in EMRs has really been justified by improved patient outcomes or quality of care. Despite these concerns, widespread adoption of EMRs is currently a national priority: in 2009 Congress and the Obama administration enacted the Health Information Technology for Economic and Clinical Health (HITECH) Act. The HITECH act provided unprecedented incentives and penalties for meaningful use of EMRs. This article describes historical and recent efforts to use EMRs to improve the quality of patient care, and provides a roadmap of EMR uses for the foreseeable future.

EARLY EFFORTS

In the 1970s and 1980s, early informatics experts envisioned computers as intellectual amplifiers that could help doctors diagnose disease. Automated history-taking, combined with statistical associations of diseases with physical and laboratory findings, could alert the physician to the most probable diagnosis, and suggest the most appropriate, safest course of action.[1] Such assistance could free up the physician to perform tasks that are uniquely human, such as bedside skills or managing emotional aspects of a patient's illness. Some experts envisioned that entire specialties, such as primary care or anesthesia, could be largely regulated to computerized automation.[1] These predictions never came to pass.

Department of Surgery, University of California, San Francisco, 521 Parnassus Avenue, C347, San Francisco, CA 94143, USA
E-mail address: Jonathan.carter@ucsf.edu

Neurosurg Clin N Am 26 (2015) 245–251
http://dx.doi.org/10.1016/j.nec.2014.11.018
1042-3680/15/$ – see front matter © 2015 Elsevier Inc. All rights reserved.

At the same time, simple computer systems were developed to automate discrete departments or processes within the hospital or clinic. Software to handle coding or billing, laboratory results, simple text reports (eg, microbiology, pathology, or radiology), or radiographic images (PACS: Picture Archiving and Communication System) became commonplace. Unfortunately, the data structures and formats of these systems were typically proprietary and protected by the vendor. This made integration between software packages difficult or impossible. In 1987, a protocol named Health Level-7 was founded to provide data standards and definitions to allow for sharing of health information. Health Level-7 was accredited in 1994 by the American National Standards Institute and created a "common language" for health systems to be able to talk to one another.

In 1999, the Institute of Medicine published "To Err is Human: Building a Safe Health System," which reported that up to 98,000 Americans died annually as a result of preventable medical errors.[2] Examples included adverse drug events, improper transfusions, wrong-site surgery, falls, pressure ulcers, and mistaken patient identities.[2] Lack of integration within the US health care system was cited as a major contributor to these errors. Shortly thereafter, systems engineering principles were applied to patient safety and medical informatics to address many of the Institute of Medicine's listed causes of patient harm. Health information systems were recognized to be more than a digital reproduction of the paper chart. Rather, they were recognized to be major actors that interact with humans to form a complex adaptive system.[3] The EMR is not an adjunct to the system of care, *it creates the system of care*.

QUICK WINS

By the early 2000s, computerized order entry systems (CPOE) were developed to address several errors reported by the Institute of Medicine. CPOE systems could eliminate handwriting errors, reduce incomplete orders, eliminate ambiguous abbreviations, force proper units, and standardize orders within an organization almost overnight. When combined with automated clinical decision support (ie, automated weight or body-surface-area dosing, drug-drug or drug-allergy interaction, order sets, and other rule-based alerts) or bar-coded medication administration (right drug, right formulation, right dose, right patient, right time), many medical errors were avoided. One study reported that such systems could reduce nonintercepted serious medication errors by 81%.[4] As a result, CPOE was heralded as a hospital "best practice" in medication safety and a litmus test of safe care.[4] Many payors

and advisory groups, such as the Leapfrog Group, pushed CPOE systems heavily in the mid-2000s.

UNINTENDED CONSEQUENCES

Although CPOE systems could overcome many of the obvious problems associated with paper-based orders, sometimes their implementation actually harmed patients. One hospital reported a doubling of the hospital mortality rate after a commercially sold CPOE system was implemented.[5] The increased mortality was attributable to usability and workflow issues: physicians could not write orders until patient arrival and registration (delaying care), no order sets were built, less provider time was spent at the bedside, and there was less communication between doctors and nurses. The designers of these systems did not anticipate the complexity of care processes within the hospital. Many physicians also pointed out the poor usability of EMR systems. Alert fatigue (defined as alerts so frequent that the physician ignores or overrides the result) was recognized as a major limitation to CPOE and decision support systems. Many hospitals did not commit adequate resources to successfully understand their own internal processes to implement EMR systems.

Despite these growing pains, by the late 2000s, most reports in the literature showed that incorporation of health technology resulted in an overall improvement in access to care, patient satisfaction, provider satisfaction, effectiveness of care, and efficiency of care.[6] By 2010, more than 50% of American office-based practices had incorporated EMRs.[7]

THE HEALTH INFORMATION TECHNOLOGY FOR ECONOMIC AND CLINICAL HEALTH ACT OF 2009

The 2008 presidential election made health care reform a major debate in the United States. After taking office, the Obama administration and Congress passed the HITECH Act under Title XIII of the American Recovery and Reinvestment Act of 2009. Under the HITECH Act, the US Department of Health and Human Services was budgeted up to $27 billion to promote and expand the adoption of health information technology. Under the act, individual provider incentive payments of up to $44,000 through Medicare and up to $63,750 through Medicaid were made available, provided clinicians could demonstrate meaningful use of EMRs in addition to simple EMR implementation. In 2010, the Department of Health and Human Services proposed meaningful use requirements and solicited public comment. The

Table 1
Centers for Medicare and Medicaid Services, 2014 Stage 2 meaningful use objectives and measures

Objective	Measure
Provide clinical summaries for patients for each office visit	Clinical summaries provided to patients within 1 business day for more than 50% of office visits
Use clinical decision support to improve performance on high-priority health conditions	1. Implement five clinical decision support interventions related to four or more clinical quality measures, if applicable, at a relevant point in patient care for the entire EHR reporting period 2. The functionality of drug-drug and drug-allergy interaction checks has been enabled for the entire EHR reporting period
Use CPOE for medication, laboratory, and radiology orders directly entered by any licensed health care professional who can enter orders into the medical record per state, local, and professional guidelines	More than 60% of medication, 30% of laboratory, and 30% of radiology orders created during the EHR reporting period are recorded using CPOE using certified EHR technology
Automatically track medications from order to administration using assistive technologies in conjunction with an eMAR	More than 10% of medication orders created by authorized providers of the eligible hospital's inpatient or emergency department during the EHR reporting period for which all doses are tracked are tracked using eMAR
Generate and transmit permissible prescriptions electronically	More than 50% of all permissible prescriptions written by the EP are compared with at least one drug formulary and transmitted electronically using certified EHR technology
Generate lists of patients by specific conditions to use for quality improvement, reduction of disparities, research, or outreach	Generate at least one report listing patients with a specific condition
Incorporate clinical laboratory test results into certified EHR technology as structured data	More than 55% of all clinical laboratory tests results ordered during the EHR reporting period whose results are either in a positive/negative or numerical format are incorporated in certified EHR technology as structured data
Perform medication reconciliation between care settings	Medication reconciliation is performed for more than 50% of transitions of care
Record the following demographics: preferred language, gender, race, ethnicity, date of birth, and date and preliminary cause of death in the event of mortality in the eligible hospital or CAH	More than 80% of all unique patients have demographics recorded as structured data
Use certified EHR technology to identify patient-specific education resources and provide those resources to the patient if appropriate	Patient-specific education resources identified by certified EHR technology are provided to patients for more than 10% of all unique patients seen during the EHR reporting period
Use secure electronic messaging to communicate with patients on relevant health information	A secure message was sent using the electronic messaging function of certified EHR technology by more than 5% of unique patients seen during the EHR reporting period

(continued on next page)

Table 1
(continued)

Objective	Measure
Use clinically relevant information to identify patients who should receive reminders for preventive/follow-up care	Use EHR to identify and provide reminders for preventive/follow-up care for more than 10% of patients with two or more office visits in the last 2 y
Protect electronic health information created or maintained by the certified EHR technology through the implementation of appropriate technical capabilities	Conduct or review a security risk analysis in accordance with the requirements under 45 CFR 164.308 (a) (1), including addressing the encryption/security of data at rest and implement security updates as necessary and correct identified security deficiencies as part of its risk management process
Record smoking status for patients 13 y old or older	More than 80% of all unique patients 13 y old or older have smoking status recorded as structured data
Capability to submit electronic data to immunization registries or immunization information systems and actual submission except where prohibited and in accordance with applicable law and practice	Successful ongoing submission of electronic immunization data from certified EHR technology to an immunization registry or immunization information system for the entire EHR reporting period
Provide summary of care record for patients referred or transitioned to another provider or setting	Summary of care record is provided for more than 50% of patient transitions or referrals Summary of care record is provided electronically for more than 10% of patient transitions or referrals Conduct an electronic summary of care exchange with either another EHR or with CMS
Provide patients the ability to view online, download, and transmit their health information within 4 business days of the information being available	i. More than 50% of all unique patients seen during the EHR reporting period are provided timely (available to the patient within 4 business days after the information is available) online access to their health information ii. More than 5% of all unique patients seen during the EHR reporting period (or their authorized representatives) view, download, or transmit to a third party their health information
Record and chart changes in vital signs: height, weight, blood pressure (age 3 and older), calculate and display BMI; plot and display growth charts for patients 0–20 y, including BMI	More than 80% of all unique patients have blood pressure (for patients age 3 and older only) and height and weight (for all ages) recorded as structured data

Menu selection objectives and measures (any three are required)

Objective	Measure
Imaging results consisting of the image itself and any explanation or other accompanying information are accessible through certified EHR technology	More than 10% of all scans and tests whose result is an image ordered for patients seen during the EHR reporting period are incorporated into or accessible through certified EHR technology
Record whether a patient 65 y old or older has an advance directive	More than 50% of all unique patients 65 y old or older admitted to the eligible hospital's or CAH's inpatient department during the EHR reporting period have an indication of an advance directive status recorded as structured data
Provide structured electronic laboratory results to ambulatory providers	Hospital laboratories send structured electronic clinical laboratory results to the ordering provider for more than 20% of electronic laboratory orders received
Capability to identify and report cancer cases to a state cancer registry, except where prohibited, and in accordance with applicable law and practice	Successful ongoing submission of cancer case information from certified EHR technology to a cancer registry for the entire EHR reporting period
Record electronic notes in patient records	Enter at least one electronic progress note created, edited, and signed by an EP for more than 30% of patients seen during the EHR reporting period
Generate and transmit permissible prescriptions electronically	More than 10% of hospital discharge medication orders are compared with at least one drug formulary and transmitted electronically using certified EHR technology
Record patient family health history as structured data	More than 20% of all unique patients seen during the EHR reporting period have a structured data entry for one or more first-degree relatives or an indication that family health history has been reviewed
Capability to identify and report specific cases to a specialized registry (other than a cancer registry), except where prohibited, and in accordance with applicable law and practice	Successful ongoing submission of specific case information from certified EHR technology to a specialized registry for the entire EHR reporting period
Capability to submit electronic syndromic surveillance data to public health agencies and actual submission except where prohibited and in accordance with applicable law and practice	Successful ongoing submission of electronic syndromic surveillance data from certified EHR technology to a public health agency for the entire EHR reporting period

Abbreviations: BMI, body mass index; CAH, critical access hospital; CMS, centers for medicare and medicaid services; CPOE, computerized provider order entry; EHR, electronic health record; eMAR, electronic medication administration record; EP, eligible professional.
Adapted from 2014 Definition Stage 1 of Meaningful Use. EHR incentive programs. Centers for Medicare and Medicaid Services. Available at: http://www.cms.gov/Regulations-and-Guidance/Legislation/EHRIncentivePrograms/Meaningful_Use.html.

meaningful use measures were chosen to maximize individual patient safety and quality, improve care coordination, and improve public and population health, while ensuring privacy and security for personal health information.[8]

The meaningful use objectives were divided into three stages, phased in over 5 years. These measures are listed in **Table 1**. Stage 1 objectives focus on simple electronic data capture and patient access. Stage 2 added objectives that focus on more advanced clinical processes: usage of clinical decision support, generating reports (ie, lists) of patients for quality improvement or outreach, or submission of digital health data to registries.[8] Stage 3 objectives have yet to be defined, but will focus on improved patient outcomes (as opposed to processes). In the next 5 years, widespread implementation of EMRs to meet meaningful use objectives will drive health care organizations and dominate patient safety efforts.

THE ELECTRONIC MEDICAL RECORD AND QUALITY IN SURGICAL CARE

Most of the process and quality initiatives described thus far apply to the care of surgical patients. But the EMR has also been applied to quality initiatives specific to surgical practice. One major example is the widespread promotion of checklists as a means to improve patient outcomes. Examples include the widespread use of timeout checklists before operative procedures,[9] best practice checklists for intensive care unit central venous catheter placement,[10] and the widespread use of order sets (which themselves are a form of a checklist). Such checklists, often integrated into EMRs, have been shown to reduce patient morbidity and mortality.[4,6,9,10]

Another good example of using EMRs to improve surgical care is the implementation of the Joint Commission's Surgical Care Improvement Project (SCIP). This campaign began in 2005 with the goal of reducing the national incidence of surgical complications by 25%.[11] The Joint Commission's SCIP measures are listed in **Table 2**. Most commercial EMR vendors have implemented modules to support SCIP compliance and documentation. For instance, at the University of California–San Francisco, the EMR was programmed to improve compliance with SCIP-Inf-9. An alert was created to the primary team that a bladder catheter was still indwelling 36 hours

Table 2
Joint Commission–2014 Surgical Care Improvement Project objectives

SCIP-Inf-1. prophylactic antibiotic preoperative timing	Preoperative prophylactic antibiotic to be administered within 1 h of incision.
SCIP-Inf-2. prophylactic antibiotic selection	Surgical patients who received prophylactic antibiotics consistent with current guidelines (specific to each type of surgical procedure).
SCIP-Inf-3. prophylactic antibiotic discontinuation within 24 h	Administration of antibiotics for more than 24 h after the anesthesia end time, offers no additional benefit to the surgical patient. Infection or suspected infection must be documented.
SCIP-Inf-4. cardiac surgery patients with controlled postoperative blood glucose	Cardiac surgery patients must have controlled postoperative blood glucose ($\leq$180 mg/dL) in the timeframe of 18–24 h after anesthesia end time.
SCIP-Inf-6. hair removal	Hair removal is documented and NO hair is removed by razor.
SCIP-Inf-9. urinary catheter removal – POD 1 or POD 2	Urinary catheter removed on postoperative day 1 or 2 or have a reason to continue Foley (documentation of reason must occur on postoperative day 1 or 2).
SCIP-card-2 β-blocker therapy	Surgery patients on β-blocker therapy before arrival who received a β-blocker during the perioperative period.
SCIP VTE 2 venous thromboembolism	Venous thromboembolism prophylaxis received within 24 h before surgical incision time to 24 h after surgery end time (see above table).

Adapted from Specifications Manual for National Hospital Inpatient Quality Measures. The Joint Commission. Available at: http://www.jointcommission.org/specifications_manual_for_national_hospital_inpatient_quality_measures.aspx.

after a surgical procedure. The physician could order its removal, or alternatively, document a reason for continuation. The physician's action could also be easily pulled into a report to document institutional SCIP compliance. Such improvements in compliance, automation, and tracking are labor intensive, costly, and almost impossible to perform without a sophisticated EMR.

Finally, EMRs have been used to improve the quality of information for transfers of care. Transfers are reported to major source of medical error, and consequently patient harm.[12] An excellent example is the use of EMRs to implement sign-out systems.[13–17] Sign-out systems pull current information, such as vital signs, fluids in and out, laboratory values, medications, active medical problems, and other clinical information, to provide the receiving physician with a concise summary of any given patient's current status, plans, and expected course. Such improvement in hand-offs is currently a major Joint Commission National Patient Safety Goal.[12]

SUMMARY

In the span of 30 years, EMRs have radically changed the practice of medicine. But it is only the beginning. Although today clinicians are using EMRs to implement meaningful use objectives and SCIP initiatives, tomorrow could bring a host of informational technologies to health care: virtual personal assistants, human augmentation, three-dimensional bioprinting systems, smart robots, prescriptive analytics, speech-to-speech translation, wearable user interfaces, big data analysis, content analytics, mobile health monitoring, cloud computing, and so on. These technologies are hyped to revolutionize medicine and surgery. The generation of surgeons born into computer technology and raised with tablet computers, social networks, and Google have yet to finish residency. When they do, they will innovate and demand technologies that will change medicine forever.

REFERENCES

1. Schwartz WB. Medicine and the computer. The promise and problems of change. N Engl J Med 1970;283(23):1257–64.
2. Kohn LT, Corrigan J, Donaldson MS. To err is human: building a safer health system. Washington, DC: National Academy Press; 2000.
3. Nemeth C, Nunnally M, O'Connor M, et al. Getting to the point: developing IT for the sharp end of healthcare. J Biomed Inform 2005;38(1):18–25.
4. Bates DW, Teich JM, Lee J, et al. The impact of computerized physician order entry on medication error prevention. J Am Med Inform Assoc 1999; 6(4):313–21.
5. Han YY, Carcillo JA, Venkataraman ST, et al. Unexpected increased mortality after implementation of a commercially sold computerized physician order entry system. Pediatrics 2005;116(6):1506–12.
6. Buntin MB, Burke MF, Hoaglin MC, et al. The benefits of health information technology: a review of the recent literature shows predominantly positive results. Health Aff 2011;30(3):464–71.
7. Available at: http://www.healthit.gov/policy-researchers-implementers/health-it-adoption-rates. Accessed August 1, 2014.
8. Available at: http://www.cms.gov/Regulations-and-Guidance/Legislation/EHRIncentivePrograms/Stage_2.html. Accessed August 1, 2014.
9. Haynes AB, Weiser TG, Berry WR, et al. A surgical safety checklist to reduce morbidity and mortality in a global population. N Engl J Med 2009;360(5):491–9.
10. Pronovost P, Needham D, Berenholtz S, et al. An intervention to decrease catheter-related blood-stream infections in the ICU. N Engl J Med 2006; 355(26):2725–32.
11. Available at: http://www.jointcommission.org/specifications_manual_for_national_hospital_inpatient_quality_measures.aspx. Accessed August 1, 2014.
12. Available at: http://psnet.ahrq.gov/primer.aspx?primerID=9. Accessed August 1, 2014.
13. Van Eaton EG, Horvath KD, Lober WB, et al. A randomized, controlled trial evaluating the impact of a computerized rounding and sign-out system on continuity of care and resident work hours. J Am Coll Surg 2005;200(4):538–45.
14. Van Eaton EG, McDonough K, Lober WB, et al. Safety of using a computerized rounding and sign-out system to reduce resident duty hours. Acad Med 2010;85(7):1189–95.
15. Sarkar U, Carter JT, Omachi TA, et al. SynopSIS: integrating physician sign-out with the electronic medical record. J Hosp Med 2007;2(5):336–42.
16. Williams RG, Silverman R, Schwind C, et al. Surgeon information transfer and communication: factors affecting quality and efficiency of inpatient care. Ann Surg 2007;245(2):159–69.
17. Palma JP, Van Eaton EG, Longhurst CA. Neonatal informatics: information technology to support hand-offs in neonatal care. Neoreviews 2011;2011(12). pii: e560.

Using Clinical Registries to Improve the Quality of Neurosurgical Care

Anthony L. Asher, MD[a],*, Scott L. Parker, MD[b], John D. Rolston, MD, PhD[c], Nathan R. Selden, MD, PhD[d], Matthew J. McGirt, MD[a]

KEYWORDS

• Registry • Database • Quality improvement • Patient outcomes

KEY POINTS

• Outcomes data are critical to achieving effective and efficient health care and can be used to guide clinical decisions, examine care outcomes, and identify opportunities for improvement.
• Clinical registries are cost-effective and scalable tools that collect uniform data evaluating specified outcomes for a population defined by a particular disease, condition, or exposure.
• Examples of successful registries are the Society of Thoracic Surgeons (STS) National Database and the National Neurosurgery Quality and Outcomes Database (N^{2}QOD), which is a prospective observational registry recording 30-day morbidity and 3- and 12-month quality data for neurosurgical patients.

INTRODUCTION

Despite rising and unsustainable US health care costs, many stakeholders feel that the quality of medical services is limited and inconsistent. Value-based reforms are touted as the key to achieving health care system sustainability. Health care value is defined as quality delivered divided by cost incurred. Unfortunately, quality in health care is difficult to accurately define, and methods to reliably assess and report health care quality are often lacking. Clinical registries have emerged as important mechanisms to define, measure, and promote health care quality. The purpose of this article is to describe the role of registries in neurosurgical quality improvement.

THE RISE OF VALUE-BASED CARE—IMPLICATIONS FOR SURGICAL EVIDENCE GENERATION

Influential reports issued by the Institute of Medicine in 1999 and 2001[1,2] generated significant public concern about the quality and safety of US medical care. Subsequent media and regulatory attention on health care cost, safety, and quality have led to calls for greater physician accountability and care optimization. The financial crisis of 2007, plus economic projections suggesting that health care expenditures may exceed 20% of the gross domestic product within another decade, has added considerable momentum to the drive for health care reform and cost control.

The research described herein was facilitated through a grant from the Neurosurgery Research and Education Foundation.
a Department of Neurological Surgery, Carolina Neurosurgery and Spine Associates, Carolinas Healthcare System Neuroscience Institute, 225 Baldwin Road, Charlotte, NC 28204, USA; b Department of Neurosurgery, Vanderbilt University Medical Center, 1211 Medical Center Drive, Nashville, TN 37232, USA; c Department of Neurological Surgery, University of California San Francisco, 505 Parnassus Avenue, San Francisco, CA 94143, USA; d Department of Neurological Surgery, Oregon Health & Science University, 3181 Southwest Sam Jackson Park Road, Portland, OR 97239, USA
* Corresponding author. 225 Baldwin Avenue, Charlotte, NC 28205.
E-mail address: asher@cnsa.com

neurosurgery.theclinics.com

Passage of the Patient Protection and Affordable Care Act also dramatically shifted the focus of national, public attention to quality and cost in health care delivery. Many resulting public and private programs make health professionals directly accountable for the overall value of care they deliver.[3–5]

Value-based care is now a permanent feature of medical practice. Health care value is measured by comparing quality delivered against expenditure (costs) and is optimally examined in the context of various consensus-based health care outcomes.[6] The acquisition of valid and reliable outcomes data is critical to achieving effective and efficient health care. Providers can use these data to guide clinical decisions, examine the care outcomes, and identify opportunities for improvement. Policy makers can use outcomes data to intelligently allocate increasingly scarce health care resources.

Demonstration of the value of surgical care is challenging because of a relative lack of high-quality data along with inadequate standardization of care across care settings and practitioners. Traditional evidence-based medicine (EBM) algorithms for clinical decision making define a hierarchy of evidence based on methodology of data collection and analysis. Randomized clinical trials (RCTs) are generally accepted as the gold standard for clinical research and evidence generation related to answering single-study questions.[7] Well-conducted RCTs are powerful evidence tools and remain the most practical method of limiting the influence of all sources of experimental bias (known and unknown). The use of RCTs to study surgical interventions, however, suffers from significant practical limitations. First, patient randomization in surgical trials is tremendously challenging due to lack of therapeutic equipoise and/or to clinical heterogeneity. Even when randomization can be performed, an ethical obligation exists to allow patients to cross over between medical and surgical therapies as clinically indicated. Subsequent intent-to-treat or as-treated analyses are often associated with confounding bias, a condition that challenges the equipoise RCTs are intended to promote. Second, group mean efficacy observed in ideal-world (controlled) clinical research settings often fails to translate into real-world (or more generalizable) clinical effectiveness when applied to patients, physicians, or health care settings dissimilar to those in tightly controlled research settings. Third, RCTs are inherently discontinuous processes that preclude use of the data collection and analysis infrastructure for other essential processes, such as measuring and improving ongoing care. Finally, RCTs are expensive, time consuming, and impractical for all but large and/or academic centers.

The need for high-quality data requires re-evaluating the traditional EBM paradigm.[8] The complexity and breadth of medical decision making preclude any realistic possibility of using RCTs to answer most causal questions.[9] Furthermore, RCTs are typically time-limited data collection efforts involving unidirectional information flow from participants to a central data repository without timely or constructive feedback to the care setting. As such, the structure of RCTs renders them inadequate to facilitate continuous quality improvement, a process that necessitates bidirectional information exchange.

Individuals from the scientific, clinical, and regulatory communities now advocate expanded use of observational techniques for developing and using medical evidence. In addition, recent advances in health information technology, such as the electronic medical record along with Web-based and mobile tools, have supported the use of observational methods for evidence generation. Statistical methodologies have increased the overall practicality, relevance, and scientific reliability of observational data, in particular patient care registries.[10]

THE ROLE OF REGISTRIES IN THE EMERGING VALUE-BASED MEDICINE PARADIGM

The majority of systematic medical data tracking is devoted to hospital or payer/purchaser claims and billing records. The resulting data sets are easily available and have low marginal collection costs. Claims-based systems can provide large-scale population assessments as well as more granular cost information. Claims data are notoriously inaccurate, however, when serving as proxies for clinical endpoints of safety or effectiveness of care.[11]

Another common large repository of patient-related data is generated by hospital-based quality programs that track compliance with a set of mandated, generally national, standards. Whether resulting process measures truly incentivize hospitals and providers to adopt best care approaches is an open question. They do not, however, provide high-level evidence for effective medical decision making. Hence, the Institute of Medicine, Agency for Healthcare Research and Quality, and Patient-Centered Outcomes Research Institute (PCORI) have called for evolution of well-designed, patient-centered outcome registries to generate evidence that will more effectively guide health care reform.[12]

Clinical registries use observational study methods to collect uniform data to evaluate specified outcomes for a population defined by a particular disease, condition, or exposure.[8] Registries are remarkably cost efficient compared with other methods of evidence development and are easily scaled. The primary advantage of well-designed registries from a scientific perspective relates to their strong external validity. This validity is achieved through an inclusive design that seeks to evaluate heterogeneous populations as opposed to the more proscriptive method of interventional analysis, which specifically strives to evaluate homogenous patient groups. As a consequence of this design, the observed outcomes from registry analyses are often more representative of what is achieved in real-world practice and can be generalized to broad patient populations or specifically to unique patient or disease subgroups. In this respect, registry data may be more relevant than clinical trials for decision-making and health care policy development. An added advantage of registries relates to their continuous nature, which allows them to adapt to innovations in care and facilitate participation in programs that require ongoing collection of quality data from practice, such as performance improvement, public and private reporting, and specialty-specific certification programs. Furthermore, registry infrastructure can be combined with other study designs to produce comprehensive hybrid approaches to evidence development.

Innovative registry-based trials may represent a disruptive technology for advancing comparative effectiveness research.[13] Well-constructed prospective registries with appropriate a priori design can produce level 1 prognostic evidence (predictive analysis) and level 2 evidence on effectiveness of care. Characteristics of quality registries are outlined in **Box 1**. A high-quality registry possesses many of the same characteristics as an RCT, including prospective data collection (as opposed to retrospectively retrieving data from administrative data sets), clinical (ie, nonclaims) sources, patient-reported outcomes (PROs) (and not process measures), high follow-up rates, quality control and data validation, and study designs that control for confounding biases.

Clinical registry uses are reviewed in **Box 2**. Four major classes of use can be described: disease and/or treatment characterization, determination of clinical/cost-effectiveness, measuring safety/harm of care, and quality improvement.[8] There has been an explosive growth in clinical registries for a variety of clinical, reporting, and scientific applications, in large part due to the relevance and versatility of this data collection method (**Box 3**).

Box 1
Characteristics of good-quality registries

- Designed specifically for conditions evaluated
- Primary data collected in a prospective fashion
- Process for monitoring quality of data (transparency in missing data)
- Patients followed long enough for outcomes to occur (appropriate time horizon)
- Independent outcome assessment
- Complete follow-up of $\geq 80\%$
- Controlling for possible confounding
- Equal follow-up times for comparative groups or for unequal follow-up times, accounting for time at risk
- Comprehensive postoperative data capture, including outside index institution
- HIPAA and IRB compliant data storage

Box 2
Overview of the potential purposes served by clinical registries

Characterization of disease and/or treatments

- Assessment of natural history, including an estimation of the magnitude of a problem of interest
- Determination of the underlying incidence or prevalence rate of a condition of interest
- Evaluation of trends in a disease over time
- Conducting surveillance of a disease over time
- Assessment of service delivery and identification of groups at high risk
- Documentation of the types of patients served by a health provider
- Describing and estimating survival of diseases of interest

Determining clinical effectiveness, cost-effectiveness, or comparative effectiveness of a test or treatment

Measuring or monitoring safety and adverse events associated with the use of specific products and treatments

- Comparative evaluation of safety and effectiveness

Measuring or improving quality of care

Box 3
Examples of current clinical registry applications

Public and private patient safety initiatives and quality reporting mandates
- Physician Quality Reporting System
- Third-party payer distinction programs
- Bariatric, orthopedic, cardiovascular, and spine registry consortia

Board certification
- American Board of Medical Specialties MOC

Specialty society–sponsored quality improvement and public reporting
- American Heart Association: Get With The Guidelines programs
- STS: voluntary performance reporting through consumer reports

Comparative effectiveness and patient-centered outcomes research
- Federal Coordinating Council for Comparative Effectiveness Research
- PCORI

Device registries
- FDA postapproval projects

Specific programs range from Food and Drug Administration (FDA) postapproval studies and Centers for Medicare and Medicaid Services (CMS) coverage determinations to specialty-based quality-improvement initiatives, certification programs, and comparative effectiveness research initiatives. Increasingly, registries are used for value-based reimbursement (such as Physician Quality Reporting System). Several of these applications are reviewed in the context of neurosurgery's national registry programs.

The Registry of Patient Registries effort is a comprehensive listing of patient registries.[14] Several specialty-based national surgical organizations have developed registries. Among these programs, the STS National Database is the most developed surgical platform and serves as a useful illustration of the value of clinical registry programs.

USING CLINICAL OUTCOMES DATABASES TO ADVANCE QUALITY CARE IN SURGERY: THE SOCIETY OF THORACIC SURGEONS EXPERIENCE

Among existing surgical registries, the STS National Database has most dramatically shown the power of national practice data collection programs in advancing patient-centered quality care[15]; 95% of all US thoracic surgery practices now use this well-established database, which is unquestionably the most established surgical registry in existence. The STS has used its database to define its own measures of quality and performance, 23 of which have been endorsed by the National Quality Forum. As a direct result, the STS has reduced the likelihood of thoracic surgeons being forced to comply with arbitrary performance standards created by outside stakeholders. For each of these measures, the STS has developed risk-adjusted national and regional benchmarks for the safety and quality of their procedures. Individual surgeons and practice groups have the tools to analyze their own morbidity and clinical outcomes in real time and compare these data with the national benchmarks, allowing surgeons to determine which areas of their practice should be targeted for quality improvement. It also allows them to satisfy public reporting requirements and develop practice-specific quality and efficiency data to support claims made to public and private payers. The STS has pioneered voluntary public reporting of outcomes data to promote accountability in care, and approximately 50% of registry sites participate in this specific program.

The STS has used aggregate national efficacy data to inform discussions with the Relative Value Scale Update Committee, private payers, and large purchasers of care. In doing so, they have successfully protected patient access to surgical care and have defended the value of their procedures. The STS has developed sophisticated risk models to determine subgroups of patients most likely to benefit from specific therapies. Finally, and perhaps most importantly, the STS National Database has been used to advance scientific discovery and improve patient care. For example, the STS database helped establish the superiority of internal thoracic artery bypass grafting and made this method standard care in thoracic surgery.

As early adopters of practice science methodologies, thoracic surgeons effectively demonstrated the value and safety of their care, increased public trust in their science, and provided other surgical specialties with a road map for pursuing their own quality-improvement efforts.

THE CASE FOR PROSPECTIVE, PATIENT-CENTERED, LONGITUDINAL SURGICAL CARE REGISTRIES

The STS National Database represents an important advance in the emerging quality care paradigm. Similar to the American College of Surgeons National Surgical Quality Improvement Project, the STS National Database relies on retrospective acquisition of clinical information from the existing medical record and a focus on short-term clinical outcomes, largely representing safety of care rather than effectiveness of care. This methodology has obviated direct patient contact and generally simplified the management of this pioneering project, thus facilitating its widespread and practical implementation.

Despite the early success of the pioneering STS National Database model, the qualitative and temporal characteristics of surgical registry design need to evolve to meet expanding data requirements. In particular, continued gaps in the evidence supporting clinical practice parameters as well as a growing emphasis on patient-centered and value-based payment approaches highlight the emerging importance of prospectively captured longitudinal data and the incorporation of more robust data elements, such as PROs.[10,16]

High-quality surgical care is both safe and effective. Both longitudinal data and PROs are fundamental to the comprehensive assessment of the quality of specific surgical interventions, in particular those typically encountered in neurosurgical practice. As such, each of these factors is critically important to accurately quantifying the numerator in the value equation (health care benefit/cost). Longitudinal data make it possible to determine the sustainability of treatment effects, which is increasingly relevant to neurosurgical subspecialties, such as spine surgery. PROs permit a more comprehensive analysis of the quality of care received, particularly in light of major discrepancies between patient and clinical estimates of symptomatic and functional treatment-related improvement. In general PROs may more accurately reflect underlying health status than physician reporting.[8]

The Blue Cross and Blue Shield Blue Distinction Program requires the collection of long-term clinical outcomes data to establish that a facility meets selected quality thresholds.[17] Many newly established surgical registries now incorporate both longitudinal and patient-focused components in their design, with the goal of tracking the extended results and cost-effectiveness of clinical care.[18,19]

CRITICAL ELEMENTS IN THE DESIGN OF PROSPECTIVE SURGICAL REGISTRIES

There are many important process-related, methodological, and endpoint measurement factors to consider when developing a high-quality surgical registry.[6,10] First, patient enrollment process needs to be transparent and unbiased. Total care

enrollment, or randomized enrollment, are among the best methods to limit introduction of confounding variables; however, costs and resources can preclude scalability. Representative sampling is a practical solution and can minimize selection bias. Clear definitions of enrollment eligibility and appropriate grouping of patients by pathology and treatment are necessary to prevent inaccuracies and ensure comparison of like patients. The incidence of missing covariate data and follow-up rates of major endpoints should be transparent and minimized. Missing data for baseline variables of disease, risk factors, or treatments reduce the reliability of registry analysis. The greatest methodological challenge to longitudinal registries is long-term follow-up. Currently, even the most successful national spine registries collecting prospective, longitudinal PROs report 12-month follow-up rates of approximately 75%. Lastly, publically transparent quality-control mechanisms are of vital importance. This can be accomplished through weekly missing data feedback reports, site visits on data accuracy validation, and site education of standardized operating procedures or case definitions.

The cost of data collection infrastructure and quality assurance poses a significant hurdle to implementation of a high-quality nationwide registry. Most national surgical registries require full-time employee data extractors and an annual subscription fee for participation. Despite this requirement, many well-designed surgical registries are proving that high PRO data can be collected on a large scale at a fraction of the cost of traditional RCTs.[6,15] As Web-based tools, such as mobile health and social networking applications, evolve to meet the demand of health care registries (particularly with respect to longitudinal patient engagement), the cost and practical challenges to registry participation are expected to improve. Nevertheless, hospital systems and surgeon groups with limited resources may initially face challenges with participating in high-quality longitudinal PRO registries.

MEETING THE QUALITY NEEDS OF MODERN NEUROSURGICAL PRACTICE
The National Neurosurgery Quality and Outcomes Database

To date, no nationally collaborative reporting mechanisms using validated outcome measures have assessed the extent to which neurosurgical procedures have an impact on pain, disability, and quality of life while adjusting for bias and influential confounders, including variances in comorbidity, surgical approach, cultural factors, region, structure, and process of health services. Furthermore, national benchmarks of surgical morbidity and effectiveness in neurosurgery, which define quality, have yet to be determined.

To help meet the quality care needs of specialty and individual surgeons, the American Association of Neurological Surgeons—in partnership with other national neurosurgical organizations, including the Congress of Neurological Surgeons, Society of Neurological Surgeons, and American Board of Neurological Surgery—developed the N²QOD.[15,20] The N²QOD is a national collaborative registry of quality and clinical outcomes reporting. This program is designed to establish, for the first time, a robust national mechanism of quality reporting, risk-adjusted benchmarking, comparative effectiveness analysis, and evidence-based practice improvement for neurosurgical procedures. Of equal importance is the inclusion of essential preoperative patient characteristics as well as prospective PROs, which will aid in identification of optimized care paradigms, refinement of surgical delivery to maximize treatment success, and objective determination of the value of neurologic surgery to the principal health care stakeholders who wish to deliver, purchase, and/or use these services.

Detailed methods of the N²QOD are described elsewhere.[15,21] Briefly, the N²QOD is a prospective observational registry recording 30-day morbidity and 3- and 12-month quality data. Site-specific data extractors/coordinators are required to undergo training on data entry and N²QOD standard operating procedures. Patient enrollment into the registry via a sampling methodology is a standardized process across all sites. Potential patients meeting eligibility criteria are identified by the on-site data coordinators from the weekly posted surgery schedule. The first 6 patients meeting inclusion criteria are contacted in person at a clinic or by phone and their health status assessed via interview. Once the first 6 surgical cases meeting inclusion criteria have answered baseline questionnaires, no further patients are enrolled for that week. Start dates for each enrollment week are standardized across all sites and span a rolling 6-day cycle. Hence, the first day of each 6-day week falls on each weekday with equal frequency. This representative sampling method prevents a disproportionate volume of enrollment on any 1 day of the week or from any 1 surgeon's schedule, thus limiting potential enrollment bias.

A standard-of-care outcomes questionnaire, using validated PRO instruments, is administered preoperatively and again at 3 and 12 months postoperatively. Information related to patient demographics, clinical presentation, diagnosis classification, perioperative medical care, and complications specific to neurosurgical procedure surgery is also collected. Recorded morbidity variables include but are not restricted to new neurologic deficit related to index surgery, surgical site infection, symptomatic hemorrhage, unanticipated return to the operating room, deep vein thrombosis/pulmonary embolism, myocardial infarction, mortality, urinary tract infection, and unanticipated readmission within 90 days. Health Insurance Portability and Accountability Act (HIPAA)-trained data coordinators/extractors at each site enter data through a secure password-protected Web-based portal (Research Electronic Data Capture) into a national aggregate database. Data analysis and site reporting are subsequently performed by epidemiologists, health services researchers, and biostatisticians at the Vanderbilt University Institute for Medicine and Public Health (VIMPH) and the Vanderbilt University Department of Biostatistics.

Data quality is maintained through a variety of methods. Data completeness and accuracy are assessed via automated and manual methods at VIMPH. Weekly missing data reports are sent to all participating N²QOD sites. Diagnostic accuracy is maintained through periodic surgeon-led self-audits, which seek to correlate entered data with radiographic and clinical records; 10% of N²QOD sites undergo random on-site audits each year. Surgical schedule logs are reviewed to ensure that appropriate case selection criteria were met and to help minimize the risk of intentional or inadvertent enrollment bias. Accuracy of diagnoses and treatment variables are confirmed via medical record audit. The accuracy of major perioperative safety endpoints with respect to morbidity and readmission is also examined.

Participating N²QOD sites receive quarterly risk-adjusted performance reports to help facilitate local focused quality-improvement programs. Aggregate data analyses allow for the description of national treatment patterns and expected outcomes in patient subpopulations.

The project is jointly funded between the American Association of Neurological Surgeons (AANS) and participating sites. The AANS provided a major grant for registry infrastructure development; N²QOD sites assist with ongoing operational and data analysis costs through a subscription system. This funding model is similar to that used by other society-based registry programs.[22,23]

The National Neurosurgery Quality and Outcomes Database Lumbar Spine Registry

Surgical therapies for spinal disorders represent a particularly important opportunity to enhance value in US health care due to the prevalence of spine conditions, the frequency with which surgical procedures involving the spine are performed, and the substantial associated costs. Given these considerations, the N²QOD lumbar spine registry was the first national neurosurgery registry program to be developed. The authors' initial experience with this program illustrates the value of comprehensive, longitudinal patient data collection in facilitating neurosurgical quality improvement.

In the lumbar spine registry, longitudinal quality data are obtained for 5 common surgical lumbar spine diagnoses: first-time surgery for disc herniation, stenosis, and spondylolisthesis as well as revision surgery for either recurrent disc herniation or adjacent segment disease. Patients undergoing lumbar surgery performed for either primary or recurrent lumbar degenerative disease are eligible for inclusion. Exclusions include spinal infection, tumor, fracture, traumatic dislocation, deformity, pseudoarthrosis, same-level(s) recurrent multilevel stenosis, neurologic paralysis due to preexisting spinal disease or injury, age less than 18 years, and incarceration. Patients whose past and/or present surgery encompasses a construct of more than 3 motion segments are also ineligible. Lumbar spine–specific PROs are collected at baseline and at 3 and 12 months and include back and leg pain (visual analog scale [VAS]),[16–19] Oswestry Disability Index (ODI),[18,24–28] EuroQol five-dimension questionnaire (EQ-5D),[29,30] and North American Spine Society Patient Satisfaction Index (PSI).

A detailed account of the first full-year operation is found elsewhere.[15] To date, more than 10,000 patients have been enrolled in the lumbar spine registry, making this one of the largest North American cooperative spine registries. Participating sites represent a broad geographic distribution and are split approximately between academic and community centers. Audited baseline data completeness and diagnostic accuracy are 98% and 95%, respectively. Twelve-month follow-up at all sites has exceeded 75%. National outcomes data show that lumbar spine surgery has generally low rates of surgical morbidity and related events. In aggregate, the mean performance in routine practice revealed sustained improvements in PROs, including ability to return to work. A majority of patients returned to work and full activity by 12 months after surgery and expressed that they were satisfied with their outcome and would have surgery again.

Despite information that points to the general safety and effectiveness of lumbar surgery, these data also point out important opportunities for care improvement. In particular, almost 10% of patients undergoing lumbar spine surgery were readmitted within 90 days of the index procedure. Additionally, 9% to 18% of patients enrolled in N²QOD do not report improvement from baseline ODI at 12 months, and 17% percent of patients state they would not have the same surgery performed for the same condition.

The most striking finding in these data is the large variation in treatment response between individual patients. Similar patterns of variability are observed for all diagnoses, in all procedures, at all centers, and for all reported outcomes (Fig. 1). Understanding the sources of this widespread variability represents the greatest opportunity for the N²QOD to improve spine care outcomes. Specifically, assessing the interactive impact of multiple clinical variables on individual patient outcomes will allow clinicians to benchmark their care against their risk-adjusted expected outcomes (Fig. 2). Similar analyses will power the development of predictive models to educate surgeons and patients on the personalized likelihood of various outcomes from spine surgery (Fig. 3). In

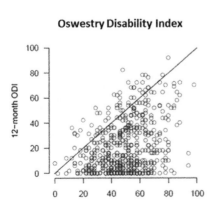 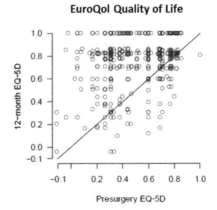

Fig. 1. Variation in 12-month reported outcomes at the individual patient level (lumbar disc herniation).

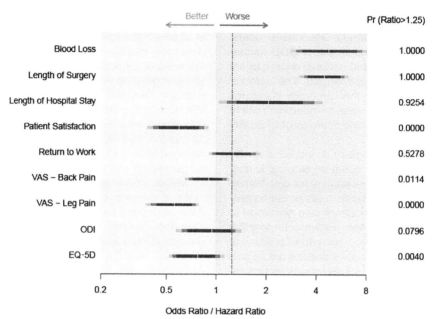

Fig. 2. Assessing the interactive impact of multiple clinical variables on individual patient outcomes will allow clinicians to benchmark their care against their risk-adjusted expected outcomes. Pr, probability.

these ways, risk-adjusted modeling will allow for targeted quality improvement, practice-based learning, shared decision making, and more effective resource utilization. To these ends, the authors are developing multivariable methodologies to evaluate the contribution of patient and environmental factors to clinical outcomes.

FUTURE DIRECTIONS

N²QOD scientific leadership is currently developing prospective registry formats appropriate to all neurosurgical subspecialty areas. In addition to the degenerative spine module, a degenerative cervical spine module is now active at approximately 30 clinical centers. A spinal deformity module created in collaboration with the Scoliosis Research Society will be activated in the autumn of 2014. A cerebrovascular module is underdevelopment and is being beta tested at large national practice sites. Tumor and other subspecialty modules are also in development.

The leadership of US national neurosurgical organizations understands the importance of

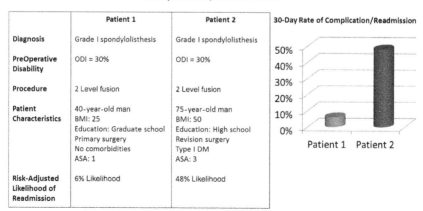

Fig. 3. Example of a predictive model that allows for surgeon and patient education on the personalized likelihood of various outcomes from spine surgery. ASA, American Association of Anesthesiologists; BMI, body mass index.

harmonizing data collection efforts and facilitating communication and cooperation among specialty groups that treat similar medical and surgical disorders. Such coordination is essential for valid outcome comparisons between various quality efforts. Furthermore, such programs will allow for the examination of comprehensive, multispecialty patient care. To that end, organized neurosurgery is committed to the creation of interconnected and cooperative national registries. The authors are currently developing a cooperative registry program with the American Society for Therapeutic Radiology and Oncology that will focus on outcomes related to the radiosurgical management of common brain tumors and vascular malformations and are working toward the development of a diagnosis-based spine disorder registry with the American Academy of Physical Medicine and Rehabilitation.

Given the increasing demands on clinicians for clinical data reporting, it is critical that any specialty-based registry program be compatible with other data collection imperatives that have an impact on the same clinicians. As an example, N^{2}QOD participants will soon be eligible to receive credit toward the practice improvement component of maintenance of certification (MOC). The N^{2}QOD has been designated a CMS qualified clinical registry and, as such, participants can now use the registry to fulfill requirements for this program. In addition, the leadership of N^{2}QOD is committed to achieving Qualified Clinical Data Registry status with CMS, which will allow for the streamlined development of specialty-specific outcomes measures in addition to providing another mechanism to facilitate public reporting requirements.

Finally, the widespread adoption of a national data collection system will dramatically increase opportunities for practice-based education and scientific collaboration within the specialty. Comprehensive Web-based services will soon link all members of the N^{2}QOD community and include programs to facilitate individual learning, the sharing of clinical experience, and cooperative knowledge generation, including comparative effectiveness research.

CHALLENGES TO REGISTRY IMPLEMENTATION

Every clinical data source and collection design has its drawbacks. Registries are subject to the limitations faced by all observational data collection methods, in particular limitations of bias. Although it is impossible to eliminate all forms of bias in the collection and analysis of registry data, challenges to data quality can be addressed through a variety of novel design and analysis tools that reduce the probability of both systematic error and errors in inference. Data collection burdens (particularly for longitudinal data) also challenge widespread implementation of registry formats. Efforts to achieve a lowest energy state for data collection, including the development of novel technologies designed to facilitate electronic medical records integration and automate longitudinal data collection, are progressing rapidly. Objective definition of value requires comprehensible cost data, which can be difficult to acquire. The N^{2}QOD is now engaged in pilot programs to merge its clinical outcomes data with administrative cost data sources.

The need for a written consent from individual patients for registry data inclusion has come under debate, based on the premise that the clinical information is used for quality improvement, not research, purposes. The US Department of Health and Human Services (HHS) Office of Human Research Protections (OHRP) has previously determined that the N^{2}QOD, as presently configured, is not research and, therefore, not subject to the jurisdiction of the Common Rule (45 CFR 46).[21] The HHS Office for Civil Rights has further determined that N^{2}QOD data methods are compliant with the Privacy Rule. Existing relevant federal regulations, however, are not specific to quality registries and varying regional interpretations of those regulations persist. For that reason, a detailed project description that outlines the proper use of protected health information, operational protocols, patient interaction, and reporting methods is routinely made available to sites for submission to their hospital's quality-improvement office or institutional review board (IRB). Registry data ultimately have to apply to clinical practice to advance value-based health care. The N^{2}QOD includes evolving mechanisms for provider education and meaningful clinical application of outcomes data through its Web-based practice-based learning network.

Finally, neurosurgery presently lacks specialty-specific, National Quality Forum–endorsed quality measures. Organized neurosurgery is now in the process of developing such measures for use in public and private reporting programs.

SUMMARY

Objective data are needed to improve the quality of health care and intelligently inform the allocation of increasingly scarce health care resources. Clinical outcomes data needs are at the heart of the ongoing national debate regarding health care reform and are in part driving the largest transformation of health care processes in modern history. The cost and rapid growth of surgical procedures for a variety of disorders have made this an area of special opportunity for enhancing the overall value of US health care. The most viable strategy for surgical practitioners in the emerging value care paradigm is to develop methods to define, measure, and produce objective value in surgical care. In this environment, prospective clinical registries have significant promise as a meaningful source of data to facilitate quality improvement and increase the overall value of surgical care.

The unique needs of patients mandate the creation of a versatile outcomes evaluation system that is relevant to all practice settings and the wide spectrum of neurosurgical disorders. It is particularly important that individual neurosurgeons have the means to assess risk-adjusted measures of the value and durability of treatment responses, understand their patients' perspectives with respect to clinical outcomes, and compare the relative effectiveness of various therapeutic interventions. From a societal perspective, it is essential that the specialty adopt sustainable, collective methods to characterize real-world neurosurgical care and identify large-scale improvement opportunities. The N^2QOD incorporates each of these capabilities, creating distinctive opportunities for neurosurgery in the era of value-based medicine.

REFERENCES

1. Institute of Medicine. Measuring the quality of health care: a statement by the National Roundtable on Health Care Quality. Washington DC: National Academy Press; 1999.
2. Institute of Medicine. Envisioning the National Health Care Quality Report. 2001.
3. Improving quality and value in the U.S. healthcare system: Bipartisan Policy Center. 2009. Available at: http://www.brookings.edu/~/media/Research/Files/Reports/2009/8/21%20bpc%20qualityreport/0821_bpc_qualityreport.PDF. Accessed June 15, 2014.
4. Accountability and health systems: overview, framework, and strategies: partners for health reformplus. 2003. Available at: http://www.who.int/management/partnerships/accountability/AccountabilityHealthSystemsOverview.pdf.
5. Zimmerli B. Improving health care value through shared accountability. Chicago: Insights Williamette Management Associates; 2013.
6. McGirt MJ, Speroff T, Godil SS, et al. Outcome science in practice: an overview and initial experience at the Vanderbilt Spine Center. Neurosurg Focus 2013;34(1):E7.
7. Burns PB, Rohrich RJ, Chung KC. The levels of evidence and their role in evidence-based medicine. Plast Reconstr Surg 2011;128(1):305–10.
8. Gliklich RE, Dreyer NA, editors. Registries for evaluating patient outcomes: a user's guide, vol. 1, 3rd edition. Washington DC: AHRQ Publication; 2014. Available at: http://www.effectivehealthcare.ahrq.gov/ehc/products/420/1897/registries-guide-3rd-edition-vol-1-140430.pdf.
9. Dahabreh IJ, Kent DM. Can the learning health care system be educated with observational data? JAMA 2014;312(2):129–30.
10. Asher AL, McCormick PC, Selden NR, et al. The National Neurosurgery Quality and Outcomes Database and NeuroPoint Alliance: rationale, development, and implementation. Neurosurg Focus 2013;34(1):E2.
11. Woodworth GF, Baird CJ, Garces-Ambrossi G, et al. Inaccuracy of the administrative database: comparative analysis of two databases for the diagnosis and treatment of intracranial aneurysms. Neurosurgery 2009;65(2):251–6 [discussion: 256–7].
12. Slutsky JR. 2012. Available at: http://www.ehcca.com/presentations/compeffective4/slutsky_1.pdf.
13. Lauer MS, D'Agostino RB Sr. The randomized registry trial–the next disruptive technology in clinical research? N Engl J Med 2013;369(17):1579–81.
14. Reinhardt UE. The disruptive innovation of price transparency in health care. JAMA 2013;310(18):1927–8.
15. McGirt MJ, Speroff T, Dittus RS, et al. The National Neurosurgery Quality and Outcomes Database (N2QOD): general overview and pilot-year project description. Neurosurg Focus 2013;34(1):E6.
16. Kelly AM. The minimum clinically significant difference in visual analogue scale pain score does not differ with severity of pain. Emerg Med J 2001;18(3):205–7.
17. Gallagher EJ, Liebman M, Bijur PE. Prospective validation of clinically important changes in pain severity measured on a visual analog scale. Ann Emerg Med 2001;38(6):633–8.
18. Hagg O, Fritzell P, Nordwall A. The clinical importance of changes in outcome scores after treatment for chronic low back pain. Eur Spine J 2003;12(1):12–20.
19. Copay AG, Glassman SD, Subach BR, et al. Minimum clinically important difference in lumbar spine surgery patients: a choice of methods using the Oswestry Disability Index, Medical Outcomes Study questionnaire Short Form 36, and pain scales. Spine J 2008;8(6):968–74.
20. Selden NR, Ghogawala Z, Harbaugh RE, et al. The future of practice science: challenges and opportunities for neurosurgery. Neurosurg Focus 2013;34(1):E8.
21. Asher AL, McGirt MJ, Glassman SD, et al. Regulatory considerations for prospective patient care registries: lessons learned from the National Neurosurgery Quality and Outcomes Database. Neurosurg Focus 2013;34(1):E5.

22. Clark RE. The development of The Society of Thoracic Surgeons voluntary national database system: genesis, issues, growth, and status. Best Pract Benchmarking Healthc 1996;1(2):62–9.

23. Ferguson TB Jr, Dziuban SW Jr, Edwards FH, et al. The STS National Database: current changes and challenges for the new millennium. Committee to Establish a National Database in Cardiothoracic Surgery, The Society of Thoracic Surgeons. Ann Thorac Surg 2000;69(3):680–91.

24. Gronblad M, Hupli M, Wennerstrand P, et al. Intercorrelation and test-retest reliability of the Pain Disability Index (PDI) and the Oswestry Disability Questionnaire (ODQ) and their correlation with pain intensity in low back pain patients. Clin J Pain 1993;9(3):189–95.

25. Moses H 3rd, Matheson DH, Dorsey ER, et al. The anatomy of health care in the United States. JAMA 2013;310(18):1947–63.

26. Fairbank JC, Couper J, Davies JB, et al. The Oswestry low back pain disability questionnaire. Physiotherapy 1980;66(8):271–3.

27. Fairbank JC, Pynsent PB. The Oswestry disability index. Spine (Phila Pa 1976) 2000;25(22):2940–52 [discussion: 2952].

28. Roland M, Fairbank J. The Roland-Morris disability questionnaire and the Oswestry disability questionnaire. Spine (Phila Pa 1976) 2000;25(24): 3115–24.

29. Jansson KA, Nemeth G, Granath F, et al. Health-related quality of life (EQ-5D) before and one year after surgery for lumbar spinal stenosis. J Bone Joint Surg Br 2009;91(2):210–6.

30. Badia X, Diaz-Prieto A, Gorriz MT, et al. Using the EuroQol-5D to measure changes in quality of life 12 months after discharge from an intensive care unit. Intensive Care Med 2001;27(12):1901–7.

Measuring Outcomes for Neurosurgical Procedures

Philip V. Theodosopoulos, MD[a],*, Andrew J. Ringer, MD[b]

KEYWORDS

- Clinical outcomes • Measuring quality • Outcome assessment • Complication rates • Outcome

KEY POINTS

- Outcomes must be measured before they can be improved.
- Improving outcomes involves understanding current levels of performance, identifying areas in need of potential improvement, initiating changes in clinical care provided, and finally, measuring the change in performance achieved.
- Secondary data (like claims data) can be used to somewhat track outcomes and quality, although there are significant problems with data validity and completeness.
- Primary data are the most accurate source of outcomes data, but require a large investment in time and money, are subject to reporter bias, and are prone to privacy concerns.

INTRODUCTION

Surgical procedures account for a large portion of health care expenditures. As such, their cost and indications have come under scrutiny at a policy level as well as on the news media. Studies of the effectiveness and efficacy of surgical interventions have been argued to be necessary in accurately assessing surgical outcomes and potentially avoiding preventable complications as it has been shown in other aspects of medical inpatient care.[1–4] The Centers for Medicare and Medicaid Services (CMS) has in the past initiated a program for the assessment of hospital performance in measures of care (www.hospitalcompare.hhs.gov), but no such programs yet exist for the assessment of surgical care provided.

Measuring surgical outcomes has been indirectly associated with improving outcomes of care. A focus on outcomes is advocated as the best way to improve outcomes. Such a process involves understanding current levels of performance, identifying areas in need of potential improvement, initiating changes in clinical care provided, and finally, measuring the change in performance achieved, a cycle that has been argued to be a powerful ally in the quest of improving quality of care.

The recent explosion of Web sites dedicated to the assessment of purported physician quality indicates an increasing public interest in the quality of their physician of choice. As most of these Internet sources rely on haphazard and potentially inaccurate data, misinformation abounds. To date, however, the lack of any official data sanctioned by the CMS, private payers, or physician professional societies has allowed for a gap of available information, often fulfilled by subpar surrogate venues.

The recently implemented Affordable Care Act promises a focus on quality and accountability of care. Although these have been concepts traditionally embedded in medical and surgical practice, few attempts have been made in quantifying those parameters as they related directly to

Disclosures: None.
[a] Department of Neurological Surgery, University of California, San Francisco, 505 Parnassus Avenue, M787, San Francisco, CA 94143, USA; [b] Department of Neurosurgery, Mayfield Clinic, University of Cincinnati, 506 Oak Street, Cincinnati, OH 45219, USA
* Corresponding author.
E-mail address: TheodosopoulosP@neurosurg.ucsf.edu

surgical procedures, in general, and neurosurgical procedures, in particular, outside the realm of research.[5,6]

Part of the difficulty in addressing quality of surgical care is the absence of a universally agreed on definition for quality. In addition, for any definition of quality used, there are limited instruments to accurately and reproducibly measure it. Although the neurosurgical literature is replete with disease-specific outcome studies using narrowly applicable scales, a more generic methodology that can be used uniformly to assess surgical outcomes does not exist.[7–11]

In this article, the important components of such a process are presented, and the possible application of a quality assessment initiative in the clinical setting is discussed. The article draws from the experience of a large similar process carried out at Mayfield Clinic and the University of Cincinnati's Department of Neurosurgery that was designed, was implemented over the past decade, and has been reported elsewhere.[5] This process has been shown to accurately record procedure-specific and disease-specific outcomes following surgical intervention in a large mixed academic and private practice setting, incorporating the entire gamut of neurosurgical interventions, both cranial and spinal.

DISCUSSION

The lack of a universally accepted definition for quality of surgical care has led to the use of several surrogates for quality, including population-derived/patient-centered data (rates of mortality, rates of major postoperative complications, and rates of type of discharge disposition as well as length of stay) and systemic indicators (data extracted from deidentified databases related to inpatient diagnoses, malpractice claims, as well as adherence to accepted standards).[12–14] Such data, although not traceable to individual patients, are nonetheless powerful because they are derived from large cohorts of patients with specific diagnoses or having undergone specific procedures.[15–17] Much of the early clinical outcomes work was performed analyzing such data.

As powerful and relatively accessible secondary data as they may be, there are several limitations that are associated with their analysis. Deidentified data that, in general, populate such databases do not allow for careful analysis of individual patient charts to assess comorbidities, additional information, or auditing of the accuracy of the data. Databases that are based on coding data are susceptible to inaccurate coding, particularly of secondary diagnoses, because the primary providers are rarely the people responsible for the coding. The almost universal adoption of electronic medical records (EMR) in most clinical settings promises to reduce the inaccuracies of coding and transcribing, but such potential benefits in studying clinical outcomes remain still unproven.

Systemic indexes, usually related to adherence to certain processes found to be effective in clinical settings, are another standard that can be used in a fairly straightforward way to assess quality of care. There have been several early data related to processes resulting in the CMS process of hospital performance evaluation (www.hospitalcompare.hhs.gov). Nonetheless, a study by Nicholas and colleagues[18] assessing the accuracy of outcomes reporting in 2000 US hospitals found a low correlation between rates of compliance with CMS preoperative process of care and perioperative outcomes.

With all the limitations of analysis of secondary data, the importance of assessing primary clinical data becomes evident. However, before the components of such an analysis are addressed, the limitations of primary outcome data study should be discussed. Primary data can be difficult to measure accurately (eg, reported postoperative pain levels), may have limited clinical utility and relevance (eg, mortality rates for most neurosurgical procedures), can be prohibitively time-consuming in their collection (eg, postoperative neuropsychological testing), are overwhelmingly operator-dependent (eg, radiologic determination of bony fusion), are often multifactorial and potentially biased by unknowable factors (eg, return to work date depending on patient social circumstances and potential for secondary gains), and are difficult to manage in a secure way that ensures against breaches of patient privacy.

Lessons from the design and implementation of an organization-wide quality improvement process that Mayfield Clinic and the Department of Neurosurgery at the University of Cincinnati undertook over a period of several years are discussed. In doing so, it is hoped that the important components of such a process are assessed and lessons learned throughout the design, trial, and implementation course of the project are shared. As the practice setting is a large mixed academic and private practice environment with more than 5000 neurosurgical procedures spanning the spectrum of cranial and spinal surgery, it is likely that parts of the authors' experience will be applicable to most neurosurgical settings.

Timeline

During the initial discussions regarding this initiative, it was decided to proceed in a graduated fashion. Once the process was designed, 3 physician champions were asked to implement a pilot trial for 3 months; this was used to identify systemic problems as well as opportunities for improving the entire process. Data generated during that time helped improve the EMR forms used to capture data, shape the process as well as identify training methods for the ancillary staff involved in the initiative. The redesigned process was then implemented system-wide, using lessons learned during the pilot phase. The entire process from beginning of design to full implementation took 6 years.

The lengthy implementation process was the result of multiple factors, including that there were no other such processes described before in the literature which could be emulated, the timing being early in the overall use of EMR for data capture in general, and the limitations in clinical practice that this entailed, as well as a purposefully cautious approach to the process to win system-wide buy-in and trust. Based on these lessons, such a full-scale implementation in a large practice may reasonably currently take as much as half of the time reported.

Components

Setting up the process for outcomes assessment is critical. Building up the culture that will support and nourish the process and developing a nuanced understanding of the level, detail, and kind of information that will be collected avoids future structural revisions to the process that can be costly and time-consuming. In the current health care environment, such a process should be EMR-based. Early design of custom forms that would include a comprehensive list of quality indicators to be collected is important. Compliance with the process can be facilitated by including the additional data fields in EMR forms already in use, such as charge sheets for procedures as well as template postoperative visit forms. Appropriate design of the additional fields should allow for information to be easily compiled and used in summative ways; therefore, free-text fields should be avoided and numeric format or preselected drop-down menus are preferable.

In general, most similar databases should include data on procedure-associated complications, length of stay, discharge disposition as well as posttreatment symptom resolution. In the authors' process, they chose to use CTCAE (National Cancer Institute Common Terminology Criteria for Adverse Effects, version 4.0, ctep.cancer.gov) grading because this has been a proven complication-reporting algorithm, with the definition of minor complication a grade 1 or 2 and major complication a grade 3 and 4. In addition, using disease-specific validated scales (eg, Karnofsky Performance Scale or Oswestry Disability Index) can add significant additional clinical information that may not be easily discernible from the general clinical data obtained during a physical examination.

It is universally accepted that any such process should be done in a prospective way to minimize biases. Furthermore, a point-of-service timing of information gathering is advisable, including data recorded at the time of patient contact, every time the patient is evaluated in an inpatient or outpatient setting. Although this may seem like an ambitious goal in most busy clinical practices, in the authors' extensive experience over several years, it is surprisingly easy to implement. This way, completeness of data collection is ensured and the end results are more robust compared with randomly chosen entry criteria that several large studies have used in other settings.[19,20]

Empowering multiple members of the health care team to record outcomes data, appropriate for their level of training and expertise, can be an important safeguard against missed information and input inaccuracies. A case in point is the accurate recording of postoperative major and minor complications that can often be missed if there is an outpatient or inpatient evaluation outside the primary health care system. Medical assistants, nurses, and nurse practitioners have proven in the authors' opinion to be better than surgeons in ensuring that such information is collected during either postoperative phone inquiries or brief office assessments. As opposed to the initial concern that such an open access to the outcome information by all members of the health care team may create more inaccuracies, the opposite was observed. It should be noted that whenever there is disagreement in different assessments, the system should allow for adjudication by the primary health practitioner.

Accuracy of data is a primary goal of such a process. Increasing daily experience with the data collection system leads to improvement in accuracy, with fewer missed data as well as fewer incorrectly coded data. Nonetheless, in most clinical practice settings, a mature outcome data collection process involves hundreds if not thousands of data fields recorded daily. As with any such large-scale process, errors are intrinsic to it and a systematic approach should be used to address this. Auditing is one of the most powerful ways to both correct errors and identify, record, and prospectively follow the rate of errors in the entire process.

Auditing can be performed in many different ways. As a safeguard for optimizing data accuracy, auditing can be performed in all data entered. In the authors' experience, this is expensive, impractical, and potentially unnecessary. The exact portion of patient records assessed is a function of manpower and level of error allowed. The authors implemented a limited audit review of 5% of the charts of patients treated each given time period and attempted to adjudicate all incongruent information recorded. Auditing consisted of generating a random list of 5% of all patients for each surgeon, and for those patients, a dedicated nurse performing a complete review of the EMR (both outpatient and inpatient) to assess for any missed data or inaccuracies in the data reported.

In using one nurse full-time equivalent (FTE) for the ongoing audit of the entire record, the authors found that not only did they develop a fair grasp on the amount of inaccuracy within the data but also they identified systemic problems with correct data gathering that in turn resulted in significant systemic improvements in minimizing erroneous information capture and missed data. An example of this improvement process was the early identification through auditing that length-of-stay information was often missing or inaccurate. This missing or inaccurate information was because when the primary surgeons were completing the immediate postoperative outcome collection forms, the exact date of discharge was not always readily available. In an attempt to improve on this, the authors shifted the date of discharge field capture to the hospital billing form completed following discharge by the coders who had the discharge date information always available, and the length-of-stay information became one of the most accurately recorded data fields.

Missing data found by auditing were noted and a rate of missed data was extrapolated from that. It should be noted that auditing results helped galvanize organization-wide support for the process and provided direct feedback along multiple vectors of performance for all involved. More generically, one should note that sharing such information among all health care providers creates an environment of positive competitive spirit that results in universal buy-in. As a result, the rates of missed information identified by the process steadily dropped for almost each successive quarter. Inaccuracies that were identified during the audit were adjudicated by the physician chair of the outcomes committee or, if need be, by the entire outcomes committee.

At the conclusion of each quarter, a report was generated that included the top 5 procedures by frequency per surgeon per quarter, with the number of procedures, complications, disposition, and length of stay for the ones the individual surgeon performed compared with the relevant aggregate numbers for the surgeon's entire career (as reported in the system) as well as for the entire organization. These reports were confidentially presented to each physician and were not shared. The chair of the committee reviewed the reports in a process designed to identify outliers (individual surgeons with outcomes more than 2 standard deviations from the mean). No such outliers were identified throughout the process.

Future Directions

Creating a prospective database wherein data on all patients are recorded in an auditable fashion is a very valuable process, but not the ultimate goal in quality improvement. Developing ways that such collected information can be channeled back to providers and system processes managers is imperative if change is to be implemented. Although this last part of the process may be difficult to carry out, the information gathered is nonetheless valuable in order for every surgeon to appreciate their outcomes and to be able to follow them in real-time throughout their practice. The Mayfield Clinic / University of Cincinnati process has not yet completed an entire cycle of implementing practice changes based on lessons learned, yet the outcomes initiative has already affected patients' outcomes by the focused attention on detailed outcome measures collected. The entire organization thus acquired a culture focused on patient-centered outcomes and that in itself is a major improvement over the antecedent anecdotal memories of complications and overall postoperative patient outcomes that most surgeons are accustomed to.

Specific improvements derived by lessons learned, particularly related to specific procedures and/or through comparisons of specific surgeons' preferences and choices, may make for a continual quality improvement process. Innovative ideas for treatment as well as new surgical technologies and techniques can in this way be tested against traditional approaches in a more nuanced way that will allow for the identification of possible opportunities for improved outcomes.

REFERENCES

1. Centers for Medicare and Medicaid Services (CMS), HHS. Medicare program; hospital inpatient prospective payment systems for acute care

hospitals and the long-term care hospital prospective payment system and Fiscal Year 2014 rates; quality reporting requirements for specific providers; hospital conditions of participation; payment policies related to patient status. Final rules. Fed Regist 2013;78. 50495–1040.

2. Kruse GB, Polsky D, Stuart EA, et al. The impact of hospital pay-for-performance on hospital and Medicare costs. Health Serv Res 2012;47:2118–36.

3. Lee GM, Kleinman K, Soumerai SB, et al. Effect of nonpayment for preventable infections in U.S. hospitals. N Engl J Med 2012;367:1428–37.

4. Miller DC, Gust C, Dimick JB, et al. Large variations in Medicare payments for surgery highlight savings potential from bundled payment programs. Health Aff (Millwood) 2011;30:2107–15.

5. Theodosopoulos PV, Ringer AJ, McPherson CM, et al. Measuring surgical outcomes in neurosurgery: implementation, analysis, and auditing a prospective series of more than 5000 procedures. J Neurosurg 2012;117:947–54.

6. Turner JA, Ersek M, Herron L, et al. Patient outcomes after lumbar spinal fusions. JAMA 1992;268:907–11.

7. Buchbinder R, Osborne RH, Ebeling PR, et al. A randomized trial of vertebroplasty for painful osteoporotic vertebral fractures. N Engl J Med 2009;361:557–68.

8. Mehta MP, Tsao MN, Whelan TJ, et al. The American Society for Therapeutic Radiology and Oncology (ASTRO) evidence-based review of the role of radiosurgery for brain metastases. Int J Radiat Oncol Biol Phys 2005;63:37–46.

9. Molyneux AJ, Kerr RS, Yu LM, et al. International subarachnoid aneurysm trial (ISAT) of neurosurgical clipping versus endovascular coiling in 2143 patients with ruptured intracranial aneurysms: a randomised comparison of effects on survival, dependency, seizures, rebleeding, subgroups, and aneurysm occlusion. Lancet 2005;366:809–17.

10. Tsao MN, Mehta MP, Whelan TJ, et al. The American Society for Therapeutic Radiology and Oncology (ASTRO) evidence-based review of the role of radiosurgery for malignant glioma. Int J Radiat Oncol Biol Phys 2005;63:47–55.

11. Wiebe S, Blume WT, Girvin JP, et al, Effectiveness, Efficiency of Surgery for Temporal Lobe Epilepsy Study Group. A randomized, controlled trial of surgery for temporal-lobe epilepsy. N Engl J Med 2001;345:311–8.

12. Longo DR, Land G, Schramm W, et al. Consumer reports in health care. Do they make a difference in patient care? JAMA 1997;278:1579–84.

13. Rolph JE, Kravitz RL, McGuigan K. Malpractice claims data as a quality improvement tool. II. Is targeting effective? JAMA 1991;266:2093–7.

14. Stevenson KS, Gibson SC, MacDonald D, et al. Measurement of process as quality control in the management of acute surgical emergencies. Br J Surg 2007;94:376–81.

15. Fu KM, Smith JS, Polly DW Jr, et al. Morbidity and mortality in the surgical treatment of 10,329 adults with degenerative lumbar stenosis. J Neurosurg Spine 2010;12:443–6.

16. Sansur CA, Reames DL, Smith JS, et al. Morbidity and mortality in the surgical treatment of 10,242 adults with spondylolisthesis. J Neurosurg Spine 2010;13:589–93.

17. Smith JS, Fu KM, Polly DW Jr, et al. Complication rates of three common spine procedures and rates of thromboembolism following spine surgery based on 108,419 procedures: a report from the Scoliosis Research Society Morbidity and Mortality Committee. Spine (Phila Pa 1976) 2010;35:2140–9.

18. Nicholas LH, Osborne NH, Birkmeyer JD, et al. Hospital process compliance and surgical outcomes in Medicare beneficiaries. Arch Surg 2010;145:999–1004.

19. Ghaferi AA, Birkmeyer JD, Dimick JB. Variation in hospital mortality associated with inpatient surgery. N Engl J Med 2009;361:1368–75.

20. Khuri SF, Daley J, Henderson W, et al. The National Veterans Administration Surgical Risk Study: risk adjustment for the comparative assessment of the quality of surgical care. J Am Coll Surg 1995;180:519–31.

Development and Implementation of Guidelines in Neurosurgery

Michael G. Fehlings, MD, PhD, FRCSC[a],*, Anick Nater, MD[b]

KEYWORDS

- Clinical practice guidelines • Guidelines • Evidence-based medicine • Best practice • Neurosurgery
- Knowledge translation • Implantation research • Quality improvement

KEY POINTS

- Clinical practice guidelines (CPGs), which involve a (1) systematic review, selection, and ranking of studies as evidence for each therapeutic option, followed by (2) achievement of a multidisciplinary panel agreement based on the analysis of the strength of the latter evidence, offer a more reliable approach to achieving quality and effectiveness than expert opinion, which is principally derived from past experience.
- CPGs are one of several tools available to improve health care delivery by assisting the decision-making process.
- All physicians should critically appraise CPGs, and determine whether the recommendations are applicable and appropriate in the case of any individual patient.
- CPGs are subject to changes as new evidence emerges, and thus are intended to be advisory statements and not standards of care.

INTRODUCTION

There is still considerable variability in therapeutic approaches for numerous neurosurgical conditions.[1–6] In addition, the rising costs of health care delivery, partly arising from the increasing use of sophisticated but expensive technology, represent significant societal financial challenges. Consequently many reform efforts around the globe, such as development and implementation of clinical practice guidelines (CPGs), aim at improving clinical outcomes in a cost-efficient manner. However, despite being endorsed by the American Association of Neurosurgical Surgeons (AANS) and the Congress of Neurosurgical Surgeons (CNS), CPGs appear not to be widely integrated as a means to assist the clinical decision-making process in neurosurgery.[7–12] Both evidence-based medicine (EBM) and CPGs have often been the source of misinterpretations and misconceptions, which could in part explain the reluctance of some neurosurgeons to apply EBM and adhere to CPGs. Indeed, some neurosurgeons believe that it is inappropriate to apply data obtained from large clinical studies to an individual patient, or that adequate EBM should exclusively rely on high-quality (level I) evidence, or, indeed, that surgery is just as much an art as it is a science. Consequently, any attempt at standardization is seen not only as a violation of surgeons' autonomy but also a potential sword of Damocles in terms of medicolegal issues.

Disclosures: None.
a Department of Surgery, Spinal Program, Krembil Neuroscience Center, 399 Bathurst Street, Suite 4W-449, Toronto, Ontario, M5T 2S8, Canada; b Division of Neurosurgery, Toronto Western Hospital, 399 Bathurst Street, WW 4-427, Toronto, Ontario, M5T 2S8, Canada
* Corresponding author.
E-mail address: michael.fehlings@uhn.on.ca

Neurosurg Clin N Am 26 (2015) 271–282
http://dx.doi.org/10.1016/j.nec.2014.11.005
1042-3680/15/$ – see front matter © 2015 Elsevier Inc. All rights reserved.

The purpose of this article is to emphasize the necessity for neurosurgeons to critically appraise their clinical and surgical decisions in the light of current available evidence. Thus, by reviewing the definition, purpose, elaboration, and appraisal of EBM and CPGs, as well as their advantages, limitations, and applicability, the authors hope to clarify their intended use and demonstrate that adequately constructed CPGs represent another tool to optimize patient care which, therefore, should be integrated into neurosurgical teaching and practice.

DEFINITION AND GENERAL PURPOSE

CPGs constitute a broad topic intertwining a plethora of concepts. The Institute of Medicine recently revised its definition of CPGs as: "statements that include recommendations intended to optimize patient care that are informed by systematic review of evidence and an assessment of the benefits and harms of alternative care options."[13(p4)] Similarly, the World Health Organization defines CPGs as "systematically developed evidence-based statements which assist providers, recipients and other stakeholders to make informed decisions about appropriate health interventions."[14(p2)] These quotations use several key words that need to be carefully considered within their background and context to fully appreciate their meaning and implications.

EVIDENCE-BASED MEDICINE AND CLINICAL PRACTICE GUIDELINES: CONTEXT OF CREATION AND APPROACH

To begin with, CPGs involve critically appraised evidence, which cannot be dissociated from the concept of EBM. In fact, the 1970s marked the convergence of pivotal movements in modern medicine that came to be called "Evidence-Based Medicine" and from which EBM and CPGs conjointly emerged.[11] Historically and traditionally, medical teaching and practice essentially depended on knowledge provided by medical leaders. Hence, clinical decisions were chiefly based on past experiences, and were thus prone to subjectivity biases and resulted in wide variability in clinical practice.[11,13,15] The actual term Evidence-Based Medicine was coined in 1991[16] by clinical epidemiologists from McMasters University, Canada, and made its first appearance in print in 1992.[17] EBM describes "the application of scientific method in determining the optimal management of the individual patient."[18(p89)] In 1992, an EBM Working Group emphasized that

"[while] clinical experience and the development of clinical instincts (particularly with respect to diagnosis) are a crucial and necessary part of becoming a competent physician [...] systematic attempts to record observations in a reproducible and unbiased fashion markedly increase the confidence one can have in knowledge about patient prognosis, the value of diagnostic tests, and the efficacy of treatment" and "the study and understanding of basic mechanisms of disease are necessary but insufficient guides for clinical practice."[17] The goal of rigorous experimentation and observation is to minimize error (bias). Clinical studies are vulnerable to 5 principal sources of bias: subject selection, subject allocation to different interventions, assessment of the effect of each intervention, analysis of the results, and how those results are reported.[11] Randomization and appropriate meticulous study design control for random and systematic error, respectively. Hence, randomized controlled trials (RCTs) are the gold standard in clinical research. Limiting bias allows greater confidence in the validity and accuracy of the results obtained and, consequently, in their interpretations and conclusions in answering specific clinical questions.[15] Sackett and colleagues[19] defined EBM as "the conscientious, explicit and judicious use of current best evidence in making decisions about the care of individual patients" [which involves] "integrating individual clinical expertise with the best available external clinical evidence from systematic research."[19]

EBM can be considered the philosophic approach from which CPGs are developed. CPGs may thus be perceived as a materialization of EBM. EBM involves 5 steps: (1) defining the question or problem; (2) searching for the evidence; (3) critically appraising the literature; (4) applying the results; and (5) auditing the outcome.[20] Critically appraising the literature (third step) essentially implies the concepts of "level of evidence" and "grades of recommendation." In fact, EBM establishes a hierarchy of strength of evidence (level of evidence) that classifies published studies based on analysis of their design and methodological rigor.[11,20] EBM favors data from studies that constitute a higher level of evidence (RCTs and meta-analysis of RCTs) in making clinical, guidelines, and health care policy decisions regarding therapy. In 1979, the Canadian Task Force on the Periodic Health Examination[21] presented organized clinical studies based solely on their study design, and derived strength of recommendation according to this system. Although the simplicity and ease of application of this approach made it attractive and popular, it

Table 1
Level of evidence and recommendation ranking

Canadian Task Force on the Periodic Health Examination		American Medical Association (AMA, 1990) and Surgical Management of TBI Author Group (2006)	
Effectiveness of Intervention		**Class of Evidence**	
I	Evidence obtained from at least one properly randomized controlled trial	I	Evidence from one or more well-designed RCTs, including overviews of such trials; Prospective RCTs
II-1	Evidence obtained from well-designed cohort or case-control analytical studies, preferably from more than one center or research group	II	Evidence from one or more well-designed comparative clinical studies, such as nonrandomized cohort studies, case-control studies, and other comparable studies; Studies in which the data were collected prospectively and retrospective studies based on clearly reliable data (eg, certain observational studies, cohort studies, prevalence studies, and case-control studies)
II-2	Evidence obtained from comparisons between times or place with or without the intervention. Dramatic results in uncontrolled experiments (such as the results of the introduction of penicillin in 1940s) could also be regarded as this type of evidence		
III	Opinions of respected authorities, based on clinical experience, descriptive studies, or reports of expert committees	III	Evidence from case series, comparative studies with historical controls, case reports, and expert opinion; most studies with retrospectively collected data (eg, clinical series, case reports, and expert opinion)
Certainty of Recommendation		**Certainty of Recommendation**	
A	There is good evidence to support the recommendation that the condition be specifically considered in a periodic health examination	*Standard*	Represent accepted principles of patient management that reflect a high degree of clinical certainty
B	There is fair evidence to support the recommendation that the condition be specifically considered in a periodic health examination	*Guideline*	Represent a particular strategy or range of management strategies that reflect a moderate degree of clinical certainty
C	There is fair evidence to support the recommendation that the condition be specifically considered in a periodic health examination	*Opinion*	Remaining strategies for patient management for which there is an unclear clinical certainty
D	There is fair evidence to support the recommendation that the condition be excluded from consideration in a periodic health examination		
E	There is good evidence to support the recommendation that the condition be excluded from consideration in a periodic health examination		

Abbreviations: RCT, randomized clinical trial; TBI, traumatic brain injury.
  Adapted from Refs.[11,15,21]

also generated significant criticisms (**Table 1**).[13] Since then, several systems to classify quality of evidence and strength of recommendations (see **Table 1**; **Tables 2** and **3**) have been elaborated to address a wider spectrum of aspects, such as research design and rigor in the methodological process, consistency of effects, clinical relevance, generalizability, audience, and clinical foci.[13] The GRADE Working Group recently elaborated a grading system that assesses 4 principal aspects: study design, study quality, consistency of effects across studies, and directness.[22]

Table 2
Level of evidence and grade of recommendation based on the type of primary clinical questions/studies

Grade of Recommendation	Study Level	Therapy/Prevention, Etiology/Harm Treatment Outcome	Prognosis Disease Outcome	Diagnosis Diagnostic Test	Differential Diagnosis/Studies on Prevalence of Symptoms	Economic and Decision Analyses Economic/Decision Model
A	1a	Homogeneous SR[a] of RCTs	Homogeneous SR[a] of inception cohort studies CDR[b] validated in different populations	Homogeneous SR[a] of level I diagnostic studies CDR[b] with 1b studies from different clinical centers	Homogeneous SR[a] of prospective cohort studies	Homogeneous SR[a] of level I economic studies
	1b	Individual RCT with narrow confidence interval	Individual inception cohort study with more than 80% follow-up CDR[b] validated in a single population	Validating[c] cohort study with good[d] reference standards CDR[b] tested within one clinical center	Prospective cohort study with good follow-up (ie, >80%) with adequate time for alternative diagnoses to emerge	Analysis based on clinically sensible costs or alternatives with multiway sensitivity analyses SR of the evidence with multiway sensitivity analyses
	1c	All or none[e]	All or none[e] case series	Absolute SpPins and SnNouts[f]	All or none[e] case series	Cost-effective studies

B					
2a	Homogeneous SR[a] of cohort studies	Homogeneous SR[a] of either retrospective cohort studies or untreated control groups in RCTs	Homogeneous SR[a] of diagnostic studies superior to level II	Homogeneous SR[a] of 2b and better studies	Homogeneous SR[a] of economic studies superior to level II
2b	Individual cohort study (including low-quality RCT (eg, <80% follow-up))	Retrospective cohort study or follow-up of untreated control patients in an RCT Derivation of CDR[b] or validated on split sample[g] only	Exploratory[h] cohort study with good[d] reference standards; CDR[b] after derivation, or validated only on split sample[g] or databases	Retrospective cohort study, or poor follow-up	Analysis based on clinically sensible costs or alternatives with multiway sensitivity analyses Limited review(s) of the evidence, or single studies with multiway sensitivity analyses
2c	Outcomes research; ecologic studies	Outcomes research		Ecologic studies	Audit or outcomes research
3a	Homogeneous SR[a] of case-control studies		Homogeneous SR[a] of 3b and better studies	Homogeneous SR[a] of 3b and better studies	Homogeneous SR[a] of 3b and better studies
3b	Individual case-control study		Nonconsecutive study or without consistently applied reference standards	Nonconsecutive cohort study or very limited population	Analysis based on limited alternatives or costs, poor-quality estimates of data, but including sensitivity analyses incorporating clinically sensible variations

(continued on next page)

Table 2
(continued)

Grade of Recommendation	Study Level	Therapy/Prevention, Etiology/Harm Treatment Outcome	Prognosis Disease Outcome	Diagnosis Diagnostic Test	Differential Diagnosis/ Studies on Prevalence of Symptoms	Economic and Decision Analyses Economic/Decision Model
C	4	Case series and poor-quality cohort and case-control studies[i]	Case series and poor-quality prognostic cohort studies[j]	Case-control study, poor, or nonindependent reference standard	Case series or superseded reference standards	Analysis with no sensitivity analysis
D	5	Expert opinion without explicit critical appraisal, or based on physiology, bench research	Expert opinion without explicit critical appraisal, or based on physiology, bench research	Expert opinion without explicit critical appraisal, or based on physiology, bench research	Expert opinion without explicit critical appraisal, or based on physiology, bench research	Expert opinion without explicit critical appraisal, or based on economic theory

Abbreviations: CDR, clinical decision rule; RCT, randomized clinical trial; SR, systematic review.

[a] Homogeneous SR is free of worrisome variations in the directions and degrees of results between individual studies. Not all systematic reviews with statistically significant heterogeneity need be worrisome, and not all worrisome heterogeneity need be statistically significant.

[b] Clinical decision rules are algorithms or scoring systems that lead to a prognostic estimation or a diagnostic category.

[c] Validating studies test the quality of a specific diagnostic test, based on prior evidence.

[d] Good reference standards are independent of the test, and applied blindly or objectively to all patients.

[e] All or none is met when all patients died before the treatment became available, but some now survive because they are taking this treatment; or when some patients died before the treatment became available, but none now die because they are taking this treatment.

[f] Absolute SpPin is a diagnostic finding whose specificity is so high that a positive result rules in the diagnosis. An Absolute SnNout is a diagnostic finding whose sensitivity is so high that a negative result rules out the diagnosis.

[g] Split-sample validation is achieved by collecting all the information in a single tranche, then artificially dividing this into "derivation" and "validation" samples.

[h] An exploratory study collects information and trawls the data (eg, using a regression analysis) to find which factors are 'significant'.

[i] A poor-quality cohort study failed to clearly define comparison groups and/or measure exposures and outcomes in the same (preferably blinded), objective way in both exposed and nonexposed individuals and/or failed to identify or appropriately control known confounders and/or failed to carry out a sufficiently long and complete follow-up of patients; a poor-quality case-control study failed to clearly define comparison groups and/or failed to measure exposures and outcomes in the same (preferably blinded), objective way in both cases and controls and/or failed to identify or appropriately control known confounders.

[j] Case series and poor-quality prognostic cohort studies have sampling biased in favor of patients who already had the target outcome, or the measurement of outcomes was accomplished in less than 80% of study patients, or outcomes were determined in an unblinded, nonobjective way, or there was no correction for confounding factors.

Produced by Bob Phillips, Chris Ball, Dave Sackett, Doug Badenoch, Sharon Straus, Brian Haynes, Martin Dawes since November 1998. Updated by Jeremy Howick March 2009. Oxford Centre for Evidence-based Medicine — Levels of Evidence (March 2009). Available at http://www.cebm.net/oxford-centre-evidence-based-medicine-levels-evidence-march-2009/. Used with permission.

Table 3
Approach to grades of recommendations[a]

Grades	Clarity of Risk/Benefit	Methodologic Strength of Supporting Evidence	Implications
1A	Clear	Randomized trials without important limitations	Strong recommendation; can apply to most patients in most circumstances without reservation
1B	Clear	Randomized trials with important limitations (inconsistent results, methodologic flaws[b])	Strong recommendation; likely to apply to most patients
1C+	Clear	No RCTs, but RCT results can be unequivocally extrapolated, or overwhelming evidence from observation studies	Strong recommendation; can apply to most patients in most circumstances
1C	Clear	Observation studies	Intermediate-strength recommendation; may change when stronger evidence is available
2A	Unclear	Randomized trials without important limitations	Intermediate-strength recommendation; best action may differ depending on circumstances or patients' or societal values
2B	Unclear	Randomized trials with important limitations (inconsistent results, methodologic flaws)	Weak recommendation; alternative approaches likely to be better for some patients under some circumstances
2C	Unclear	Observation studies	Very weak recommendations; other alternative may be equally reasonable

[a] Since studies in categories B and C are flawed, it is likely that most recommendations in these classes will be Level 2. The following considerations will bear on whether the recommendation is Grade 1 or Grade 2: the magnitude and precision of the treatment effect, patients' risk of the target event being prevented, the nature of the benefit, the magnitude of the risk associated with treatment, variability in patient preferences, variability in regional resource availability and health-care delivery practices, and cost considerations. Inevitably, weighing these considerations involves subjective judgment.
[b] These situations include RCTs with both lack of blinding and subjective outcomes, where the risk of bias in measurement of outcomes is high. and with large loss to follow-up.
From Fisher CG, Wood KB. Introduction to and techniques of evidence-based medicine. Spine (Phila Pa 1976) 2007;32 (19 Suppl):S66–72.

These systems, based on the level of evidence and consistency of findings, allow the grading of studies, which distils down to a strategy for rating evidence and identifying the strength of recommendations for a specific treatment according to an ordinal scoring scheme.[11,20]

In 1973, Wennberg and Gittelsohn[3] reported that practice patterns of local provider communities, that is, hospital market areas, varied markedly despite having similar patient populations. As stated by Health Canada, "Quality health care is about delivering the best possible care and achieving the best possible outcomes for people every time they deal with the health care system or use its services. Essentially, it means doing the best possible job with the resources available."[23] The eclecticism and disparities in health practices associated with the escalating use of technology and concomitant costs prompted the instigation of mechanisms to evaluate and ascertain the quality of care delivery.[15] Indeed, in 1989

in the United States, Congress amended the Public Health Service Act to form the Agency for Health Care Policy and Research (AHCPR), whose aims were to support research and other activities to increase the quality, appropriateness, and effectiveness of health care services, largely in reaction to rising public and private concerns regarding health care delivery and expenditure. Those concerns mainly emerged from mounting health care costs, the great variability and questionable value of some health services and clinical practices, and the idea that diverse types of financial, educational, and organizational incentives could reduce inappropriate utilization of the health service.[24] In fact, given the astronomical growth in the number of publications in clinical research, it is nowadays impossible to keep up to date with the current evidence, even in a specialized field such as neurosurgery. Therefore, acquiring knowledge through the process of EBM, thereby establishing the value of different clinical practices and developing CPGs, is, in principle, a potentially powerful means to build confidence in a limited set of established practices, and consequently to enhance the quality of health care.

CURRENT PRACTICE GUIDELINES: EXPECTATIONS, LIMITATIONS, AND CRITICAL APPRAISAL

CPGs are based on the model that "scientific evidence and clinical judgment can be systematically combined and produce clinically valid, operational recommendations for appropriate care that can and will be used to persuade clinicians, patients, and others to change their practices in ways that lead to better health outcomes and lower health care costs."[25(p19)] This model relies on 6 expectations: (1) there is a sufficient quantity and quality of scientific evidence from which CPGs can be built; (2) CPGs are developed by organized, funded, and effectively managed programs exempted from any conflicts of interests, which produce reliable and applicable recommendations about appropriate care options for clinically and financially significant health conditions or technologies; (3) most clinicians, patients, and other stakeholders have the opportunity, support, and incentives to search, comprehend, and adopt these recommendations in ways that change patterns of clinical practice, health behavior, or payments for health care services, thus enhancing consistency of care; (4) these changes are appreciable, so they change patient outcomes; (5) overall, CPGs support cost-controlling rather than cost-magnifying behavior in clinicians, patients, and health care systems; and (6) the body of CPGs continually enlarges to include more sectors and limit the overall increase in health care costs.[25]

Today, EBM and CPGs still raise numerous apprehensions within the neurosurgical and the medical community at large. Indeed, clinicians and other stakeholders are mainly concerned with the limitations of the scientific evidence from which CPGs are elaborated, lack of transparency in the methodology involved in developing CPGs, conflicts of interest between developers and funders, and contradiction between guidelines.[8,10,11,13] First, it must be stressed that, as the EBM Working Group and other investigators asserted, unfounded claims of certainty are made in an uncertain world.[11,13,17] Nonetheless, the Institute of Medicine[24] described 7 attributes that can assist the concerned individual in identifying reliable recommendations and CPGs: (1) the available scientific literature should be searched using appropriate and comprehensive search terminology; (2) a thorough review of the scientific literature

should precede guideline development; (3) the evidence should be evaluated and weighted, reflecting the scientific validity of the methodology used to generate the evidence; (4) there should be a link between the available evidence and the recommendations, with the strength of the evidence being reflected in the strength of recommendations, reflecting scientific certainty (or lack thereof); (5) empirical evidence should take precedence over expert judgment in the development of guidelines; (6) expert judgment should be used to evaluate the quality of the literature and formulate guidelines when the evidence is weak or nonexistent; and (7) guideline development should be a multidisciplinary process, involving key groups affected by the recommendations.[15] Moreover, similarly to quality checklists for RCTs (CONSORT), Cochrane-style systematic reviews (PRISMA), quality improvement studies (SQUIRE), and observational studies in epidemiology (STROBE), CPGs also have quality checklists and reporting standards to help with (1) designing high-quality CPGs and (2) assessing the validity and reliability of existing CPGs. Siering and colleagues[26] identified 40 assessment aids for CPGs, among the best known of which is the Appraisal of Guidelines for Research and Evaluation II (AGREE II). AGREE II is an updated and validated appraisal tool for CPGs that evaluates CPGs with regard to 23 items grouped into 6 domains of quality: scope and purpose, stakeholder involvement, rigor of development, clarity of presentation, applicability, and editorial independence.[27] A quality score for each AGREE II domain is then calculated from the individual item scores given by each evaluator. The AGREE II Consortium states that the domain scores can be used for comparing guidelines and guideline recommendations, and that quality CPGs should be based on the context in which the AGREE II is used. Consequently, the consortium has not determined a threshold score to help distinguish between poor-quality and high-quality CPGs. However, a score superior to 60% in at least 3 domains has been used to define high-quality CPGs in several critical appraisals of CPGs.[28–30]

CURRENT PRACTICE GUIDELINES IN NEUROSURGERY: HISTORY, CONCERNS, POTENTIAL IMPACT, AND FUTURE DIRECTIONS

In 1993, the Brain Trauma Foundation (BTF) and the American Academy of Neurology suggested to the AANS to join forces, inaugurating the primary guidelines effort in organized neurosurgery in the United States. Two years later, the BTF/AANS

Guidelines for the Management of Severe Traumatic Brain Injury was the first offspring of this collaboration.[31] Although multiple projects were initiated, only 5 were completed and approved by the AANS/CNS from 1993 to 2005: Management of Severe Traumatic Brain Injury (1995); Cervical Spine and Spinal Cord Injury Guidelines (2002); Severe Traumatic Brain Injury in Infants, Children, and Adolescents (2003); Lumbar Fusion Guidelines (2005); and Surgical Management of Traumatic Brain Injury (2006).[31] Furthermore, the official society journals did not accept any of these CPGs for publication until 2002.[31] Today, 8 CPGs figure in the *Guidelines Repository for Neurosurgery* on the AANS Web site[32] while the CNS Web site[33] counts 7 internally and 8 externally produced CNS-endorsed guidelines, totaling 19 CPGs between these 2 major neurosurgical organizations (**Table 4**).

The elaboration of CPGs requires 2 challenging steps: (1) systematic review, selection, and ranking of studies as evidence for each intervention; and (2) based on this analysis of strength of evidence, achievement of multidisciplinary panel agreement.[34] Therefore, CPGs may formulate recommendations that are lower in strength than the levels of evidence they are based on, but not the opposite: levels of strength of recommendation cannot exceed the levels of evidence supporting them.[31] This notion is essential, as it not only minimizes bias but also preserves physician autonomy of clinical judgment.[34] Levels of evidence and critical appraisal are based on a medical model that does not necessarily take into consideration the unique challenges of the neurosurgical field, such as selection and observer bias, blinding, learning curve, generalizability, incidence of the disorder, and patient and surgeon equipoise.[20] Indeed, RCTs are lengthy and expensive; they generally require multiple disciplines and institutions. Moreover, ethical issues often make them an inappropriate study design in neurosurgery.[35] Over the past 15 years, the neurosurgical literature has disclosed only a limited and static number of level I evidence–based studies.[35] Moreover, in 2005 the CNS conducted a feasibility study, which revealed that each guideline effort: (1) may cost up to $100,000 to produce, before the consideration of any publication costs; (2) relying uniquely on volunteer work of the physician writing group, takes on average 3 years to complete, and (3) has a relatively short shelf life given that the average validity of EBM CPGs is about 5 to 7 years.[34]

It must be highlighted that although CPGs are meant to be formal advisory statements, they do not necessarily equate to standards of care.[36]

However, CPGs have been used in both an exculpatory and inculpatory manner in medicolegal issues.[37] In 1989, James Todd, who was then the president of the American Medical Association, warned that "you cannot restrict physicians to one procedure or series of procedures for a specific condition (…) no two patients are exactly alike and no two conditions are exactly alike. What we must do is provide physicians with parameters that give them the flexibility to use their own skills within an acceptable range of options."[38]

Nonetheless, as in most medical fields, there is a great need to reduce variability in neurosurgery. For instance, lumbar fusion is drastically increasing, and there are significant variations in spinal surgery both internationally and across states in the United States with little medical, clinical, or surgical evidence to explain this heterogeneity. In fact, rates of lumbar fusion were the highest in Idaho Falls, Idaho (4.6 per 1000 Medicare enrollees) and lowest in Bangor, Maine (0.2 per 1000), representing a rate variation factor superior to 20.[39] In the case of traumatic brain injury (TBI), Gerber and colleagues[7] recently reported that the marked decrease in TBI mortality in the state of New York between 2001 and 2009 was associated with an increase in adherence to the recommendations for intracranial pressure monitoring and cerebral perfusion pressure management provided in the Guidelines for the Management of Severe TBI but no substantial changes in observance of other Guidelines recommendations, suggesting that this adherence improved outcomes. In addition, a cost-benefit analysis estimated that the implementation of the latter guideline would translate into US$3,837,577,538 in total societal cost savings.[40]

In conclusion, the relative dearth of high-powered evidence in neurosurgery, somewhat idealistic expectations, relatively short shelf life, and potential usage in medicolegal litigations should be perceived as working grounds to improve the development, evaluation, implementation, and adherence to CPGs. CPGs can be powerful tools at various levels. Indeed, they have the potential to optimize patient care by providing recommendations about the various treatment options available and their respective strengths based on best current evidence. CPGs can assist patients, the general public, groups, organizations, and societies in addition to health care practitioners, administrators, and policy makers in the therapeutic decision-making process, and limit variation in care between providers, institutions, and geographic regions without hindering physician autonomy and clinical judgment.[8,13,14,31,34,36,41] The authors are convinced

Table 4
Clinical practice guidelines appearing on organized neurosurgery Web sites: AANS and/or CNS

Guideline	Latest Copyright Year	Sponsor—Publisher	Organized Neurosurgery Web Site
Guidelines for the Management of Severe Traumatic Brain Injury, 3rd edition	2007	Brain Trauma Foundation—Brain Trauma Foundation	AANS and CNS
Guidelines for Acute Medical Management of Severe Traumatic Brain Injury in Infants, Children, and Adolescents, 2nd edition	2012	Brain Trauma Foundation—*Pediatric Critical Care Medicine*	AANS and CNS
Guidelines for the Management of Acute Cervical Spine and Spinal Cord Injuries	2013	AANS/CNS Joint Section on Disorders of the Spine and Peripheral Nerves—*Spine Universe/Neurosurgery*	AANS and CNS
Lumbar Fusion Guideline	2014	AANS/CNS Joint Section on Disorders of the Spine and Peripheral Nerves—*Journal of Neurosurgery: Spine*	AANS and CNS
Guidelines for Field Management of Combat-Related Head Trauma	2006	Brain Trauma Foundation—*Neurosurgery*	AANS
Guidelines for the Surgical Management of Traumatic Brain Injury	2006	Brain Trauma Foundation—*Neurosurgery*	AANS
Society of Critical Care guidelines		Society of Critical Care Medicine (Sponsor)	AANS
American Pain Society guidelines		American Pain Society (Sponsor)	AANS
Guidelines for the Management of Newly Diagnosed Glioblastoma	2008	CNS/AANS Joint Section on Tumors—*Journal of Neuro-Oncology*	CNS
Clinical Guideline on the Treatment of Carpal Tunnel Syndrome	2008	American Academy of Orthopaedic Surgeons (AAOS)—AAOS	CNS
Guideline for the Surgical Management of Cervical Degenerative Disease	2009	CNS/AANS Joint Section on Spine—*Journal of Neurosurgery*	CNS
Evidence-Based Clinical Practice Parameter Guidelines for the Treatment of Patients with Metastatic Brain Tumor	2009	CNS/AANS Joint Section on Tumor, in collaboration with McMaster Evidence-Based Practice Center—*Journal of Neuro-Oncology*	CNS
Guidelines for the Prevention of Stroke in Patients with Stroke and Transient Ischemic Attack (Secondary Stroke Prevention)	2010	American Heart Association/American Stroke Association—AHA/ASA	CNS
Guideline for the Management of Spontaneous Intracerebral Hemorrhage in Adults	2010	American Heart Association/American Stroke Association/American College of Cardiology—*Stroke* (Journal of the American Heart Association)	CNS

(continued on next page)

Table 4
(continued)

Guideline	Latest Copyright Year	Sponsor—Publisher	Organized Neurosurgery Web Site
Guideline on the Management of Patients with Extracranial Carotid and Vertebral Artery Disease	2011	American Heart Association/ American Stroke Association/ American College of Cardiology—*Journal of the American Heart Association*	CNS
Guidelines for the Management of Aneurysmal Subarachnoid Hemorrhage	2012	American Heart Association/ American Stroke Association/ American College of Cardiology—*Stroke*	CNS
Guideline on Radiotherapeutic and Surgical Management for Brain Metastases	2012	American Society for Radiation Oncology—*Practical Radiation Oncology*	CNS
Guidelines for the Management of Progressive Glioblastoma	2014	CNS/AANS Joint Section on Tumors—*Journal of Neuro-Oncology*	CNS
Deep Brain Stimulation for Obsessive-Compulsive Disorder (OCD)	2014	American Society for Stereotactic and Functional Neurosurgery (ASSFN)—*Neurosurgery*	CNS

Abbreviations: AANS, American Association of Neurosurgical Surgeons; CNS, Congress of Neurosurgical Surgeons.

that surgery is an art, and good clinical and surgical practice builds on personal experiences, individual skills, and current available evidence rather than personal, departmental, or institutional dogmas. CPGs promote consistency, efficacy (consequences of an intervention under ideal and controlled circumstances[42]), and effectiveness (consequences of an intervention under usual clinical setting, ie, real-world conditions[42]), and thus can enhance the quality of health care by supporting therapeutic options offering the best risk-benefit ratio while minimizing unnecessary, ineffective, or potentially harmful neurosurgical interventions.

REFERENCES

1. Irwin ZN, Hilibrand A, Gustavel M, et al. Variation in surgical decision making for degenerative spinal disorders. Part II: cervical spine. Spine (Phila Pa 1976) 2005;30(19):2214–9.
2. Irwin ZN, Hilibrand A, Gustavel M, et al. Variation in surgical decision making for degenerative spinal disorders. Part I: lumbar spine. Spine (Phila Pa 1976) 2005;30(19):2208–13.
3. Wennberg J, Gittelsohn J. Small area variations in health care delivery. Science 1973;182(4117):1102–8.
4. Marcus HJ, Price SJ, Wilby M, et al. Radiotherapy as an adjuvant in the management of intracranial meningiomas: are we practising evidence-based medicine? Br J Neurosurg 2008;22(4):520–8.
5. Santarius T, Lawton R, Kirkpatrick PJ, et al. The management of primary chronic subdural haematoma: a questionnaire survey of practice in the United Kingdom and the Republic of Ireland. Br J Neurosurg 2008;22(4):529–34.
6. Bernstein M, Khu KJ. Is there too much variability in technical neurosurgery decision-making? Virtual Tumour Board of a challenging case. Acta Neurochir (Wien) 2009;151(4):411–2 [discussion: 412–3].
7. Gerber LM, Chiu YL, Carney N, et al. Marked reduction in mortality in patients with severe traumatic brain injury. J Neurosurg 2013;119(6):1583–90.
8. Bandopadhayay P, Goldschlager T, Rosenfeld JV. The role of evidence-based medicine in neurosurgery. J Clin Neurosci 2008;15(4):373–8.
9. Luijsterburg PA, Verhagen AP, Braak S, et al. Neurosurgeons' management of lumbosacral radicular syndrome evaluated against a clinical guideline. Eur Spine J 2004;13(8):719–23.
10. Vachhrajani S, Kulkarni AV, Kestle JR. Clinical practice guidelines. J Neurosurg Pediatr 2009;3(4):249–56.
11. Linskey ME. Evidence-based medicine for neurosurgeons: introduction and methodology. Prog Neurol Surg 2006;19:1–53.
12. Bar M, Mikulik R, Skoloudik D, et al. Decompressive surgery for malignant supratentorial infarction

remains underutilized after guideline publication. J Neurol 2011;258(9):1689–94.

13. Committee on Clinical Practice Guidelines (Institute of Medicine), Graham RM, Mancher M, et al, editors. Institute of Medicine: clinical practice guidelines we can trust. Washington, DC: National Academic Press; 2011.

14. World Health Organization. Guidelines for WHO guidelines. 2003. Available at: http://whqlibdoc.who.int/hq/2003/EIP_GPE_EQC_2003_1.pdf. Accessed August 7, 2014.

15. Bullock MR, Chesnut R, Ghajar J, et al. Surgical management of TBI author group. Neurosurgery 2006;58(3 Suppl). s2.i–s2.iV.

16. Guyatt GH. Evidence-based medicine. Ann Intern Med 1991;114(ACP J Club Suppl 2):A16.

17. Evidence-Based Medicine Working Group. A new approach to teaching the practice of medicine. JAMA 1992;268(17):2420–5.

18. Daly J. Evidence-base medicine and the search for a science of clinical care. Berkeley (CA): University of California Press; 2005.

19. Sackett DL, Rosenberg WM, Gray JA, et al. Evidence based medicine: what it is and what it isn't. BMJ 1996;312(7023):71–2.

20. Fisher CG, Wood KB. Introduction to and techniques of evidence-based medicine. Spine (Phila Pa 1976) 2007;32(19 Suppl):S66–72.

21. The periodic health examination. Canadian task force on the periodic health examination. Can Med Assoc J 1979;121(9):1193–254.

22. Atkins D, Best D, Briss PA, et al. Grading quality of evidence and strength of recommendations. BMJ 2004;328(7454):1490.

23. Health Canada. Quality of care: health care system. 2011. Available at: http://www.hc-sc.gc.ca/hcs-sss/qual/index-eng.php. Accessed August 10, 2014.

24. Committee to Advise the Public Health Service on Clinical Practice Guidelines (Institute of Medicine), Field MJ, Lohr KN, editors. Clinical practice guidelines: directions for a new program. Washington, DC: National Academy Press; 1990.

25. Committee on Clinical Practice Guidelines (Institute of Medicine), Field MJ, Lohr KN, editors. Guidelines for clinical practice: from development to use. Washington, DC: National Academic Press; 1992.

26. Siering U, Eikermann M, Hausner E, et al. Appraisal tools for clinical practice guidelines: a systematic review. PLoS One 2013;8(12):e82915.

27. Brouwers MC, Kho ME, Browman GP, et al. AGREE II: advancing guideline development, reporting, and evaluation in health care. Prev Med 2010;51(5):421–4.

28. Acuna-Izcaray A, Sanchez-Angarita E, Plaza V, et al. Quality assessment of asthma clinical practice guidelines: a systematic appraisal. Chest 2013; 144(2):390–7.

29. Brosseau L, Rahman P, Poitras S, et al. A systematic critical appraisal of non-pharmacological

management of rheumatoid arthritis with Appraisal of Guidelines for Research and Evaluation II. PLoS One 2014;9(5):e95369.

30. Ou Y, Goldberg I, Migdal C, et al. A critical appraisal and comparison of the quality and recommendations of glaucoma clinical practice guidelines. Ophthalmology 2011;118(6):1017–23.

31. Linskey ME. Defining excellence in evidence-based medicine clinical practice guidelines. Clin Neurosurg 2010;57:28–37.

32. American Association of Neurological Surgeons. Education and meetings: guidelines repository for neurosurgery. Available at: http://www.aans.org/Education%20and%20Meetings/Clinical%20Guidelines.aspx. Accessed August 7, 2014.

33. Congress of Neurological Surgeons. Education and University of Neurosurgery: completed guidelines. 2014. Available at: http://www.cns.org/guidelines/completed.aspx. Accessed August 7, 2014.

34. Linskey ME, Kalkanis SN. Evidence-linked, clinical practice guidelines-getting serious; getting professional. J Neurooncol 2010;96(1):1–5.

35. Sami Walid M, Robinson JS 3rd, Robinson JS. Shortfalls in published neurosurgical literature. J Clin Neurosci 2012;19(7):942–5.

36. Hollon SD, Arean PA, Craske MG, et al. Development of clinical practice guidelines. Annu Rev Clin Psychol 2014;10:213–41.

37. Hyams AL, Brandenburg JA, Lipsitz SR, et al. Practice guidelines and malpractice litigation: a two-way street. Ann Intern Med 1995;122(6):450–5.

38. Mehlman MJ. Medical practice guidelines as malpractice safe harbors: illusion or deceit? J Law Med Ethics 2012;40(2):286–300.

39. Weinstein JN, Lurie JD, Olson PR, et al. United States' trends and regional variations in lumbar spine surgery: 1992–2003. Spine (Phila Pa 1976) 2006;31(23):2707–14.

40. Faul M, Wald MM, Rutland-Brown W, et al. Using a cost-benefit analysis to estimate outcomes of a clinical treatment guideline: testing the Brain Trauma Foundation guidelines for the treatment of severe traumatic brain injury. J Trauma 2007; 63(6):1271–8.

41. Davis D, Goldman J, Palda VA. Handbook on clinical practice guidelines. Toronto (Canada): Canadian Medical Association; 2007. Available at: https://www.cma.ca/Assets/assets-library/document/en/clinical-resources/CPG%20handbook-e.pdf.

42. Gartlehner G, Hansen RA, Nissman D, et al. Criteria for distinguishing effectiveness from efficacy trials in systematic reviews. Technical review 12 (Prepared by the RTI-International–University of North Carolina Evidence-based Practice Center under Contract No. 290-02-0016.) AHRQ Publication No. 06-0046. Rockville (MD): Agency for Healthcare Research and Quality; 2006.

The Role of Neurosurgery Journals in Evidence-Based Neurosurgical Care

Jordan P. Amadio, MD, MBA[a],[*],
Nelson M. Oyesiku, MD, PhD[b]

KEYWORDS

- Review • Evidence-based medicine • Neurosurgery publishing • Reporting guidelines
- Meta-analysis • Clinical practice guidelines • Peer review

KEY POINTS

- Journals have played a key role in improving the quality of neurosurgical care over the past several decades, in part by endorsing an evidence-based view of neurosurgery practice.
- Reporting guidelines have emerged as a key tool for strengthening the quality of neurosurgery literature.
- Neurosurgery journals promote the organization of knowledge into clinically useful forms via the publication of systematic reviews, meta-analyses, and clinical practice guidelines.
- Peer review continues to be a core feature of neurosurgery publishing that serves to safeguard the quality of the literature.
- Through several initiatives, neurosurgery journals have undertaken a leadership position for the future of medical publishing.

INTRODUCTION

Throughout the past several decades, the neurosurgery publishing community has undertaken an active role in improving the quality of the neurosurgery literature. Notably, in recent years, neurosurgery journals have provided the main conduit through which the techniques of evidence-based medicine, originating outside the field, have illuminated the data produced by neurosurgery researchers. In particular, journals have promoted improvements in patient care by endorsing an evidence-based view of neurosurgery practice and actively safeguarding the quality of the review process.

In the early twentieth century, as neurosurgery matured, Osler's "medico-chirurgical neurologists" split from general surgery to form their own discipline.[1] The Society of Neurologic Surgeons was founded in 1920, followed by the Harvey Cushing Society (now the American Association of Neurologic Surgeons [AANS]) in 1931. With these professional accretions, a gradual awareness of the need for neurosurgery-specific journals dawned on that burgeoning community. The *Journal of Neurosurgery* (1944), *Surgical Neurology* (1975), and *Neurosurgery* (1977) were among the earliest and most influential journals devoted to neurosurgery in North America.[2,3] The emergence of such periodicals stemmed from the recognition that despite sharing subject matter with related fields, such as neurology and general surgery, the peculiar complexities of neurosurgical care and its reliance on new science demanded discipline-focused venues for publication. Harvey

a Department of Neurosurgery, Emory University School of Medicine, 1365B Clifton Road, Northeast, Atlanta, GA 30322, USA; b Neurosurgery Residency Program, Department of Neurosurgery, Emory Pituitary Center, Emory University School of Medicine, 1365B Clifton Road, Northeast, Atlanta, GA 30322, USA
* Corresponding author.
E-mail address: jamadio@emory.edu

Neurosurg Clin N Am 26 (2015) 283–294
http://dx.doi.org/10.1016/j.nec.2014.11.001
1042-3680/15/$ – see front matter © 2015 Elsevier Inc. All rights reserved.

Cushing, writing in 1929, famously recognized the binding influence of scientific publications in cultivating disciplinary consensus.[4] The promulgation of independent neurosurgery journals over the course of the twentieth century reflects, in microcosm, the evolution of neurosurgery itself as a self-governing specialty with its own set of professional mores and standards.

Over the past century, the quantity of scientific information available to neurosurgeons has expanded dramatically. Neurosurgery journals have proliferated at an exponential rate, reflecting a trend seen across all scientific disciplines. This has been accompanied by a concomitant increase in the number of published articles, and increased pressures to organize that knowledge into useful forms for the clinical practitioner. At the same time, as the sea change of evidence-based medicine swept through the medical world in the 1990s, exhortations for achieving an "evidence-based neurosurgery" resulted from convincing arguments that the insistence on evidence-based patient care is applicable to neurologic surgery.[5] Quality and quantity of the data have become paramount.[6]

Organizing the ever-expanding mass of research data into the kind of knowledge that can guide clinical practice has proved a demanding feat. On this front, neurosurgery journals have been responsible for spearheading or facilitating many of the key initiatives. With assistance from professional societies, such as the AANS and Congress of Neurologic Surgeons (CNS), journals have improved the quality of neurosurgical knowledge by enforcing reporting standards, promoting meta-analysis, disseminating evidence-based clinical practice guidelines, and governing the process of peer review.

NEUROSURGERY JOURNALS AND PROLIFERATION OF SCIENTIFIC INFORMATION

The proliferation of neurosurgery journals and their quantitative impact over time is not well described in the primary literature, in part because categorizing scientific periodicals by discipline can be a deceptively difficult task. However, irrespective of which method is applied, it is clear that over several decades the number of neurosurgery journals has increased dramatically. In the mid-1970s, three major journals dominated the field. Today, there are dozens in the English language alone. One popular neurosurgery community World Wide Web portal lists 35 neurosurgical journals, rank-ordered by impact factor, in its resources section.[7] Another source identified 182

neurosurgery-related journals and found 2522 distinct journals cited by neurosurgical literature during a 3-month period.[8] New neurosurgery journals have been incepted de novo from professional interest groups, by evolution from preexisting journals (eg, the continuation of *Surgical Neurology* as *World Neurosurgery*), or by splitting from a parent journal. The latter mechanism is represented, for example, by the recent spinoff of *Operative Neurosurgery* from its parent journal, *Neurosurgery*.[9]

The importance of a periodical within its field is classically measured by metrics based on citation analysis.[10] For example, the impact factor is defined as the average number of citations per paper published in that journal over the preceding 2 years. The *h* index reflects number of publications and citations; a journal with an *h* index of N has published N papers that have each been cited a minimum of N times. Both the impact factor and the *h* index have been applied to individual authors and to journals, although their dominance as metrics of scientific importance has been debated.[10–13] Citations in neurosurgical literature have been described as following a clear clustering pattern, with a recent analysis identifying the six "core" neurosurgery journals, in order of citations for a given time period, as *Journal of Neurosurgery*, *Neurosurgery*, *Spine*, *Acta Neurochirurgica*, *Stroke*, and *Journal of Neurotrauma*.[8]

In modern neurosurgery publishing, several safeguards are put in place to ensure the quality of research publications and, by consequence, the contribution of literature to the quality of patient care.

REPORTING GUIDELINES AS A TOOL FOR LITERATURE QUALITY

Around the turn of the twenty-first century, there emerged a growing awareness of the poor quality of reporting in medical research literature.[14–16] Selective reporting of data, incomplete listing of interventions, problematic conclusions, and unclear methodologies plagued many papers. In neurosurgery, these deficiencies were particularly profound. Despite the well-known preeminence of randomized controlled trials (RCTs),[17] these were scarce in the neurosurgery literature even when compared with general surgery or other surgical subspecialties.[18–20] Moreover, under close examination, neurosurgical RCTs as a group showed many flaws. In a survey of 108 RCTs on neurosurgery procedures during a 36-year span, underpowered trials and inadequate design reporting were widespread.[21] Another survey of 159 neurosurgical RCTs found, among other pitfalls, that nearly half of trials had inadequate reporting of allocation concealment, a core feature of proper RCT design.[22]

Beginning in the 1990s, the advent of consensus reporting guidelines from internationally recognized working groups has revolutionized the ability to objectively qualify clinical studies. The most widely accepted of these, introduced in 1996 and last revised in 2010, is known as the CONSORT statement (Consolidated Standards of Reporting Trials)[16] and centers on a 25-item checklist for RCT reporting. CONSORT has been recognized as an important tool for ensuring the quality RCTs in the literature. Because RCTs are uncommon in neurosurgery, the variety of guidelines developed for other study designs are of considerable importance. Prominent examples include GRADE (2004)[23] for formal grading of evidence, AMSTAR (2007)[24] for systematic reviews, PRISMA (2009)[25] for systematic reviews and meta-analyses, and MOOSE for meta-analyses that include observational studies. Collectively, these reporting guidelines have standardized and strengthened the organization of clinical knowledge.

The first publicized effort by a major neurosurgical journal to improve the quality of its literature by applying internationally recognized guidelines took place in 2011, when *Neurosurgery* endorsed and began requiring several of these guidelines.[26] This followed comparable initiatives by top-tier journals in other biomedical disciplines, and endorsements of CONSORT by the International Committee of Medical Journal Editors (www.icjme.org) and other associations.

Today, *Neurosurgery* endorses and requires authors to adhere to several key reporting guidelines. Research articles that must be submitted according to the appropriate reporting guidelines include, but are not limited to, randomized trials, systematic reviews, meta-analyses of interventions, meta-analyses of observational studies, diagnostic accuracy studies, and observational epidemiologic studies (eg, case series, cohort, case-control, and cross-sectional studies). For manuscripts that report statistics, the journal requires that authors provide evidence of statistical consultation or expertise. As of October 2014, *Neurosurgery* explicitly requires the reporting guidelines listed in **Table 1**.[27]

Myriad resources exist to assist authors and reviewers in the task of understanding and meeting reporting guideline requirements. Authors are referred to the EQUATOR Network, which was established in 2006 to promote transparent and accurate reporting of research studies by providing an up-to-date list of guidelines.[31] These include reporting guidelines for niche topics, such as neuro-oncology trials, and other nonrequired checklists and consensus statements designed to ensure research quality.

ORGANIZATION OF KNOWLEDGE: SYSTEMATIC REVIEWS AND META-ANALYSES

In tandem with efforts to improve the reporting and methodology of primary research, such as RCTs, renewed emphasis has been placed on secondary analyses of primary data, such as systematic reviews and meta-analyses.[15] This attention is justified by the fact that meta-analyses can represent powerful levels of evidence.[26] Current initiatives to improve the quality of meta-analyses and systematic reviews in the neurosurgery literature have mirrored efforts in the larger world of medical publishing. The most successful of these has been the Cochrane Database of Systematic Reviews, established in 1993 as an electronic collection of "living documents" representing systematic

Table 1
Clinical reporting guidelines applicable to neurosurgery publishing

Type of Submission	Reporting Guideline	Online Information
Randomized trials	Revised Consolidated Standards of Reporting Trials (CONSORT)[16]	http://www.consort-statement.org
Systematic reviews and meta-analyses	Preferred Reporting Items for Systematic Reviews and Meta-Analyses (PRISMA)[25]	http://www.prisma-statement.org
Systematic reviews and meta-analyses of observational studies	Meta-Analysis of Observational Studies in Epidemiology (MOOSE)[28]	http://bit.ly/MOOSEstatement
Studies of diagnostic accuracy	Standards for the Reporting of Diagnostic Accuracy Studies (STARD)[29]	http://www.stard-statement.org
Observational research	Strengthening the Reporting of Observational Studies in Epidemiology (STROBE)[30]	http://www.strobe-statement.org

Data from Refs.[16,25,28–30]

reviews of primary research in health care and health policy. In 2011, the Cochrane Database of Systematic Reviews was recognized with a seat on the World Health Organization's World Health Assembly. Although the Cochrane Database of Systematic Reviews contains more than 5000 reviews, a keyword search of that database for "neurosurgery" yielded only 13 reviews.[32] This validates the need for more neurosurgery-specific efforts to organize data from clinical studies into systematic reviews.

Attempts to quantify the quality of evidence in the neurosurgical literature have yielded varying results. A recent study found that higher levels of evidence (levels I and II) represented only 1 in 10 clinical papers from the top neurosurgical journals.[33] Publications with larger sample size were significantly associated with a higher level of evidence. The authors of that study compared their data with that obtained for the year 1999,[34] concluding that the proportion of high-quality evidence in neurosurgery journals had not significantly changed.

In the realm of methodologic and reporting quality for neurosurgery studies, there remains significant room for improvement. By some measures, the quality of meta-analyses in the neurosurgical literature seems to be improving.[18,35] However, among 72 papers in neurosurgery journals self-described as meta-analyses, one study found that on average only 53% of PRISMA items and 31% of AMSTAR items were completed.[35] Only 15% of the papers mentioned using a content checklist, and none mentioned using a methodology checklist. According to an editorial accompanying that study, these results demonstrated that neurosurgery had one of the worst quality meta-analyses of any medical field.[36] Concerns about literature quality have emerged not only for meta-analyses, but also for observational study designs, which are more numerous. A 2014 study found that most papers in the neurosurgical literature self-identifying as "case-control studies" are labeled incorrectly, with several attendant concerns in methodology.[37] In evaluating those papers that met the definition as case-control studies, the authors applied the Strengthening the Reporting of Observational Studies in Epidemiology Checklist and found examples of reporting deficiencies, such as reporting of bias (28%), missing data (55%), and funding (44%). Evidence is emerging, however, that the intervention of enforcing reporting guidelines may measurably improve the quality of published literature. In at least one editorial position statement,[26] this has been noted as a promising way forward for quality of the neurosurgery literature. For instance,

comparison of RCTs published before and after the advent of CONSORT,[38–40] and of RCTs in journals that do or do not endorse CONSORT reporting,[39,41–43] supported a beneficial effect of the CONSORT statement on literature quality.[44,45]

ORGANIZATION OF KNOWLEDGE: CLINICAL PRACTICE GUIDELINES

Initiatives to improve the quality of primary and secondary clinical research studies have been accompanied by coordinated efforts to develop comprehensive clinical practice guidelines for specific conditions. Neurosurgery journals have often worked in conjunction with professional societies to develop and disseminate the guidelines produced via these efforts. The CNS has formalized an in-house infrastructure to curate clinical practice guidelines, which it defines as including recommendations intended to optimize patient care and informed by a systematic review of evidence along with an assessment of benefits and harms.[46]

The most concentrated large-scale efforts to develop evidence-based clinical practice guidelines in neurosurgery have occurred over the past 15 years. In chronologic order of their date of publication, **Table 2** lists clinical practice guidelines publicly endorsed by the CNS[46] and other neurosurgery-related guidelines.

In addition to the guidelines listed in **Table 2**, ongoing work of interest to neurosurgeons has led to the development of clinical practice guidelines for deep brain stimulation,[70] lumbar radiculopathy,[71] normal pressure hydrocephalus,[72] neuro-oncology (eg, low-grade glioma, new glioblastoma, progressive glioblastoma, metastasis),[73] and concussion.[74]

The impact of clinical practice guidelines on patient care is difficult to assess directly, because the mere publication of guidelines does not guarantee their adoption or provide mechanisms to record outcomes. Adoption of guidelines will likely be reflected by long-term changes in neurosurgery patient management. In their introduction to the 2013 cervical spine injury guidelines, Hadley and Walters[57] describe the role and limitations of evidence-based guidelines from the standpoint of a practicing neurosurgeon:

Medical evidence-based guidelines, when properly produced, represent a contemporary scientific summary of accepted management, imaging, assessment, classification, and treatment strategies on a focused series of medical and surgical issues. They are an evidence-based hierarchal ranking of the scientific literature produced to date...

Medical evidence-based guidelines are not meant to be restrictive or to limit a clinician's practice. They chronicle multiple successful treatment options (for example) and stratify the more successful and the less successful strategies based on scientific merit. They are not absolute, "must be followed" rules...

Guidelines documents are not tools to be used by external agencies to measure or control the care provided by clinicians. They are not medical-legal instruments or a "set of certainties" that must be followed in the assessment or treatment of the individual pathology in the individual patients we treat. While a powerful and comprehensive resource tool, guidelines and the recommendations contained therein do not necessarily represent "the answer" for the medical and surgical dilemmas we face with our many patients.

The concept of guidelines based on evidence- and expert-based consensus has influenced neurosurgery not only in the realm of clinical decision-making, but also in the realm of clinical education. Inspired in part by the growing body of clinical practice guidelines, a collaborative curriculum of educational guidelines was developed for neurosurgery trainees, based on the Self-Assessment in Neurologic Surgery educational tool.[75–77] The Self-Assessment in Neurologic Surgery curriculum is now available as a free resource template to aid program directors in defining a body of knowledge to be attained by neurosurgical trainees.

PEER REVIEW

Peer review continues to be a core feature of neurosurgery publishing that serves to safeguard the quality of the literature. A historical perspective shows that peer review has long been a venerated aspect of the neurosurgery publication process.[78] To maintain community standards, the neurosurgery editorial community has sought to provide guidance to peer reviewers in published form.[79] All original material published by *Neurosurgery* undergoes "rigorous multi-factorial double-blind peer-review by carefully selected panels of knowledgeable and dedicated individuals who are highly versed in the academic process and the given topic."[27] The *JNS* Publishing Group journals (*Journal of Neurosurgery, Journal of Neurosurgery: Spine, Journal of Neurosurgery: Pediatrics,* and *Neurosurgical Focus*) share a similar requirement.[80]

The generally accepted methodology of peer review has been sustained despite several controversies, including those that are ethical and cultural in nature. Sources of controversy and potential pitfalls in peer review have received much scrutiny.[78,81–84] The validity of the modern peer review process itself has been questioned by investigators, such as John Ioannidis, who have suggested that most clinical studies published in prestigious peer-reviewed journals are ultimately proved false.[85] The problem of articles retracted because of scientific misconduct muddies these waters still further. The journals with the highest impact factor tend to have the highest incidence of articles retracted because of scientific fraud, and in one study, only 6% of downstream citations were found to mention the cited article's retraction.[86] When these retracted articles continue to be cited, a worrisome cycle is set in motion. Conflicts of interest also represent a potentially pernicious source of reviewer bias.[81–83] It has become commonplace for journals and meetings to mitigate conflicts of interest, financial or otherwise, by mandating disclosures.[84,87,88] A concise definition of such conflicts is provided by the *Journal of Neurosurgery* submission guidelines: "a situation in which a person has competing loyalties or interests—financial, personal, or professional—that may make it difficult to fulfill his or her duties impartially."[80] To reduce bias and potential conflicts in analysis, both *Neurosurgery* and the *JNS* Publishing Group journals extend the strict requirement of disclosure to authors and peer reviewers.

As a whole, neurosurgery journals have maintained the peer review process as a cornerstone of literature quality, with a constantly evolving appreciation of ethical and procedural safeguards.

NEUROSURGERY JOURNALS AND FUTURE INNOVATIONS

In the past decade, neurosurgery journals have responded proactively to the technological and cultural changes sweeping the publishing industry. Business model innovations in publishing have led to opportunities and grave challenges. Among the most significant of these developments is the introduction of open access publishing, with the annual volume of articles published in open access journals increasing from 20,702 in 2000 to 340,130 in 2011, or 17% of all articles published.[89–91] Controversies over open access publishing have centered on concerns about endangering scholarly institutions and unethical behavior by investigators and journals alike.[91] Although open access publishing has not been significantly adopted within the world of neurosurgery, the globalization of neurosurgery has made it increasingly important to make evidence-based

Table 2
Notable neurosurgery guidelines and consensus statements

	Year	Publisher	Sponsor
Guidelines Endorsed by CNS			
Guidelines for the Management of Severe Traumatic Brain Injury (Third Edition)	2007	Journal of Neurotrauma[47]	Brain Trauma Foundation, AANS, CNS
Guidelines for the Treatment of Newly Diagnosed Glioblastoma	2008	Journal of Neuro-Oncology[48]	CNS/AANS Joint Section on Tumors
Clinical Guideline on the Treatment of Carpal Tunnel Syndrome	2008	American Academy of Orthopedic Surgeons[49]	American Academy of Orthopedic Surgeons
Evidence-Based Clinical Practice Parameter Guidelines for the Treatment of Patients with Metastatic Brain Tumor	2009	Journal of Neuro-Oncology[50]	CNS/AANS Joint Section on Tumors, in collaboration with McMaster Evidence-Based Practice Center
Guideline for the Surgical Management of Cervical Degenerative Disease	2009	Journal of Neurosurgery: Spine[51]	CNS/AANS Joint Section on Spine
Guidelines for the Management of Spontaneous Intracerebral Hemorrhage in Adults	2010	Stroke[52]	American Heart Association/American Stroke Association/American College of Cardiology
Guidelines for the Prevention of Stroke in Patients with Stroke and Transient Ischemic Attack (Secondary Stroke Prevention)	2011	Stroke[53]	American Heart Association/American Stroke Association
Guideline on the Management of Patients with Extracranial Carotid and Vertebral Artery Disease	2011	Circulation[54]	American Heart Association/American Stroke Association/American College of Cardiology and others
Guidelines for the Acute Medical Management of Severe Traumatic Brain Injury in Infants, Children, and Adolescents	2012	Pediatric Critical Care Medicine[55]	Brain Trauma Foundation
Guidelines for the Management of Aneurysmal Subarachnoid Hemorrhage	2012	Stroke[56]	American Heart Association/American Stroke Association/American College of Cardiology
Guidelines for the Management of Acute Cervical Spine and Spinal Cord Injuries	2013	Neurosurgery[57]	AANS/CNS Section on Disorders of the Spine and Peripheral Nerves
Guideline Update for the Performance of Fusion Procedures for Degenerative Disease of the Lumbar Spine	2014	Journal of Neurosurgery: Spine[58]	AANS/CNS Section on Disorders of the Spine and Peripheral Nerves

Consensus Statements Endorsed by CNS

Title	Year	Journal	Organization
Position Statement on Percutaneous Vertebral Augmentation	2007	Journal of Vascular and Interventional Radiology[59]	Multiple including AANS, CNS, American Society of Interventional and Therapeutic Neuroradiology
Reporting Standards for Angioplasty and Stent-Assisted Angioplasty for Intracranial Atherosclerosis	2010	Journal of NeuroInterventional Surgery[60]	Society of Interventional Radiology
Reporting Standards for Endovascular Repair of Saccular Intracranial Aneurysms	2010	American Journal of Neuroradiology[61]	Society of Interventional Radiology
Diagnosis and Management of Cerebral Venous Thrombosis	2011	Stroke[62]	American Heart Association/American Stroke Association/American College of Cardiology
Key Data Elements and Definitions for Peripheral Atherosclerotic Vascular Disease	2012	Journal of the American College of Cardiology[63]	American College of Cardiology/American Heart Association
An Updated Definition of Stroke for the 21st Century: A Statement for Healthcare Professionals from the American Heart Association/American Stroke Association	2013	Stroke[63]	American Heart Association/American Stroke Association

Guidelines and Statements Reviewed but not Endorsed by CNS

Title	Year	Journal	Organization
Occupational Medicine Practice Guidelines, Low Back Disorders	2007	American College of Occupational and Environmental Medicine[64]	American College of Occupational and Environmental Medicine
Evaluation and Management of Adult Patients Presenting to the Emergency Department With Acute Headache	2008	Annals of Emergency Medicine[65]	American College of Emergency Physicians
Occupational Medicine Practice Guidelines, Chronic Pain	2008	American College of Occupational and Environmental Medicine[64]	American College of Occupational and Environmental Medicine
Occupational Medicine Practice Guidelines, Hand, Wrist, and Forearm Disorders	2009	American College of Occupational and Environmental Medicine[64]	American College of Occupational and Environmental Medicine
Treatment of Symptomatic Osteoporotic Spinal Compression Fractures	2011	Journal of the American Academy of Orthopedic Surgeons[66]	American Academy of Orthopedic Surgeons

Other Notable Neurosurgery-Related Guidelines[a]

Title	Year	Journal	Organization
Guidelines for Field Management of Combat-Related Head Trauma	2005	Brain Trauma Foundation[67]	Brain Trauma Foundation
Guidelines for the Surgical Management of Traumatic Brain Injury	2006	Neurosurgery[68]	N/A
Guidelines for Prehospital Management of Traumatic Brain Injury, Second Edition	2007	Journal of Neurotrauma[69]	Brain Trauma Foundation, AANS/CNS Joint Section on Neurotrauma and Critical Care

[a] The list of "other" neurosurgery-related guidelines is adapted from AANS - Clinical Guidelines Repository. Available at: http://www.aans.org/Education and Meetings/Clinical Guidelines.aspx. Accessed October 2, 2014, after omission of duplicates.
Data from Refs. [47–69]

information available to those in developing nations. Alternatives to journals as sources of clinical information—once limited to professional conferences and books—now include Web sites, social media, and nontraditional publishing models based on the early examples of ArXiv.org and Wikipedia, which have achieved some success by supplementing editor-mediated peer review with crowd intelligence. Free online initiatives by professional societies, such as the CNS University of Neurosurgery,[92] NeuroWiki,[93] AANS Operative Grand Rounds,[94] and the AANS Neurosurgery YouTube channel,[95] have now expanded the reach of global neurosurgery education.

In the context of these technological and business model challenges, neurosurgery journals have stayed competitive and relevant. Amid an ocean of non–peer reviewed information, journals have found themselves in the position of being arbiters of authenticity. They have been early adopters of new technologies to disseminate their original research publications, such as podcasting, QR codes, videos, electronic editions formatted for tablets, and mobile applications. The ubiquity of Internet access has changed neurosurgery publishing in beneficial ways, including facilitating more widespread access to content.

Perhaps most importantly, this ready availability of evidence-based information at the point of care, particularly in electronic format and on mobile devices, has allowed it to become a day-to-day element of neurosurgery training. The feasibility of teaching evidence-based practice to residents in neurosurgery and other surgical subspecialties has previously been confirmed.[96–98] Building on the long tradition of the academic journal club in neurosurgery training,[99,100] in 2012 *Neurosurgery* launched a Neurosurgery Journal Club enabling residents and fellows to perform critical commentaries on previously published original research.[101] Structured as a competition, this quarterly feature is designed to hone the next generation of peer reviewers and editors by engaging neurosurgery trainees in the editorial process, and to contribute to trainees' understanding of statistical evidence.

SUMMARY

Since their rise to prominence in the twentieth century, neurosurgery journals have played an active role in improving the quality of the neurosurgical literature. Over the past two decades, as the number and variety of journals devoted to neurosurgery has increased, this role has expanded to improve the quality of care by incorporating an evidence-based view of neurosurgery practice. The explicit endorsement of reporting guidelines, such as CONSORT and PRISMA, promises to generate much-needed improvements in the quality of neurosurgery research articles. Reflecting secular trends in the world of evidence-based medicine, neurosurgery journals have facilitated the organization of knowledge into clinically useful forms via the publication of meta-analyses and dissemination of clinical practice guidelines. Peer review continues to be a core feature of neurosurgery publishing, with attendant ethical and procedural safeguards. Finally, neurosurgery journals have spearheaded innovative responses to cultural and technological changes, including initiatives to deliver high-quality research in electronic formats and support the education of future neurosurgery investigators.

REFERENCES

1. Feindel W. Osler and the "medico-chirurgical neurologists": Horsley, Cushing, and Penfield. J Neurosurg 2003;99(1):188–99. http://dx.doi.org/10.3171/jns.2003.99.1.0188.
2. Laws ER. The binding influence of the *Journal of Neurosurgery* on the evolution of neurosurgery. J Neurosurg 1994;81(2):317–21.
3. Wilkins RH. Birth of a journal: the origin and early years of *Neurosurgery*. Neurosurgery 1982;10(6):820–6.
4. Cushing H. The binding influence of a library on a subdividing profession. Science 1929;70(1821):485–91. http://dx.doi.org/10.1126/science.70.1821.485.
5. Haines SJ, Hodge CJ, Chakrabarti I, et al. Evidence-based neurosurgery. Neurosurgery 2003;52:36–47. http://dx.doi.org/10.1097/00006123-200301000-00004.
6. Bandopadhayay P, Goldschlager T, Rosenfeld JV. The role of evidence-based medicine in neurosurgery. J Clin Neurosci 2008;15:373–8. http://dx.doi.org/10.1016/j.jocn.2007.08.014.
7. NEUROSURGIC.com (Resources: Neurosurgical journals). Available at: http://www.neurosurgic.com/index.php?option=com_content&view=category&layout=blog&id=101&Itemid=465. Accessed October 2, 2014.
8. Madhugiri VS, Ambekar S, Strom SF, et al. A technique to identify core journals for neurosurgery using citation scatter analysis and the Bradford distribution across neurosurgery journals. J Neurosurg 2013;119:1274–87. http://dx.doi.org/10.3171/2013.8.JNS122379.
9. Oyesiku N. Operative neurosurgery: a new beginning. Neurosurgery 2013;73(1):2013.
10. Garfield E. The history and meaning of the journal impact factor. JAMA 2006;295:90–3. http://dx.doi.org/10.1001/jama.295.1.90.

11. Vanclay JK. Impact factor: outdated artefact or stepping-stone to journal certification? Scientometrics 2012;92:211–38. http://dx.doi.org/10.1007/s11192-011-0561-0.

12. Ponce FA, Lozano AM. Highly cited works in neurosurgery. Part I: the 100 top-cited papers in neurosurgical journals. J Neurosurg 2010;112(2):223–32. http://dx.doi.org/10.3171/2009.12.JNS091599.

13. Ponce FA, Lozano AM. Highly cited works in neurosurgery. Part II: the citation classics. J Neurosurg 2010;112(2):233–46. http://dx.doi.org/10.3171/2009.12.JNS091600.

14. Chan A-W, Hróbjartsson A, Haahr MT, et al. Empirical evidence for selective reporting of outcomes in randomized trials: comparison of protocols to published articles. JAMA 2004;291:2457–65. http://dx.doi.org/10.1001/jama.291.20.2457.

15. Page MJ, McKenzie JE, Kirkham J, et al. Bias due to selective inclusion and reporting of outcomes and analyses in systematic reviews of randomised trials of healthcare interventions. Cochrane Database Syst Rev 2014;(10). http://dx.doi.org/10.1002/14651858.MR000035.pub2. MR000035.

16. Schulz KF, Altman DG, Moher D. CONSORT 2010 statement: updated guidelines for reporting parallel group randomised trials. BMJ 2010;340:c332. Available at: http://www.pubmedcentral.nih.gov/articlerender.fcgi?artid=2844940&tool=pmcentrez&rendertype=abstract. Accessed August 17, 2014.

17. Patsopoulos NA, Analatos AA, Ioannidis JP. Relative citation impact of various study designs in the health sciences. JAMA 2005;293:2362–6. http://dx.doi.org/10.1097/01.AOG.0000173954.21555.b6.

18. Gnanalingham KK, Tysome J, Martinez-Canca J, et al. Quality of clinical studies in neurosurgical journals: signs of improvement over three decades. J Neurosurg 2005;103:439–43. http://dx.doi.org/10.3171/jns.2005.103.3.0439.

19. Tiruvoipati R, Balasubramanian SP, Atturu G, et al. Improving the quality of reporting randomized controlled trials in cardiothoracic surgery: the way forward. J Thorac Cardiovasc Surg 2006;132:233–40. http://dx.doi.org/10.1016/j.jtcvs.2005.10.056.

20. Horton R. Surgical research or comic opera: questions, but few answers. Lancet 1996;347:984–5. http://dx.doi.org/10.1016/S0140-6736(96)90137-3.

21. Vranos G, Tatsioni A, Polyzoidis K, et al. Randomized trials of neurosurgical interventions: a systematic appraisal. Neurosurgery 2004;55:18–25. http://dx.doi.org/10.1227/01.NEU.0000126873.00845.A7.

22. Scholler K, Licht S, Tonn JC, et al. Randomized controlled trials in neurosurgery: how good are we? Acta Neurochir (Wien) 2009;151:519–27. http://dx.doi.org/10.1007/s00701-009-0280-y.

23. Atkins D, Best D, Briss PA, et al. Grading quality of evidence and strength of recommendations. BMJ 2004;328(7454):1490. http://dx.doi.org/10.1136/bmj.328.7454.1490.

24. Shea BJ, Grimshaw JM, Wells GA, et al. Development of AMSTAR: a measurement tool to assess the methodological quality of systematic reviews. BMC Med Res Methodol 2007;7:10. http://dx.doi.org/10.1186/1471-2288-7-10.

25. Moher D, Liberati A, Tetzlaff J, et al. Preferred reporting items for systematic reviews and meta-analyses: the PRISMA statement. PLoS Med 2009;6(7):e1000097. http://dx.doi.org/10.1371/journal.pmed.1000097.

26. Barker FG, Oyesiku N. The registrar: improving the quality of research reports in neurosurgery. Neurosurgery 2011;68(1):1–5.

27. Neurosurgery: instructions for authors. Available at: http://journals.lww.com/neurosurgery/Documents/Files and Resources/For Authors/Instructions for Authors (Effective Jan 1 2011).pdf. Accessed October 3, 2014.

28. Stroup DF, Berlin JA, Morton SC, et al. Meta-analysis of observational studies in epidemiology: a proposal for reporting. Meta-analysis Of Observational Studies in Epidemiology (MOOSE) group. JAMA 2000;283(15):2008–12. Available at: http://www.ncbi.nlm.nih.gov/pubmed/10789670. Accessed July 11, 2014.

29. Bossuyt PM, Reitsma JB, Bruns DE, et al. Towards complete and accurate reporting of studies of diagnostic accuracy: the STARD initiative. BMJ 2003;326(7379):41–4. Available at: http://www.pubmedcentral.nih.gov/articlerender.fcgi?artid=1124931&tool=pmcentrez&rendertype=abstract. Accessed September 17, 2014.

30. Von Elm E, Altman DG, Egger M, et al. The Strengthening the Reporting of Observational Studies in Epidemiology (STROBE) statement: guidelines for reporting observational studies. PLoS Med 2007;4(10):e296. http://dx.doi.org/10.1371/journal.pmed.0040296.

31. The EQUATOR Network. Available at: http://www.equator-network.org/. Accessed October 2, 2014.

32. Cochrane Reviews (The Cochrane Collaboration). Available at: http://www.cochrane.org/cochrane-reviews. Accessed October 2, 2014.

33. Yarascavitch BA, Chuback JE, Almenawer SA, et al. Levels of evidence in the neurosurgical literature: more tribulations than trials. Neurosurgery 2012;71(6):1131–7. http://dx.doi.org/10.1227/NEU.0b013e318271bc99 [discussion: 1137–8].

34. Rothoerl RD, Klier J, Woertgen C, et al. Level of evidence and citation index in current neurosurgical publications. Neurosurg Rev 2003;26:257–61. http://dx.doi.org/10.1007/s10143-003-0270-0.

35. Klimo P, Thompson CJ, Ragel BT, et al. Methodology and reporting of meta-analyses in the neurosurgical literature: response. J Neurosurg 2014;

120(4):794–5. Available at: http://www.ncbi.nlm.nih.gov/pubmed/24809077.

36. Sampson JH, Barker FG. Methodology and reporting of meta-analyses in the neurosurgical literature [editorial]. J Neurosurg 2014;120(4):791–5. http://dx.doi.org/10.3171/2013.10.JNS13724.

37. Nesvick CL, Thompson CJ, Boop FA, et al. Case-control studies in neurosurgery. J Neurosurg 2014;121(2):285–96. http://dx.doi.org/10.3171/2014.5.JNS132329.

38. Sánchez-Thorin JC, Cortés MC, Montenegro M, et al. The quality of reporting of randomized clinical trials published in *Ophthalmology*. Ophthalmology 2001;108:410–5. http://dx.doi.org/10.1016/S0161-6420(00)00500-5.

39. Hewitt C, Hahn S, Torgerson DJ, et al. Adequacy and reporting of allocation concealment: review of recent trials published in four general medical journals. BMJ 2005;330:1057–8. http://dx.doi.org/10.1136/bmj.38413.576713.AE.

40. Hill CL, LaValley MP, Felson DT. Secular changes in the quality of published randomized clinical trials in rheumatology. Arthritis Rheum 2002;46:779–84. http://dx.doi.org/10.1002/art.512.

41. Kane RL, Wang J, Garrard J. Reporting in randomized clinical trials improved after adoption of the CONSORT statement. J Clin Epidemiol 2007;60:241–9. http://dx.doi.org/10.1016/j.jclinepi.2006.06.016.

42. Montori VM, Bhandari M, Devereaux PJ, et al. In the dark: the reporting of blinding status in randomized controlled trials. J Clin Epidemiol 2002;55:787–90. http://dx.doi.org/10.1016/S0895-4356(02)00446-8.

43. Devereaux PJ, Manns BJ, Ghali WA, et al. The reporting of methodological factors in randomized controlled trials and the association with a journal policy to promote adherence to the Consolidated Standards of Reporting Trials (CONSORT) checklist. Control Clin Trials 2002;23:380–8. http://dx.doi.org/10.1016/S0197-2456(02)00214-3.

44. Moher D, Jones A, Lepage L. Use of the CONSORT statement and quality of reports of randomized trials: a comparative before-and-after evaluation. JAMA 2001;285:1992–5. http://dx.doi.org/10.1001/jama.285.15.1992.

45. Plint AC, Moher D, Morrison A, et al. Does the CONSORT checklist improve the quality of reports of randomised controlled trials? A systematic review. Med J Aust 2006;185:263–7. pii:pli11098_fm.

46. Guidelines | Congress of Neurological Surgeons. Available at: https://www.cns.org/guidelines. Accessed October 2, 2014.

47. Bullock MR, Povlishock JT. Guidelines for the management of severe traumatic brain injury. J Neurotrauma 2007;24(Suppl 1):S1–106. http://dx.doi.org/10.1089/neu.2007.9999.

48. Olson JJ, Ryken T. Guidelines for the treatment of newly diagnosed glioblastoma: introduction. J Neurooncol 2008;89(3):255–8. http://dx.doi.org/10.1007/s11060-008-9595-4.

49. Keith MW, Masear V, Chung KC, et al. American Academy of Orthopaedic Surgeons clinical practice guideline on the treatment of carpal tunnel syndrome. J Bone Joint Surg Am 2010;92(1):218–9. http://dx.doi.org/10.2106/JBJS.I.00642.

50. Kalkanis SN, Linskey ME. Evidence-based clinical practice parameter guidelines for the treatment of patients with metastatic brain tumors: introduction. J Neurooncol 2010;96(1):7–10. http://dx.doi.org/10.1007/s11060-009-0065-4.

51. Matz PG, Anderson PA, Kaiser MG, et al. Introduction and methodology: guidelines for the surgical management of cervical degenerative disease. J Neurosurg Spine 2009;11(2):101–3. http://dx.doi.org/10.3171/2009.1.SPINE08712.

52. Morgenstern LB, Hemphill JC, Anderson C, et al. Guidelines for the management of spontaneous intracerebral hemorrhage: a guideline for healthcare professionals from the American Heart Association/American Stroke Association. Stroke 2010;41(9):2108–29. http://dx.doi.org/10.1161/STR.0b013e3181ec611b.

53. Kernan WN, Ovbiagele B, Black HR, et al. Guidelines for the prevention of stroke in patients with stroke and transient ischemic attack: a guideline for healthcare professionals from the American Heart Association/American Stroke Association. Stroke 2014;45(7):2160–236. http://dx.doi.org/10.1161/STR.0000000000000024.

54. Brott TG, Halperin JL, Abbara S, et al. 2011 ASA/ACCF/AHA/AANN/AANS/ACR/ASNR/CNS/SAIP/SCAI/SIR/SNIS/SVM/SVS guideline on the management of patients with extracranial carotid and vertebral artery disease. A report of the American College of Cardiology Foundation/American Heart Association Task Force. Circulation 2011;124(4):e54–130. http://dx.doi.org/10.1161/CIR.0b013e31820d8c98.

55. Kochanek PM, Carney N, Adelson PD, et al. Guidelines for the acute medical management of severe traumatic brain injury in infants, children, and adolescents–second edition. Pediatr Crit Care Med 2012;13(Suppl 1):S1–82. http://dx.doi.org/10.1097/PCC.0b013e31823f435c.

56. Connolly ES, Rabinstein A, Carhuapoma JR, et al. Guidelines for the management of aneurysmal subarachnoid hemorrhage: a guideline for healthcare professionals from the American Heart Association/American Stroke Association. Stroke 2012;43(6):1711–37. http://dx.doi.org/10.1161/STR.0b013e3182587839.

57. Hadley MN, Walters BC. Introduction to the guidelines for the management of acute cervical spine and spinal cord injuries. Neurosurgery 2013;

72(Suppl 2):5–16. http://dx.doi.org/10.1227/NEU.0b013e3182773549.

58. Kaiser MG, Eck JC, Groff MW, et al. Guideline update for the performance of fusion procedures for degenerative disease of the lumbar spine. Part 1: introduction and methodology. J Neurosurg Spine 2014;21:2–6. http://dx.doi.org/10.3171/2014.4.SPINE 14257.

59. Jensen ME, McGraw JK, Cardella JF, et al. Position statement on percutaneous vertebral augmentation: a consensus statement developed by the American Society of Interventional and Therapeutic Neuroradiology, Society of Interventional Radiology, American Association of Neurological Surgeons/Congress. J Vasc Interv Radiol 2007;18(3):325–30. http://dx.doi.org/10.1016/j.jvir.2007.01.014.

60. Schumacher HC, Meyers PM, Higashida RT, et al. Reporting standards for angioplasty and stent-assisted angioplasty for intracranial atherosclerosis. J Neurointerv Surg 2010;2(4):324–40. http://dx.doi.org/10.1136/jnis.2010.002345.

61. Meyers PM, Schumacher HC, Higashida RT, et al. Reporting standards for endovascular repair of saccular intracranial cerebral aneurysms. Stroke 2009;40(5):e366–79. http://dx.doi.org/10.1161/STROKEAHA.108.527572.

62. Saposnik G, Barinagarrementeria F, Brown RD, et al. Diagnosis and management of cerebral venous thrombosis: a statement for healthcare professionals from the American Heart Association/American Stroke Association. Stroke 2011;42(4):1158–92. http://dx.doi.org/10.1161/STR.0b013e31 820a8364.

63. Sacco RL, Kasner SE, Broderick JP, et al. An updated definition of stroke for the 21st century: a statement for healthcare professionals from the American Heart Association/American Stroke Association. Stroke 2013;44(7):2064–89. http://dx.doi.org/10.1161/STR.0b013e318296aeca.

64. American College of Occupational and Environmental Medicine (ACOEM). Available at: http://www.acoem.org/default.aspx. Accessed October 7, 2014.

65. Edlow JA, Panagos PD, Godwin SA, et al. Clinical policy: critical issues in the evaluation and management of adult patients presenting to the emergency department with acute headache. Ann Emerg Med 2008;52(4):407–36. http://dx.doi.org/10.1016/j.annemergmed.2008.07.001.

66. Esses SI, McGuire R, Jenkins J, et al. The treatment of symptomatic osteoporotic spinal compression fractures. J Am Acad Orthop Surg 2011;19:176–82.

67. Knuth T, Letarte PB, Ling G, et al. Guidelines for the field management of combat-related head trauma. New York: The Brain Trauma Foundation 2005.

68. Bullock MR, Chesnut R, Ghajar J, et al. Introduction (guidelines for surgical management of traumatic brain injury). Neurosurgery 2006;58(Suppl). http://dx.doi.org/10.1227/01.NEU.0000210361.83548.D0.S2-1–S2-3.

69. Badjatia N, Carney N, Crocco TJ, et al. Guidelines for prehospital management of traumatic brain injury, 2nd edition. Prehosp Emerg Care 2007;12(Suppl 1):S1–52.

70. Hamani C, Pilitsis J, Rughani AI, et al. Deep brain stimulation for obsessive-compulsive disorder: systematic review and evidence-based guideline sponsored by the American Society for Stereotactic and Functional Neurosurgery and the Congress of Neurological Surgeons (CNS) and endorsed by the CNS. Neurosurgery 2014;75(4):327–33. http://dx.doi.org/10.1227/NEU.000000000 0000499.

71. Kreiner DS, Hwang SW, Easa JE, et al. An evidence-based clinical guideline for the diagnosis and treatment of lumbar disc herniation with radiculopathy. Spine J 2014;14(1):180–91. http://dx.doi.org/10.1016/j.spinee.2013.08.003.

72. Marmarou A, Bergsneider M, Relkin N, et al. Development of guidelines for idiopathic normal-pressure hydrocephalus: introduction. Neurosurgery 2005;57(3). http://dx.doi.org/10.1227/01.NEU.0000168188.25559.0E. S2-1–S2-3.

73. Linskey ME, Olson JJ, Mitchell LS, et al. Clinical practice guidelines in the AANS/CNS section on tumors: past, present and future directions. J Neurooncol 2014;119(3):557–68. http://dx.doi.org/10.1007/s11060-014-1497-z.

74. Carney N, Ghajar J, Jagoda A. Executive summary of concussion guidelines step 1: systematic review of prevalent indicators. Neurosurgery 2014;75(Suppl 1):S1–2. http://dx.doi.org/10.1227/NEU.0000000000000434.

75. Ragel BT, Asher AL, Selden N, et al. Self-assessment in neurological surgery: the SANS wired white paper. Neurosurgery 2006;59:759–65. http://dx.doi.org/10.1227/01.NEU.0000232864.73007.38.

76. SANS Resident Curriculum Guidelines for Neurosurgery. Available at: http://w3.cns.org/education/resCur/index2.asp. Accessed October 2, 2014.

77. Sheehan J, Starke RM, Pouratian N, et al. Identification of knowledge gaps in neurosurgery through analysis of responses to the Self-Assessment in Neurological Surgery (SANS). World Neurosurg 2014;81(2):229–33. http://dx.doi.org/10.1016/j.wneu.2012.05.033.

78. Apuzzo ML. Peer-review: a citadel under siege. Neurosurgery 2008;63(5):821. http://dx.doi.org/10.1227/01.NEU.0000339200.39507.A7.

79. Apuzzo ML. Ideas regarding developing, submitting, reviewing, and publishing a scientific manuscript: an editor's perspective. World Neurosurg 2014;81(3–4):443–6. http://dx.doi.org/10.1016/j.wneu.2014.01.013.

80. Editorial and Publishing Policies of the JNS Publishing Group (JNSPG). Available at: http://jns.msubmit.net/html/JNSPG_Editorial_and_Publishing_Policies.pdf. Accessed October 3, 2014.

81. Firlik KS, Firlik AD. The peer-review process of the *Journal of Neurosurgery*. J Neurosurg 1999; 90:364–70. http://dx.doi.org/10.3171/jns.1999.90.2.0364.

82. Curfman GD, Morrissey S, Annas GJ, et al. Peer review in the balance. N Engl J Med 2008;358(21): 2276–7.

83. Adler JR. A new age of peer reviewed scientific journals. Surg Neurol Int 2012;3:145. http://dx.doi.org/10.4103/2152-7806.103889.

84. Ferris LE, Fletcher RH. Conflict of interest in peer-reviewed medical journals: the World Association of Medical Editors (WAME) position on a challenging problem. Neurosurgery 2010;66(4): 629–30. http://dx.doi.org/10.1227/01.neu.0000369904.38343.e4.

85. Ioannidis J. Why most published research findings are false. PLoS Med 2005;2:e124. http://dx.doi.org/10.1371/journal.pmed.0020124.

86. Budd JM, Coble ZC, Anderson KM. Retracted publications in biomedicine: cause for concern. Assoc Coll 2011;390–5. Available at: https://surgery.med.uky.edu/sites/default/files/retracted_publicatio.pdf. Accessed October 3, 2014.

87. Patel AA, Whang PG, White AP, et al. Pitfalls in the publication of scientific literature: a road map to manage conflict of interest and other ethical challenges. J Neurosurg 2011;114:21–6. http://dx.doi.org/10.3171/2010.8.JNS091834.

88. Lundh A, Barbateskovic M, Hróbjartsson A, et al. Conflicts of interest at medical journals: the influence of industry-supported randomised trials on journal impact factors and revenue - cohort study. PLoS Med 2010;7. http://dx.doi.org/10.1371/journal.pmed.1000354.

89. Beall J. Predatory publishers are corrupting open access. Nature 2012;489(7415):179. http://dx.doi.org/10.1038/489179a.

90. Frank M. Open but not free: publishing in the 21st century. N Engl J Med 2013;368(9):787–9. http://dx.doi.org/10.1056/NEJMp1211410.

91. Apuzzo MLJ. Acquiring wisdom in the information age. World Neurosurg 2013;79(5–6):595–6. http://dx.doi.org/10.1016/j.wneu.2013.03.041.

92. Education | Congress of Neurological Surgeons. Available at: https://www.cns.org/education. Accessed October 4, 2014.

93. Congress of Neurological Surgeons NeuroWiki. Available at: http://wiki.cns.org/wiki/index.php/Main_Page. Accessed October 4, 2014.

94. AANS Operative Grand Rounds. Available at: http://www.aans.org/Education and Meetings/Master Series/AANS Operative Grand Rounds.aspx. Accessed October 4, 2014.

95. AANS Neurosurgery Channel on YouTube. Available at: https://www.youtube.com/user/AANSNeurosurgery. Accessed October 4, 2014.

96. Burneo JG, Jenkins ME. Teaching evidence-based clinical practice to neurology and neurosurgery residents. Clin Neurol Neurosurg 2007;109(5):418–21. http://dx.doi.org/10.1016/j.clineuro.2007.03.001.

97. Haines SJ, Nicholas JS. Teaching evidence-based medicine to surgical subspecialty residents. J Am Coll Surg 2003;197:285–9. http://dx.doi.org/10.1016/S1072-7515(03)00114-5.

98. Ahmadi N, McKenzie ME, MacLean A, et al. Teaching evidence based medicine to surgery residents: is journal club the best format? A systematic review of the literature. J Surg Educ 2012;69:91–100. http://dx.doi.org/10.1016/j.jsurg.2011.07.004.

99. Rajpal S, Resnick DK, Başkaya MK. The role of the journal club in neurosurgical training. Neurosurgery 2007;61:397–402. http://dx.doi.org/10.1227/01.NEU.0000280003.49319.F1.

100. Mobbs RJ. The importance of the journal club for neurosurgical trainees. J Clin Neurosci 2004;11:57–8. http://dx.doi.org/10.1016/S0967-5868(03)00074-2.

101. Amadio J. Introducing Neurosurgery's Journal Club. Neurosurgery 2012;71(5):907–8. http://dx.doi.org/10.1227/NEU.0b013e3182759804.

Comanagement Hospitalist Services for Neurosurgery

Hugo Quinny Cheng, MD

KEYWORDS

- Comanagement • Medical consultation • Hospitalists • Physician satisfaction • Cost effectiveness
- Care coordination • Perioperative management

KEY POINTS

- Comanagement is a rapidly growing care model that lets the hospitalist share the responsibility, authority, and accountability for the care of the surgical patient.
- Features of comanagement include advance negotiation of an agreement between hospitalists and surgeons, criteria for automatic hospitalist engagement, and broad scope of practice and for the hospitalist.
- Implementation of comanagement enhances provider satisfaction and the efficiency of care, but has not been shown to improve clinical outcomes.
- Potential pitfalls of comanagement include fragmented care and disengagement of the surgeon; careful planning prior to implementation of comanagement can reduce these risks.

INTRODUCTION

Surgeons have long depended on medical specialists (either general internists or subspecialists) to provide advice and assistance in caring for their patients. In this traditional consultation relationship, medical specialists have limited roles and responsibilities. They saw patients only at the surgeon's request and focused on the narrow topic of the consultation question. They left recommendations for care but deferred to the surgeon to implement them. While traditional consultation still exists, a more collaborative comanagement model is gaining popularity.

EMERGENCE OF HOSPITALIST COMANAGEMENT
Growth of Comanagement

Comanagement is a negotiated relationship that lets the medical specialist share the responsibility, authority, and accountability for the care

of the surgical patient. Although any medical specialty can comanage surgical patients, this role has largely fallen to hospitalists. Hospital medicine emerged in the 1990s and has become the fastest growing medical specialty.[1] Because of their availability to care for inpatients, familiarity with the hospital's operations, and capability of managing a broad range of medical problems, hospitalists are the natural providers of perioperative care. As a result, comanagement of surgical patients by hospitalists increased by over 11% per year between 2001 and 2006.[2] Factors contributing to this growth include:

- Patients once deemed too old or medically complicated to undergo elective surgery are now routinely having operations. This requires more frequent and intensive involvement of physicians able to provide perioperative medical care.
- Competing responsibilities and financial incentives reduce the time surgeons can spend

Division of Hospital Medicine, University of California, San Francisco, UCSF Box 0131, 533 Parnassus Avenue, Suite U-101, San Francisco, CA 94143-0131, USA
E-mail address: quinny@medicine.ucsf.edu

Neurosurg Clin N Am 26 (2015) 295–300
http://dx.doi.org/10.1016/j.nec.2014.11.004
1042-3680/15/$ – see front matter © 2015 Elsevier Inc. All rights reserved.

taking care of postoperative patients on the wards. In teaching hospitals, duty hour restrictions also limit resident availability.

- Surgeons are more willing to share responsibility for the management of their patients' medical problems. A 2007 study found only a minority of surgeons believed that consultations should be limited to a specific question or that consultants should not write orders without prior discussion. A majority of surgeons desired a comanagement relationship.[3]
- Medical centers have promoted hospitalist comanagement, hoping to improve efficiency and patient safety, as hospitalists have demonstrated in the care of medical patients.[4]

Features of Comanagement

The specific features of a hospitalist comanagement service depend on the needs of the surgeons and resources available to the hospital medicine group. However, comanagement differs from consultation in several aspects (**Table 1**).

Comanagement relationships are negotiated in advance

The surgeon and hospitalist must have a prior understanding of their respective roles and responsibilities. These are described in a comanagement agreement. This is particularly important for management issues that require shared responsibility, such as discharge planning.

Comanaging hospitalists can select which patients to see and what problems they will manage

The hospitalist can automatically see patients who meet predetermined clinical criteria, which were negotiated as part the comanagement agreement. These might include admitting diagnoses (eg, all patients with subarachnoid or subdural hemorrhage), medical comorbidities (eg, coronary artery disease or diabetes), or demographic features (eg, age over 70 years or admission to a critical care unit). Instead of depending on the surgeon to formulate a specific question, comanaging hospitalists have broad latitude to address most medical issues they identify.

Comanagement allows the hospitalist to write most orders without the surgeon's approval

Exceptions to the hospitalist's order writing privileges, such as initiation of anticoagulation, are delineated in the comanagement agreement.

Comanagement may include nonclinical collaboration

Although comanagement focuses on direct patient care, a successful relationship often evolves into a broader alliance between surgeons and hospitalists. Hospital medicine groups often play key roles in patient safety and hospital quality improvement endeavors. Surgeons who may have less experience or availability to address these concerns have collaborated with hospitalists to optimize their systems of care. Surgeons and hospitalists may also provide reciprocal education through conferences. In academic settings, comanagement relationships have also yielded joint research and publication.

Comanagement can occur whether a patient is under the care of the surgeon or hospitalist as the attending physician of record. In teaching hospitals, the surgeon typically remains the primary attending physician, with the hospitalist charting and billing as a consultant. In community hospitals, however, these roles are sometimes reversed. The hospitalist may have primary

Table 1
Differences between consultation and comanagement

	Traditional Consultation	Comanagement
Relationship between surgeon and consultant	Informal, ad hoc	Formal, negotiated in advance
Patient selection	Only at surgeon's request	Hospitalist sees all patients who meet predetermined clinical criteria
Consultant's focus	Narrow consultation question chosen by surgeon	Comprehensive care of medical issues determined by surgeon or hospitalist
Consultant's scope of practice	Leave recommendations	Write orders without prior approval in most circumstances
Discharge planning	Surgeon's responsibility	Shared responsibility
Nonclinical roles	None	Surgeon and hospitalist may collaborate on quality improvement, research, and education projects

responsibility for the patient, and the surgeon's role is limited to performing the operation and managing care directly related to the surgical diagnosis.

COMANAGEMENT EXPERIENCE FOR NEUROSURGICAL PATIENTS

A 2010 study found that comanagement by a generalist was most common among general and orthopedic surgery patients, among whom the incidence was 29% and 28% respectively.[2] The incidence of comanagement among neurosurgical patients is unknown. Compared with orthopedic surgery in particular, there have been few published descriptions of comanagement services for these patients.

Description of a Hospitalist Comanagement with Neurosurgery Service

In 2007, the Department of Neurologic Surgery and the Department of Medicine's Division of Hospital Medicine at the University of California, San Francisco (UCSF) collaborated to create the Comanagement with Neurosurgery Service (CNS). The service is staffed 365 days per year by faculty hospitalists, without the involvement of medicine trainees. In the first 18 months after implementation, CNS hospitalists provided care to 988 (29%) of the 3393 adult patients admitted to the neurologic surgery service.[5]

Patient selection
In addition to seeing patients at the request of the neurosurgeons, the CNS hospitalist screens the chart of all patients within 24 hours of admission. Patients with any of the following conditions are automatically evaluated by the hospitalist: coronary artery disease, heart failure, chronic obstructive lung disease, chronic kidney disease, cirrhosis, dementia, diabetes requiring insulin, and treatment with anticoagulants. The hospitalist may also manage other patients without prior invitation based on their clinical judgment.

Scope of practice
The CNS hospitalist is generally responsible for their patients' chronic or acute medical problems that are not directly related to the neurosurgical diagnosis. Some exceptions include hyponatremia, due to differences in management strategies between internal medicine and neurosurgery, and diabetes insipidis following transsphenoidal operations, which neurosurgical residents are trained to manage with the assistance of a neuroendocrinologist. Similarly, antiepileptic and glucocorticoid therapy remain the purview of the surgery team.

The hospitalist writes orders directly and may consult other specialists without prior approval. Initiation of anticoagulant or antiplatelet therapy and invasive procedures require discussion with the surgical attending physician.

Care coordination
The CNS hospitalist routinely engages with ancillary staff, including rehabilitation therapists, clinical pharmacists, and case managers to provide advice and learn about their concerns. Completion of discharge materials remains the responsibility of the neurosurgical service, with input from the hospitalist as needed.

Other collaboration
Subsequent to the implementation of the CNS, neurosurgeons and hospitalists have conducted clinical research and published numerous manuscripts together. One hospitalist receives salary support from the Department of Neurosurgery to direct quality and safety efforts. In addition to having hospitalists participate in neurosurgery educational conferences, neurosurgery residents have rotated on the CNS to gain experience with perioperative medicine.

OUTCOMES OF COMANAGEMENT

Despite the rapid growth of comanagement, relatively few data exist on its effect on outcomes compared with more traditional medical consultation. Published studies include only 1 randomized trial and several retrospective cohort studies comparing comanagement with consultation (**Table 2**). At UCSF, outcomes on the neurosurgical surgery service before and after implementation of the CNS were examined and can be compared with reports from other comanagement services.[5]

Clinical Outcomes

Overall mortality and 30-day readmission rates did not change after creation of the CNS. This finding is consistent with other published descriptions of comanagement services, where important clinical outcomes were unaffected by the care model. Comanagement by pediatric hospitalists did not reduce the readmission rate in pediatric neurosurgical patients compared with a historical control group.[6] In orthopedic surgery patients undergoing elective arthroplasty, randomization to care by a comanagement team reduced the incidence of minor complications (urinary tract infection, electrolyte abnormalities, fever). However, the mortality and readmission rates and incidence of more serious complications (eg, myocardial infarction, and venous thromboembolism) remained the

Table 2
Outcomes from surgeon and hospitalist comanagement

Population	Clinical Outcomes	Economic Outcomes
Neurosurgery[5]	No effect on mortality or readmission	LOS unchanged Costs reduced
Neurosurgery (pediatric)[6]	No effect on readmission	LOS reduced
Elective arthroplasty[7]	Minor complications reduced No effect on major complications, mortality, or readmission	Adjusted LOS reduced Costs unchanged
Hip fracture[8]	No effect on mortality or readmission	LOS reduced
Spinal fusion (pediatric)[9]	NA	LOS reduced
Orthopedic[10]	NA	LOS reduced
Hip fracture[11]	NA	LOS reduced Costs reduced

Abbreviations: LOS, Length of stay; NA, not assessed or reported.
Data from Refs.[5–11]

same.[7] In patients with hip fracture, comanagement did not improve mortality rates or 30-day readmission rates.[8]

Economic Outcomes

Unlike the case with clinical outcomes, several studies suggest that comanagement can improve the efficiency of care, as measured by length of stay and direct care costs. Implementation of the CNS was associated with a $1439 reduction in costs per admission across the entire neurosurgical surgery service. Although length of stay did not decrease after implementation of the CNS, it did fall in association with comanagement in several other studies.[6–11]

Satisfaction with Comanagement

Several studies looked at provider satisfaction with comanagement. Over 90% of neurosurgeons and nurses said they felt the CNS improved the quality of patient care and made it easier for them to provide care to neurosurgical patients. There was a marked increase in the perception that unstable patients were promptly identified and treated; medical problems were addressed after discharge, and communication between providers was optimal. These finding are again in line with other studies showing broad support for comanagement among surgeons and nurses.[6,7] Less is known about patient satisfaction with comanaged care. Two studies failed to demonstrate meaningful changes in patient satisfaction.[5,7]

PITFALLS OF COMANAGEMENT

Enthusiasm for comanagement must be tempered by concern for potential pitfalls of this care model. Without careful planning, the shared clinical responsibilities under comanagement can fragment patient care and promote the disengagement of the surgeon. In addition, it may harm career satisfaction, particularly among hospitalists.

Fragmentation of Care

Under traditional consultation, all responsibilities for management remain with the surgeon. Comanagement fragments these responsibilities between different providers. In some cases, the delineation of roles is obvious (the surgeon manages the external ventricular drain while the hospitalist manages diabetes). However, in many situations, there may be considerable overlap, leading to omission or duplication of care unless there is coordination of efforts. For example, the surgeon and hospitalist may both fail to order antibiotics for a septic patient as each has assumed the other would do so. Even when roles are clear, failure to review the other provider's plans can lead to harm. For example, the hospitalist ordering insulin can induce hypoglycemia after the surgeon's order to discontinue dexamethasone goes unnoticed.

Fragmented care can also hinder communication. Under comanagement, the surgeon and hospitalist may each be privy to clinical information the other physician requires. Also, nurses and other providers may not know which physician to contact with concerns or questions. The comanagement relationship may also confuse patients, who might then be unable to direct their concerns to the appropriate provider.

Disengagement of the Surgeon

Comanagement relieves surgeons of some of the burden of caring for ward patients, allowing them to spend more time in clinic or the operating room. Taken to the extreme, this can promote the surgeon's disengagement from their responsibilities.[12] The risk may be greater in comanagement arrangements in which the hospitalist serves as the attending physician of record. The surgeon's absence leaves hospitalists in the precarious position of having to manage problems that are beyond their training or experience.

Risks to the Hospitalist

Hospitalist's attitudes toward comanagement are mixed. Some hospitalists argue in favor of comanagement relationships as a natural extension of their skills; others have urged caution.[12,13] Concerns include the disengagement of the surgeon, loss of prestige if there is inequality in the relationship, and the sustainability of the workload.

MAKING COMANAGEMENT WORK

Creation of a successful comanagement service requires considerable advance planning. Developing the CNS required 6 months of planning and negotiation, including the recruitment of 2.5 full-time faculty equivalents. A Society of Hospital Medicine task force examining comanagement of the lists 5 keys to success for creating a service, which will be addressed in the following sections.[14]

Select Champions

Both the surgeons and the hospitalists should select representatives committed to the success of a comanagement service. While they will represent their party's interests in negotiations, champions must be willing to compromise and act as a voice of moderation to ensure that the comanagement agreement is acceptable to all providers. Champions must promote the service to their colleagues. They should expect to meet after the service's implementation to review outcomes and resolve problems.

Identify Obstacles and Challenges

Both surgical and medical champions must understand their group's limitations, as well as the obstacles, challenges, and risks that stand in the way of a successful service. Some common concerns include: disagreements on treatment strategies, hospitalists' unfamiliarity with surgical issues, adequacy of staffing to handle patient load, and professional respect. For example, because of differences in philosophy on treating hyponatremia, the CNS hospitalist defers management of this issue to the neurosurgeons. When negotiating the comanagement agreement, providers should establish a process for working through disagreements. Champions should also identify other institutional stakeholders and determine how a comanagement service will affect their interests.

Clarify Roles and Responsibilities

To mitigate against the fragmented care that comanagement can cause, the service agreement should specify which aspects of care each provider will manage. Questions to address will include

- Who will be the attending of record?
- How will patients be selected for comanagement?
- Which issues will be managed by the hospitalist, and which will remain the responsibility of the surgeon?
- What limits will be imposed on the hospitalist's permission to write orders?

In addition, communication protocols should be established, both between surgeons and hospitalists and with nurses and other providers.

Measure Performance

Mortality and the 30-day readmission rate are the most commonly and easily measured clinical outcomes. When measuring the rates of complications that a hospitalist might be able to prevent (eg, pneumonia or myocardial infarction), the data must be interpreted with caution. One study reported the incidence of postoperative delirium increased under comanagement, but this may be because of enhanced detection and documentation of delirium by hospitalists.[7] Thus, it may be more appropriate to measure process outcomes that reflect quality of care, such as use of venous thromboembolism prophylaxis.

Provider satisfaction and efficiency of care improve more consistently under comanagement than clinical outcomes. Both physicians and nurses should be surveyed prior to implementation of comanagement to establish a baseline and then reassessed 6 to 12 months later. Typical questions inquire about perceived quality of medical care, promptness of physicians in addressing concerns, effectiveness of communication, and the impact of comanagement on the provider's ability to deliver care. Patient satisfaction is commonly measured using existing consumer surveys, such as the Hospital Consumer Assessment of Healthcare Providers and Systems (HCAHPS).[15] Some common measurements of efficiency of care include length of stay, direct costs per admission, and surgical cancellation rates.

Address Financial Issues

In many cases, the greatest barrier to implementation of hospitalist comanagement is lack of financial support. Hospitalists are usually unable to support their salaries solely through professional fee collections. In 2012, the median subsidy provided by hospitals to hospital medicine groups was over $140,000 per full-time hospitalist.[16] Thus, hospital medicine groups will be reluctant to recruit additional physicians without guarantees of support.

SUMMARY

As perioperative care grows in complexity, the traditional model of the surgeon being the sole physician in charge of the patient's care is being supplanted by arrangement of shared responsibility. Comanagement between surgeons and hospitalists provides an opportunity to enhance care of neurosurgical patients by allowing each provider to focus on their area of expertise. For the hospitalist, this means identifying and caring for patients at risk of medical complications. This model is not without pitfalls, however, and given that research has yet to demonstrate improved clinical outcomes, physicians are urged to exercise care when developing and implementing comanagement services.

REFERENCES

1. Kuo YF, Sharma G, Freeman JL, et al. Growth in care of older patients by hospitalists in the United States. N Engl J Med 2009;360:1102–12.
2. Sharma G, Kuo YF, Freeman J, et al. Comanagement of hospitalized surgical patients by medicine physicians in the United States. Arch Intern Med 2010;170:363–8.
3. Salerno SM, Hurst FP, Halvorson S, et al. Principles of effective consultation: an update for the 21st-century consultant. Arch Intern Med 2007; 167:271–510.
4. White HL, Glazier RH. Do hospitalist physicians improve the quality of inpatient care delivery? A systematic review of process, efficiency and outcome measures. BMC Med 2011;9:58.
5. Auerbach AD, Wachter RM, Cheng HQ, et al. Comanagement of surgical patients between neurosurgeons and hospitalists. Arch Intern Med 2010;170:2004–10.
6. Sullivan CB, Skurkis CM, McKay K, et al. Pediatric hospitalist co-management of neurosurgical patients leads to decreased length of stay. Poster presented at AAP Experience. American Academy of Pediatrics National Conference and Exhibition. Orlando, October 25–29, 2013.
7. Huddleston JM, Long KH, Naessens JM, et al. Medical and surgical comanagement after elective hip and knee arthroplasty: a randomized, controlled trial. Ann Intern Med 2004;141:28–38.
8. Phy MP, Vanness DJ, Melton LJ III, et al. Effects of a hospitalist model on elderly patients with hip fracture. Arch Intern Med 2005;165:796–801.
9. Simon TD, Eilert R, Dickinson LM, et al. Pediatric hospitalist comanagement of spinal fusion surgery patients. J Hosp Med 2007;2:23–30.
10. Pinzur MS, Gurza E, Kristopaitis T, et al. Hospitalist–Orthopedic co-management of high-risk patients undergoing lower extremity reconstruction surgery. Orthopedics 2009;32:495.
11. Roy A, Heckman MG, Roy V. Associations between the hospitalist model of care and quality-of-care-related outcomes in patients undergoing hip fracture surgery. Mayo Clin Proc 2006;81:28–31.
12. Siegel EM. Just because you can, doesn't mean that you should: a call for the rational application of hospitalist comanagement. J Hosp Med 2008; 3:398–402.
13. Whinney C, Michota F. Surgical comanagement: a natural evolution of hospitalist practice. J Hosp Med 2008;3:394–7.
14. Society of Hospital Medicine. Hospitalist comanagement with surgeons and specialists. Available at: http://www.hospitalmedicine.org/Web/Practice_Management/Co-Management/Hospitalist_Co-Management.aspx. Accessed August 29, 2014.
15. Center for Medicare and Medicaid Services. HCAHPS Patients' Perspectives of Care Survey. Available at: http://www.cms.gov/Medicare/Quality-Initiatives-Patient-Assessment-Instruments/Hospital-QualityInits/HospitalHCAHPS.html. Accessed August 29, 2014.
16. Fuller D. Financial support increases for hospital medicine programs. 2012. Available at: http://www.the-hospitalist.org/details/article/3783081/Financial_Support_Increases_for_Hospital_Medicine_Programs.html. Accessed August 29, 2014.

Recent Advances in the Patient Safety and Quality Initiatives Movement
Implications for Neurosurgery

Isaac Yang, MD*, Nolan Ung, BS, Daniel T. Nagasawa, MD, Panayiotis Pelargos, MD, Winward Choy, BA, Lawrance K. Chung, BS, Kim Thill, BA, Neil A. Martin, MD, Nasim Afsar-Manesh, MD, Brittany Voth, BA, MPH

KEYWORDS

- Quality initiatives • Quality • Safety • Cost • Neurosurgery

KEY POINTS

- A large proportion of morbidity and mortality due to medical errors contribute to unnecessary medical costs within the United States health care system.
- Quality initiatives and cost control can be improved if started from within individual departments on the local scale.
- Neurosurgery has the opportunities to become a leader in quality improvement, cost control, and patient satisfaction.

INTRODUCTION

It is widely recognized that the United States' (US) healthcare system faces a number of challenges in medical errors, leading to increasing costs, which are unsustainable and threaten the national economy. In November 1999, the Institute of Medicine (IOM) published the landmark report, *To Err is Human*,[1] which placed the issues of patient safety and medical errors in the US health care system under the national spotlight. This report estimated that medical errors were responsible for up to 98,000 deaths annually in hospitals across the nation, at a cost of $17 billion to $29 billion per year.[1] However, this conservative estimate did not include outpatient medical errors or morbidities from lapses in the quality of medical care.

Quality improvement initiatives must be implemented and reformed at the local level within individual departments, understanding the challenges of health care at a national scale with the challenging movements for large-scale reform. It is imperative that our physician leaders understand the need to reform health care from within, beginning from their own departments, to improve quality and control cost. In this article, we review the quality improvement initiative and analyze the opportunities within the field of neurosurgery for individual neurosurgery departments to integrate initiatives

Disclosures: The authors have no conflicts of interest to disclose.
I. Yang (senior author) was partially supported by a Visionary Fund Grant, an Eli and Edythe Broad Center of Regenerative Medicine and Stem Cell Research UCLA Scholars in Translational Medicine Program Award, the Jason Dessel Memorial Seed Grant, the UCLA Honberger Endowment Brain Tumor Research Seed Grant, and the STOP CANCER Research Career Development Award.
Department of Neurological Surgery, University of California Los Angeles, Los Angeles, CA, USA
* Corresponding author. Department of Neurological Surgery, University of California Los Angeles, 300 Stein Plaza, Ste. 562 5th Floor Wasserman Bldg, Los Angeles, CA 90095-6901.
E-mail address: iyang@mednet.ucla.edu

Neurosurg Clin N Am 26 (2015) 301–315
http://dx.doi.org/10.1016/j.nec.2014.11.017
1042-3680/15/$ – see front matter © 2015 Elsevier Inc. All rights reserved.

promoting quality improvement and patient safety into their institutional and departmental priorities.

THE NATIONAL PROBLEM

Although the United States is a leader in creating innovative technologies and treatments, the progress has not translated to overall higher quality health care. Since the release of the IOM report in 1999, the National Institutes of Health has doubled its budget and invested more than $32.2 billion to advance medical research.[2,3] Recently, the McKinsey Global Institute and the Kaiser Family Foundation report that the United States spends more per capita and spends a higher percentage of its national gross domestic product (GDP) on health care than any other country listed under the Organization for Economic Cooperation and Development.[4–6] In 2007, US health expenditures increased to $2.3 trillion, accounting for nearly 17% of the nation's GDP, and are expected to reach more than 20% of the nation's GDP by the end of 2015.[7,8] Despite these increasing expenditures, the United States fairs poorly compared with other nations in multiple health metrics. The World Health Report 2000 states that despite spending the highest percentage of its GDP on health care, the United States is ranked 37th for its health care performance.[9] The United States fares worse than 46 countries in infant mortality and 48 countries in life expectancy.[10] In a 2003 study by McGlynn and colleagues,[11] roughly only half of all recommended preventative, acute, and chronic care were received by Americans with significant variability based on the medical condition, ranging from 11% to 79% of recommended care. There is a large discrepancy between the quality of care that Americans receive and their cost.

Medical errors and system inefficiencies not only decrease the quality of health care that patients receive but also come at a huge cost to the nation by compromising the nation's economy, limiting access to health care, and threatening the security of present and future generations. Increasing health care costs threaten the sustainability of government programs like Medicare and force employers to cut coverage or shift part of the financial burden onto their employees. The increasing costs are shifting health care patterns, and hospitals are seeing decreases in admissions and increases in uncompensated care.[12,13] However, some estimates project that almost 30% of health care costs can be decreased without compromising the quality of health care delivered.[7,14] Thomson Reuters[4] estimate that wasted health care expenditures account for between $600 million and $850 billion annually, with 40% of wasteful spending attributed to the overuse of unnecessary services or procedures. Of the 6 categories of waste identified in this report, medical errors and unsafe clinical practices accounted for $25 billion to $50 billion annually, an increase from the IOM's initial annual figure of $17 billion to $29 billion.[1] However, medical errors negatively affect more than mere health care costs and may lead to further readmissions, additional procedures, complications that compromise quality of life, and increase overall mortality.[4,15,16]

Now, more than a decade after the IOM *To Err is Human* report, there seems to be little progress in patient safety reform and quality control to make health care safer, more cost effective, and more assessable for the American public. The obstacles to controlling costs, ensuring patient safety, and improving health care quality are rooted in a highly fragmented and complicated health care system.[17] In addition, the unsustainable health care expenditure growth is fueled by several factors, including technological innovations, for which cost-effectiveness and comparative clinical usefulness and evidence are not readily available, and an expanding aging population with chronic medical conditions who require costlier end-of-life care.[7] With more than 40 million Americans uninsured,[2] equitable access to quality and efficient care also remains elusive.

NATIONAL INITIATIVES: LEGISLATIVE REFORM AND THEIR CHALLENGES

Some national initiatives have been initiated, and several system-wide solutions have been proposed to address health care safety and quality. One of the key recommendations in the IOM's *To Err is Human* report[1] included creating a comprehensive national reporting system that is mandatory, validated, and public. In light of the ongoing deficits in patient safety and quality initiatives, there is a need for an adequate and universal system of metrics that can track and follow progress. However, there is still no consensus on which metrics should be focused on or what should be measured. One potential metric is patient outcomes, which examines aspects including patient mortality and morbidity. Another aspect of quality improvement is processes of care: the services and therapies that physicians or hospitals provide to their patients. For example, patients with myocardial infraction treated with aspirin, which has been correlated to improve patient survival, could be a process measure.

With this aim, several different groups have made fragmented progress toward creating process measures to assess a provider's performance.

With more assessable quality metrics, patients will have the ability to identify safer providers, and payers could refuse to reimburse substandard care, pushing providers to prioritize higher quality of care.[17] The National Quality Forum (NQF) uses a consensus development process that lists hundreds of performance metrics, safe practices, and quality frameworks to assess the overall quality of health care.[18] In their 2008 Physician Quality Reporting Initiative (PQRI), the Center for Medicare and Medicaid Services[19] collected data on and proposed 119 different quality metrics of physician performance, ranging from adhering to guidelines for chemotherapy and radiation therapy to blood glucose control for diabetic patients. Another arm of the government, the US Department of Health and Human services, through its Hospital Compare Web site, publishes hospital-specific process of health care quality metrics for surgical, cardiac, and pneumonia treatment (http://www.hospital-compare.hhs.gov/). In addition to these national organizations, various states and independent groups have also begun collecting and publishing quality metrics,[17] but these efforts remained complicated and fragmented, as shown here.

Despite the move toward improved metrics in patient safety, health care quality metrics have certain limitations. Outcome measures are confounded by the health of a hospital's patient population. There are also issues of statistical power, because outcome measures may not adequately reflect quality of care between physicians if the comparative sample sizes are too small.[20] Process measures and metrics cannot account for the unquantifiable but still important clinical decisions made in providing quality health care.[21] Some studies show only a weak correlation between process measures and improved clinical outcomes.[20]

National reform is needed to create a uniform and mandatory national reporting system, which promotes accountability through transparency. There have been only fragmented efforts on the state level to require reporting. Throughout the past few years, an increasing number of hospitals have been required to report incidence of medical errors under different state laws. Only 28 states require hospitals to make annual infection rates available to the public.[22] Several states have passed their own safety reform laws to hold hospitals accountable for medical errors, but implementation has been slow. In 2006, California passed patient safety legislation requiring the California Department of Public Health to complete several patient safety provisions. However, in a recent Consumer's Union report, the California Department of Public Health has been slow to

accomplish several key requirements, including creating a hospital-acquired infection protection program, collecting and reporting infection rates from hospitals, reporting medical errors to the public, and conducting inspections to ensure that hospitals are following patient safety policies.[23,24] The Agency for Healthcare Research and Quality (AHRQ) is the closest national agency that comprehensively aggregates and tracks national progress based on claims from Medicare, hospital data from states, and other sources. However, these data are often dated and presented as a national and state aggregate rather than for specific providers, limiting their usefulness.[24]

Other national priorities have been to introduce payment reform that places a financial incentive for health care quality reform. Through implementing pay-for-performance and bundling payment, the government can provide economic incentives for hospitals to provide better quality care at a lower cost, rather than merely the quantity of procedures.[17] Furthermore, Medicare, as one of the largest payers into the US health care system, is reducing and removing reimbursements for several avoidable hospital-acquired conditions. Although Medicare has made efforts such as these reimbursement changes to realign financial incentives with clinical quality and safety goals, progress has been slow and challenging without clear evidence that these efforts are resulting in improved patient safety and health care quality. For example, the Tax Relief and Health Care Act of 2006 created the 2007 PQRI, a voluntary, Medicare provider quality reporting program. This program offers a bonus payment of up to 1.5% of total Medicare reimbursements for physicians who report various quality measures through medical registries. However, the PQRI has been criticized as "insufficiently funded and overly burdensome," poorly crafted, without input from all stakeholders, and improperly incentivized, because the rewards do not balance the costs to implement such a reporting program.[25,26]

With the implementation of the Affordable Care Act (ACA), the United States has shifted the national spotlight to a triple aim focusing on improving quality, experience of care, and decreasing costs. A component of the ACA penalizes hospitals for acquired infection rates and readmission rates to improve the quality of care delivered. Medicare also uses the Value-Based Payment Modifier program to reward or fine physicians based on their quality data. As a provision, the ACA requires the use of PQRI by 2015, and physicians are mandated to report 138 different quality practice measures; those who are unable to comply will face payment reductions. Furthermore, Accountable Care Organizations, which were created to provide financial incentives for provider networks who are able to improve outcomes without higher costs, have increased since the passage of the ACA. Because the ACA is still in its infancy, data on its effectiveness are still being tracked. More time and evidence are needed to elucidate the full effects of the ACA on the quality and cost of health care in the United States.

THE LOCAL INITIATIVE: HEALTH CARE REFORM FROM THE INSIDE

Issues of patient safety and health care quality initiatives have been under the national spotlight for more than a decade, yet progress has been slow, unwieldy, and challenging. Although the national movement toward patient safety and quality initiatives should be a multidisciplinary endeavor, progress in this movement can and should be initiated locally. As legislators struggle to create patient safety reform on a state and national scale, we as clinicians and leaders in medicine and neurosurgery have our part to improve and reinvent health care. The significant and critical components needed for comprehensive restructuring of the US health care system may be achieved only through the creative insights, interventions, and leadership of the physicians and health care providers working every day in the trenches of the operating room and on the frontlines of medicine. The IOM, in their subsequent report *Ensuring Quality Cancer Care*, noted that "for many Americans with cancer, there is a wide gulf between what could be construed as the ideal and the reality of their experience with cancer care."[27] In the same report, the National Cancer Policy Board further addresses the decentralization at the patient and illness level, noting that the "fragmented cancer care system does not ensure access to care, lacks coordination, and is inefficient in its use of recourse" and concluded that "efforts to improve cancer care in many cases will therefore be local or regional and could feasibly originate in a physician's practices, [or] in a hospital." With 83% of all national health expenditures categorized under direct clinical care,[28] reform within regional hospitals and individual departments, led by physicians and hospital leaders through a health care reform from within approach, is especially promising, with great potential. The Institute for Healthcare Improvement (IHI), New England Healthcare Institute (NEHI), and Thomson Reuters have all recently published studies addressing specific waste and

inefficiencies in clinical care and provided a detailed review of various categories of waste and opportunities to cut spending.[4,7,12]

In *The Fragmentation of US Healthcare*, Elhauge[17] identifies 4 levels of fragmentation. In the broadest level, coverage and access are fragmented across different patient groups. Care for patients can be fragmented over time, when beneficiaries move among different insurers. Similarly, care for a particular patient can be fragmented if there is miscommunication between different hospitals and providers treating the same patient for different conditions. In the narrowest level, care for a certain illness can be fragmented as a patient visits different professions during the course of a hospital stay. For example, care for a patient with a brain tumor may move from a neurosurgeon to the intensive care unit (ICU) hospitalist to a neurooncologist and then to a radiation oncologist. Addressing fragmentation at the patient and illness levels can be most effectively addressed at the local level of improving patient safety and developing quality initiatives.

One of the largest costs of national health care spending originates from great regional variations in care and services that are not correlated to significant differences in overall clinical outcomes.[7,29–32] Depending on geography, Medicare beneficiaries have been documented to receive wide variations in the intensity of medical care, which includes greater referrals to specialists, office visits, diagnostic tests, and procedures.[33] There is an especially high variation in spending on chronic medical conditions, end-of-life treatment, and medical care delivered at academic medical centers.[7,34] For example, Medicare spending per patient in 2005 ranged from $5358 in Oregon to greater than $14,000 in Florida.[31,32] A study of 226 California hospitals revealed that Medicare spending varied from $24,722 to $106,254 per patient per year during the last 2 years of life.[4,35] However, many studies have found that the variation in demography and health status does not account for the variation in health care expenditures.[31,32] Many studies have found that increased health care spending is not positively correlated to improved clinical outcomes at the level of states and Hospital Referral Regions.[30,33,36–38] Instead, higher costs are correlated with higher intensities of medical care, including longer ICU stays and more frequent tests and procedures, and, at times, result in decreased quality of medical care based on process-of-care measures and less patient satisfaction.[30,33] A study analyzing hospital performance for 2712 national hospitals and their spending intensity showed either a zero or negative correlation between quality of care (through process-of-care measures) and spending both among and within regions.[33] Further-more, a NEHI report[7] estimates that 30% of national health care expenditure or $600 billion in annual savings can be reduced without compromising health care quality, because of unnecessary care.

These challenges and opportunities present an opportunity for improving patient safety, quality initiatives, and efficiency of care on a local and regional level if providers, health care profes-sionals, and individual departments work to imple-ment evidence-based medicine to eliminate avoidable costs within their respective hospitals and departments. Quality initiatives at this narrow local scale within individual departments have huge potential for significant gains, because prog-ress is more easily measured, and efforts are more quickly focused in responding to patient needs and improving safety.

Neurosurgery is in an optimal position in this movement toward improving patient safety, qual-ity initiatives, and health care reform from within. Neurosurgery has always been at the forefront of clinical and technological advances and should continue to lead in this realm of safety and quality. Neurosurgery is inherently high risk, with a low margin of error, and possesses a real potential for catastrophic outcomes. Neurosurgery also re-quires the close collaboration between a myriad of services, departments, and professionals within every hospital. A single neurosurgical patient may require multiple costly scans and tests,[4,39–60] require the coordinated care of a multidisciplinary team, and represent a multitude of opportunities to lead improvements in patient safety and quality initiatives. Because of the high degree of com-plexity and risks involved, neurosurgery stands in a unique position to incur significant risks and costs, affect many medical processes, and have a significant impact on the quality and safety of medical care. As leaders in the growing move-ment for patient safety and quality improvements, neurosurgery can make significant contributions in making health care a more integrated, efficient, and safe process. Although there are few pub-lished studies that specifically address compre-hensive quality improvements in neurosurgery, there are many reports on specific areas in which neurosurgeons can lead health care reform from the inside.

SCOPE OF LOCAL QUALITY INITIATIVES
Systems Approach

In both the IOM's reports, *Crossing the Quality Chasm* and *To Err is Human*, deficits in the safety and quality of the US health care system are attrib-uted to system failures, rather than to the fault of a single physician or department.[1,2] Challenges arise from the lack of proper metrics, reporting systems to track progress, and coordinated multi-disciplinary effort that prioritizes safety and quality. Consequently, efforts at the hospital and depart-ment level to improve clinical quality should focus on the systems of medical care.[61]

A report summarizing lessons learned from the NSQIP's 15-year experience in the Veterans Affairs and private sector promoted a new concep-tual framework, encouraging providers to consider surgical safety as safety from all adverse events, not merely preventable errors or sentinel events as addressed by IOM's *To Err is Human* and *The Joint Commission*, respectively.[62] This new frame-work suggests that not all preventable errors are easily identifiable and places the focus on system failures, rather than individual's errors.[61] These re-sults, along with reports from the National Surgical Risk Study, highlight the importance of systems that facilitate clear communication and coordina-tion among all professionals involved in surgical care.[61,63–65]

Tracking Progress

Quality efforts using metrics, including thorough process-of-care measures and risk-adjusted outcomes, are critical in identifying system prob-lems and tracking progress. The NSQIP initially originated with the Veterans Administration in 1991 and has now grown into the private sector in collaboration with the ACS.[66] As the only "multi-specialty, clinically based, prospectively collected, quality improvement program,"[66] the NSQIP is working toward improving surgical quality and safety through rigorous collection and reporting outcome data.[61,67–69] The main metrics on which the ACS-NSQIP focuses are risk-adjusted 30-day surgical outcomes in mortality and morbid-ities, further classified into areas ranging from wound and urinary tract to central nervous system. Quality improvement is achieved by providing hos-pitals with timely, outcomes-based, risk-adjusted data and patient risk factors to empower providers to accurately track and improve clinical safety.

In a recent study analyzing the progress of 118 hospitals participating in ACS-NSQIP from 2006 to 2007, Hall and colleagues[66] found marked improvements in surgical quality, with 66% of participating hospitals improving in risk-adjusted mortality and 82% improving in risk-adjusted complication rates. These improvements pro-vide a strong precedent that local process-of-care improvements can result in clinical outcome improvements. In addition, embracing a culture that values metrics can pave the way for evidence-based medicine, in which the best practices are identified to minimize variations in practice among physicians and ensure that the quality of care is held to a proper standard.

Quality Through Evidence-Based Medicine

The scope of quality initiatives must include cost efficiency and medical waste. Traditionally, motives for quality improvement focused on patient safety, and resulting financial savings were considered secondary benefits. However, the IHI recently reported changing economic pressures and mounting evidence that better care can come from lower costs, and this has paved a new approach for quality improvement: "the systematic identification and elimination of waste, while maintaining or improving quality."[12]

In 2008, the National Priorities Partnership, a collaboration between the NQF and 28 other health organizations, published a report detailing 9 priorities to cut wasteful health care spending. During the same year, the NEHI published a comprehensive review on a system-wide approach toward improving quality and efficiency, which focused on cutting out waste, which was defined as "healthcare spending that can be eliminated without reducing the quality of care."[12] The variation in the intensity of clinical care can also be attributed to several factors. Some argue that variations arise not from a medical need but from supply-side forces and practice-style variations, such that facilities with more beds, specialists, and resources tend to have more services and procedures.[30,31,36,57,70–72] Variations may also be caused by patient demands.[31,73,74] Patient safety is intimately tied to cost, and a movement toward greater reliance on evidence-based medicine will help reduce variation through reducing uncertainty and identifying the best practices that are most cost effective.

A clear and thorough understanding of best practices supported by evidence-based reports in the literature will empower physicians to make informed, patient-centered decisions that minimize the use of excess procedures, tests, and medications may unnecessarily expose patients to further health risks and complications. Given the increased risks inherent in neurosurgery, an assessment of the risk factors, prognosis, clinical outcomes, and impact on quality of life of a potential treatment is especially important. This understanding, combined with personal experiences, will help physicians make clinical decisions that maximize safety and quality by providing a guideline for the best practices with the best outcomes.[75] During the Congress of Neurological Surgeons (CNS) 2009 Annual Meeting, the American Association for Neurological Surgeons and CNS led neurosurgeons in this patient safety and quality initiatives movement and released the nation's first evidence-based, multidisciplinary treatment guidelines for patients with brain metastases.[76] These guidelines provide up-to-date and best treatment practices that produce optimal clinical outcomes and incorporates the latest research through evaluating the myriad of treatments available, including surgical resection, stereotactic radiosurgery, whole brain radiation therapy, partial brain radiation, and chemotherapy.[76,77]

However, clinical practice guidelines created from evidence-based medicine may have unclear medical-legal ramifications during malpractice suits. In addition, there is a concern for the slow replacement of the art of medicine, based on a neurosurgeon's own clinical experience and expertise, by the rigid science of evidence-based medicine: a movement that may reduce the practice of medicine to a set of protocols.[77,78] However, evidence-based medicine is a tool that is meant to complement a physician's own clinical knowledge, not a means to deny a patient's or physician's choice of treatment, stifle the intimacy of the physician-patient relationship, or hinder innovation of new methods and protocols.[79]

OPPORTUNITIES IN NEUROSURGERY
Quality and Safety in Neurosurgical Care

The most immediate area for quality improvement is to address issues of patient safety and medical errors, because these cost savings have been well documented.[4,39,80–88] In the 2008 National Healthcare Quality report,[89] avoidable hospitalizations from errors in 2005 cost the nation $29.6 billion. A 2009 report by the Healthcare Cost and Utilization Project[90] estimated that avoidable complications cost hospitals 30.8 billion, roughly 10% of total hospital expenditures. Nearly 18% of Medicare's reimbursements are for preventable hospitalizations.[86] The elimination of these factors can significantly contribute to the improvement of safety, quality, and cost.

Surgical errors
Despite the widespread implementation of the Universal Protocol since its introduction by the Joint Commission in 2004,[91–94] wrong-site and wrong-patient surgeries still occur with uncomfortable frequency.[91,95–105] The 3 steps of the protocol, which included a preprocedure verification, surgical site marking, and a presurgical time-out, were designed to ensure that the correct surgical procedure was performed for the correct patient

on the indicated side every time. Although such errors, often termed never-events, are considered 100% avoidable given proper safety protocols and procedures, a 2007 study of Pennsylvania hospitals over a 30-month period[91,97] reported 427 accounts of wrong-site, wrong-patient, and wrong-procedure operations. The study also noted that a formal time-out was unsuccessful in preventing 31 of these accounts. However, reports of the prevalence of wrong-site procedures have been mixed. A review of the National Practitioner Data Bank and other claims databases[91] showed that wrong-site surgeries in the United States occurred with a frequency of 1300 to 2700 per year. A study by Kwaan and colleagues[106] reviewing cases of wrong-site surgery reported to a malpractice insurer showed only 25 accounts of wrong-site surgery from almost 3 million procedures over a 20-year period. Critics suggest that this study is a gross underestimate of the errors, because many wrong-site surgeries never result in a malpractice claim,[91,103] and surgeons are often reluctant to disclose errors because of legal and professional repercussions.[96,107–109]

Of all surgical fields, neurosurgery is third highest risk in wrong-site surgeries, after orthopedic and general surgery.[110,111] The complexity of neurosurgery and the required coordination of several surgeons are contributing factors for the increased risk.[110] Jhawar and colleagues[96] conducted a national survey of 138 practicing neurosurgeons to examine the prevalence of wrong-site and wrong-level craniotomies and diskectomies. Based on the self-reported data from 4695 lumbar diskectomies, 2640 cervical diskectomies, and 10,203 craniotomies, the frequency of wrong-level lumbar surgery and incorrect-site cervical diskectomies and craniotomies was 4.5, 6.8, and 2.2 per 10,000, respectively. Of all participating neurosurgeons, 25% reported cutting skin at the wrong site at least once in their careers, and 32% reported removing lumbar disk material at the wrong level at least once in their careers.[96] This study, along with others,[96,104,110] also showed that incidence of wrong-site surgery varied with number of surgeries performed rather than the number of years of practicing, suggesting that experience alone does not guarantee a reduction of errors.

Despite the increasing attention given to wrong-site surgeries and new safety protocols, these never-events still occur.[100,112,113] Many experts suggest that these avoidable errors are largely caused by communication errors.[110,114–120] In a systematic review of 35 cases of wrong-site craniotomy,[110] the leading and common cause was human error. Four cases resulted from the surgeons'

inaccurate assumptions, and 7 cases were attributed to time pressures and fatigue.[110] Other main causes for wrong-site craniotomies in the study include communication breakdowns within surgical teams and among departments, inadequate preoperative checks that led to failed site marking, mixing of the identities of patients with similar names, improper surgical time-outs, mixing of scans, technical factors, imaging that included mislabeled images, and unconventional operating room setup.[110] Causes of wrong-site errors in spine surgery included odd patient anatomy and inadequate use of radiographic verification of surgical site.[96]

Although some investigators recognize that wrong-site surgeries will not be completely eliminated, rigorous adherence to systems of prevention at various stages[96] of a patient's treatment can reduce error incidence. Several of the risk factors, including communication breakdown and inadequate checks, can be addressed through proper protocols and checklists. Makary and colleagues[121] found that operating room briefings improved team communication and significantly reduced wrong-site surgeries. An 8-year experience with a neurosurgical checklist at the Mayo Clinic[115] observed high compliance among neurosurgeons and reported increased awareness of safety of surgical teams. Connolly and colleagues[122] reported on the effective clinical usefulness of a neurosurgery operational checklist for movement disorder surgery because of the ease of implementation of the checklist and the consistent ability to identify errors over time. However, protocols and checklists have limited efficacy without a culture of safety and the coordination of the entire team.[91,110,123] Neurosurgeons need to not only lead the use of appropriate checks and safety protocols but, more importantly, lead in the adoption of an improved culture of safety and communication to improve the systems delivery of the inherently high-risk field that is neurosurgery.[15,124–128]

Nosocomial infections

Nosocomial infections also comprise another area of opportunity in improving clinical safety and efficiency. Nosocomial infections, or hospital-acquired infections, result in an estimated 90,000 deaths and a cost of 4.5 to 5.7 billion dollars annually.[7,80] However, a study by the Pennsylvania Health Care Cost Containment Council reported a greater incidence.[7] Hospitals in Pennsylvania alone reported 11,668 hospital-acquired infections in 2004, 15.4% of which led to death, with an overall cost of $2 billion.

The US Centers for Disease Control and Prevention (CDC) National Nosocomial Infections

Surveillance system noted that in participating acute care hospitals in the United States, surgical site infections (SSI) comprised 38% of all nosocomial infections in surgical patients.[129] The National Healthcare Safety Network and the National Center for Health Statistics[130] estimate that 250,000 to 1 million cases of SSI occur each year in the United States. Patients facing SSIs are at least 60% more likely to be admitted to an ICU, 15 times as likely for readmission within 30 days of discharge,[130] and stay in hospitals an average of 7.5 days longer.[129] Beyond costing $1.6 billion in avoidable health care expenditures, SSIs can lead to increased morbidity, mortality, and compromised quality of life.[131] The University of Pennsylvania Medical Center[12] reported savings of 1.2 million over 2 years from reducing hospital-acquired infections.

Although rare compared with other surgical specialties,[132] neurosurgical cases of surgical infections may have devastating consequences, including meningitis, permanent functional and cognitive deficits, and pseudarthrosis.[132–134] For example, nearly 75% of patients with diskitis from a surgical complication or infection may experience chronic back pain and functional deficits.[132,135] Developing safety protocols to address SSI requires a thorough understanding of prevalence, incidence, and risk factors. There have been several reports proposing best practices and identifying risks for SSIs from neurosurgical procedures.

In a 2010 retrospective case study of 103 patients undergoing craniotomies, Cha and colleagues[136] identified increased length of stay and low level of consciousness, among other risk factors, as causes for increased incidence of SSI. Studies of infections resulting from spine surgery cite several risk factors for surgical infections, including patient age, previous surgical infection, diabetes, malnutrition, obesity, operation length, and operation complexity.[132–134,137,138] Inamasu and colleagues[139] examined the differing efficacies of bone flap storage methods in reducing the incidence of SSI after decompressive craniotomy followed by cranioplasty. The study found that temporary storage in a subcutaneous pocket for traumatic brain injury could be beneficial over cryopreservation, although both methods seem to be equal for nontraumatic brain injury causes.

Cerebrospinal fluid (CSF) shunts are commonly used to treat hydrocephalus and other intracranial conditions to relieve intracranial pressure. However, shunt infections cost an average of $50,000 per hospital treatment and billions of dollars nationally[140] and are the single most expensive implant-related infection in the United States.[141] Rates of reported shunt infection range from 0% to 39%.[142] Many published studies exist, documenting proper techniques, different preventive and safe practices, and antibiotic treatment options, yet, infections still occur.[143,144] Risk factors include presence of CSF leak, patient age (<40 weeks' gestation), and improper handling of the shunt system.[145] Safe practices include using antibiotic-impregnated shunts (AISs),[140,144,146,147] antibiotic prophylaxis,[144,148–151] limited hardware and skin edge manipulation,[152] and using the double gloving technique.[144,153] After implementing AISs, Johns Hopkins Hospital reduced shunt infection rates from 12% to 3.2% and reduced infection-related costs.[141] Many other studies[144,154–158] have shown that adherence to safe protocols for shunt surgery is successful in reducing shunt infections and controlling costs. Neurosurgeons must use the evidence-based medicine in the literature to lead in the implementation of protocols and culture to improve patient safety and decrease surgical errors.

Use of an external ventricular drain (EVD) is a common approach for monitoring and controlling intracranial pressure while treating brain tumors and hydrocephalus and is used in emergency neurosurgery.[159] However, the most common complication from EVDs is CSF infection, which is associated with morbidity, including bacterial meningitis and ventriculitis, and mortality.[160] Frequency of CSF infections resulting from ventriculostomy has been reported within a range of 2.2% to 10.4%.[161–168] Several studies have documented several risk factors, including craniotomy, depressed cranial fracture, intraventricular hemorrhage, systemic infection, CSF leakage, operation length, and inadequate closure of skin or dura.[163,165,169–176] Other risk factors, including duration of catheter use, use of antibiotics, and EVD exchange, have been noted, but associations are still controversial.[162,165,177–180]

In implementing safety initiatives to control nosocomial infections and minimize antibiotic resistance, neurosurgeons should implement safety protocols that consider evidence-based strategies on infection prevention and risk factors identified in the literature. Although reducing nosocomial infections remains a challenge, several successes have been reported. In 2006, the Michigan Health and Hospital Association Quality Keystone ICU project[181] reported its state-wide success in decreasing catheter-related bloodstream infections in 103 participating ICUs. An estimated 80,000 catheter-related blood stream infections occur each year, resulting in up to 28,000 deaths, costing hospitals an average of $45,000 per patient and costing the nation $2.3 billion annually.[181] Through leadership, team training and education, consistent data reporting, a culture of patient safety, and adherence to a safety checklist of evidence-based procedures from the CDC's recommendations, hospitals observed up to 66% reduction in catheter-related bloodstream infections. Within 3 months, the median infection rate was 0, and remained at 0 through an additional 15 months of follow-up.[181] Implementation of the safety program was simple, inexpensive, and cost effective.

In a 2006 study, Dasic and colleagues[182] reported a significant reduction in EVD infections, from 27% to 12% over a 2-year period, through the adoption of an evidence-based protocol. A 2010 study from Leverstein-van Hall and colleagues[160] observed a reduction in external ventricular and lumbar drain–related infections from 37% to 9% through a multidisciplinary effort that focused on 5 pillars, which included increased vigilance, standardized operation protocols, and a diagnostic and therapeutic algorithm. Classen and colleagues[183] reported $0.7 million annual savings from reducing deep surgical wound infections, from 1.8% to 0.4%, through a protocol that included proper prophylactic administration of antibiotics.[184] Neurosurgeons must lead in the development of team training and education, consistent data reporting, a culture of patient safety, and adherence to safety checklist to develop a simple, inexpensive, and cost-effective practice to prevent EVD and shunt infections to dramatically improve patient outcomes and reduce neurosurgery care costs.

Improvements in neurosurgery processes for patient safety and quality

There have also been several studies on process improvements specific to neurosurgery.[185] After implementing a protocol that included 3 clinical pathways for patients with CSF shut malfunctions at the Texas Children's Hospital, total time for completion of emergency department physician evaluation and initiating diagnostic imaging was reduced from 147 to 104 minutes.[186] The department's ability to triage and treat more severe cases improved, and patients in the expedited pathway experienced a shorter hospital stay.[186] In 1990, the University of Michigan Medical Center[187] implemented a critical pathway for lumbar laminectomy and transphenoidal pituitary tumor resection, as part of a hospital-wide multidisciplinary effort to standardize processes of care, cut costs, and maintain clinical quality. During the first 14 months, the center observed a decrease in length of stay at the ICU and routine care unit. Similarly, Arriaga and colleagues[188] reported a decrease in length of ICU and hospital stays after implementing a clinical pathway for

acoustic neuroma surgery. Recently, a study of 106 patients on the implementation of a clinical pathway for lumbar laminectomy[189] found an average reduction in hospital stay, decreased variability in length of stay, and improved patient satisfaction. The use of process improvements presents as an opportunity for neurosurgery to provide a more streamlined care to augment overall quality care and lower costs.

SUMMARY

Since the IOM published its seminal study on medical errors in 1999, minimal progress has been made on a national scale to address issues of patient safety and clinical quality. Furthermore, increasing costs of national health care expenditure have compromised and will continue to compromise the national economy and limit health care access. National efforts, including the ACA, payment reform that prioritizes quality, passing legislation requiring accountability and transparency, and creating a centralized regulatory agency for clinical quality, have been slow and challenging. Neurosurgeons have an obligation to expand their clinical priorities to include quality initiatives, patient safety, and cost efficiency. In tackling these issues, neurosurgeons possess the necessary agility and clinical insight from working at the frontlines of health care delivery to provide the ingenuity and leadership necessary for the increasing movement of local and regional changes to reform health care from the inside.

Given the potential and scope of quality improvement initiatives at the local level within individual departments and hospitals, neurosurgery is in an optimal position to lead this patient safety and quality initiatives movement. Neurosurgery has always been a field of innovators, at the forefront of clinical and technological advances, and should continue to lead in clinical quality and patient safety. As a high-risk field, neurosurgery can make the most impact and significant gains in improving patient safety, quality initiatives, and cost efficiency.

The authors of this review will serve as a catalyst and foundation for the planning and execution of quality improvement initiatives, departmental efforts, and neurosurgical cost efficiencies. The goal is to contribute to the increasing dialogue concerning patient safety, quality initiatives, and cost efficiency within the neurosurgery community, the medical profession, and for the health care of our nation. Efforts will be challenging and will require a change in organizational culture; however, given the severity of the current health care challenges, this patient safety and quality initiatives movement in neurosurgery is an imperative. As neurosurgeons, we have the option of being either active leaders or reactionary participants in this movement.

REFERENCES

1. Kohn LT, Corrigan J, Donaldson MS. To err is human: building a safer health system. Washington, DC: National Academy Press; 2000.
2. Institute of Medicine (US), Committee on Quality of Health Care in America. Crossing the quality chasm: a new health system for the 21st century. Washington, DC: National Academy Press; 2001.
3. Summary of the FY 2011 President's Budget. National Institute of Health; 2010.
4. Kelley R. Where can $700 billion in waste be cut annually from the US Healthcare System. Thomson Reuters; 2009.
5. Trends in healthcare costs and spending. 2009.
6. Accounting for the cost of US healthcare: a new look at why Americans pay more. McKinsey Global Institute; 2008. Available at: http://www.mckinsey.com/mgi/reports/pdfs/healthcare/US_healthcare_Executive_summary.pdf. Accessed November 18, 2010.
7. Waste and inefficiency in the US healthcare system, clinical care: a comprehensive analysis in support of system-wide improvements. New England Healthcare Institute; 2008.
8. Borger C, Smith S, Truffer C, et al. Health spending projections through 2015: changes on the horizon. Health Aff (Millwood) 2006;25:w61–73.
9. The World Health Report 2000: health systems: improving performance. 2000.
10. Robertson MP, Miller SL. Prebiotic synthesis of 5-substituted uracils: a bridge between the RNA world and the DNA-protein world. Science 1995; 268:702–5.
11. McGlynn EA, Asch SM, Adams J, et al. The quality of health care delivered to adults in the United States. N Engl J Med 2003;348:2635–45.
12. Martin LA, Meuman CW, Mountford J, et al. Increasing efficiency and enhancing value in health care: ways to achieve savings in operating costs per year. Institute for Healthcare Improvement; 2009.
13. Report on the economic crisis: initial impact on hospitals. 2008.
14. Reducing the cost of poor quality heath care through responsible purchasing leadership. Midwest Business Group on Health; 2003.
15. Agarwal R, Sands DZ, Schneider JD. Quantifying the economic impact of communication inefficiencies in US hospitals. J Healthc Manag 2010; 55:265–81 [discussion: 281–2].
16. Clemmer TP, Spuhler VJ, Oniki TA, Horn SD. Results of a collaborative quality improvement program on outcomes and costs in a tertiary critical care unit. Crit Care Med 1999;27:1768–74.
17. Elhauge E. The fragmentation of US health care: causes and solutions. New York: Oxford University Press; 2010.
18. Noller HF. Ribosomes. Drugs and the RNA world. Nature 1991;353:302–3.
19. Lahav N. Prebiotic co-evolution of self-replication and translation or RNA world? J Theor Biol 1991; 151:531–9.
20. Jha AK. Measuring hospital quality: what physicians do? How patients fare? Or both? JAMA 2006;296:95–7.
21. Pronovost PJ, Miller MR, Wachter RM. Tracking progress in patient safety: an elusive target. JAMA 2006;296:696–9.
22. Jennings T. Health care reform targets hospital-acquired infections. The New Mexico Independent; 2010.
23. McCauley M. Consumers Union finds slow progress on patient safety in California: California Department of Public Health has failed to carry out key requirements of recent patient safety laws. Consumers Union; 2010.
24. To err is human–to delay is deadly: ten years later: a million lives lost, billions of dollars wasted: safe patient project. Consumers Union; 2009.
25. Medicare's physician quality improvement program: neurosurgery works toward meaningful quality improvement system. American Association of Neurological Surgeons; 2007. Available at: http://www.aans.org/Media/Article.aspx?ArticleId=45767. Accessed November 20, 2010.
26. Callcut RA, Breslin TM. Shaping the future of surgery: the role of private regulation in determining quality standards. Ann Surg 2006;243:304–12.
27. Hewitt ME, Simone JV, National Cancer Policy Board (US). Ensuring quality cancer care. Washington, DC: National Academy Press; 1999.
28. Catlin A, Cowan C, Heffler S, et al. National Health Spending in 2005: the slowdown continues. Health Affairs 2007;26:142–53.
29. Wennberg J, Cooper M, editors. The quality of medical care in the United States: a report on the Medicare program, the Dartmouth Atlas of Health Care in the United States. Chicago: 1999.
30. Fisher ES, Wennberg DE, Stukel TA, et al. The implications of regional variations in Medicare spending. Part 1: the content, quality, and accessibility of care. Ann Intern Med 2003;138:273–87.
31. Anthony DL, Herndon MB, Gallagher PM, et al. How much do patients' preferences contribute to resource use? Health Aff (Millwood) 2009;28:864–73.
32. Wennberg JE. Tracking the care of patients with severe chronic illness: the Dartmouth Atlas of Health Care 2008. The Dartmouth Institute for Health Policy & Clinical Practice; 2008.

33. Yasaitis L, Fisher ES, Skinner JS, et al. Hospital quality and intensity of spending: is there an association? Health Aff (Millwood) 2009;28:w566–72.

34. Wennberg JE, Fisher ES, Stukel TA, et al. Use of Medicare claims data to monitor provider-specific performance among patients with severe chronic illness. Health Aff (Millwood) 2004;Suppl Web Exclusives:VAR5–18.

35. Supply sensitive care. A Dartmouth Atlas Project Topic Brief. 2007.

36. Fisher ES, Wennberg DE, Stukel TA, et al. The implications of regional variations in Medicare spending. Part 2: health outcomes and satisfaction with care. Ann Intern Med 2003;138:288–98.

37. Baicker K, Chandra A. Medicare spending, the physician workforce, and beneficiaries' quality of care. Health Aff (Millwood) 2004;Suppl Web Exclusives:W184–97.

38. Chandra A, Staiger DO. Productivity spillovers in healthcare: evidence from the treatment of heart attacks. J Polit Econ 2007;115:103–40.

39. Ensuring quality through appropriate use of diagnostic imaging. America's Health Insurance Plans; 2008.

40. Colliver V. Curbing costs of medical scans: insurers seek to rein in fast-growing use of pricey high-tech MRIs and CTs. San Francisco Chronicle 2005.

41. William W. Conversation with a leader: Curt Thorne. Nashville City Paper 2007.

42. Krizner K. Special report: one eye on the image and the other on the wallet. Managed HealthCare Executive 2006.

43. Jablokow A. Radiology seen as next cost battleground between health plans and physicians. HealthLeaders/InterStudy; 2006.

44. Keehan S, Sisko A, Truffer C, et al. Health spending projections through 2017: the baby-boom generation is coming to Medicare. Health Aff (Millwood) 2008;27:w145–55.

45. Farr C. Oncologic imaging: growth forecast for a cancer management fundamentals. Imaging Economics 2006.

46. Dehn T, O'Connell B, Hall RN, et al. Appropriateness of imaging examinations: current state and future approaches. Imaging Economics 2000.

47. Brenner DJ, Hall EJ. Computed tomography–an increasing source of radiation exposure. N Engl J Med 2007;357:2277–84.

48. Meko J. A tool box for medical management. Healthcare Savings Chronicle 2007.

49. Rothenberg B. Medical technology as a driver of healthcare costs: diagnostic imaging. BlueCross BlueShield Association; 2003.

50. Angrisano C. Accounting for the cost of health care in the United States. McKinsey Global Institute; 2007.

51. Mullaney T. This man wants to heal health care. Business Week 2005.

52. Kaplan D. A new way to manage radiology utilization could help limit costs. Managed Healthcare Executive 2006.

53. Kowalczyk L. Radiation risk: doctors concerned about the exploding use of CT scanners. The Boston Globe 2007.

54. Cohen D. Radiology 2005: state of the industry. Imaging Economics 2005.

55. Fisher ES, Staiger DO, Bynum JP, et al. Creating accountable care organizations: the extended hospital medical staff. Health Aff (Millwood) 2007;26: w44–57.

56. Baker L, Birnbaum H, Geppert J, et al. The relationship between technology availability and health care spending. Health Aff (Millwood) 2003;Suppl Web Exclusives:W3-537-51.

57. Wennberg JE, Fisher ES, Skinner JS. Geography and the debate over Medicare reform. Health Aff (Millwood) 2002;Suppl Web Exclusives:W96–114.

58. Studdert DM, Mello MM, Sage WM, et al. Defensive medicine among high-risk specialist physicians in a volatile malpractice environment. JAMA 2005; 293:2609–17.

59. Health reform's taboo topic: defensive medicine. Washington Post 2009.

60. Prat G, Lefevre M, Nowak E, et al. Impact of clinical guidelines to improve appropriateness of laboratory tests and chest radiographs. Intensive Care Med 2009;35:1047–53.

61. Khuri SF. Safety, quality, and the National Surgical Quality Improvement Program. Am Surg 2006;72: 994–8 [discussion: 1021–30, 33–48].

62. Leung SW, Apponi LH, Cornejo OE, et al. Splice variants of the human ZC3H14 gene generate multiple isoforms of a zinc finger polyadenosine RNA binding protein. Gene 2009;439:71–8.

63. Young GJ, Charns MP, Daley J, et al. Best practices for managing surgical services: the role of coordination. Health Care Manage Rev 1997;22: 72–81.

64. Young GJ, Charns MP, Desai K, et al. Patterns of coordination and clinical outcomes: a study of surgical services. Health Serv Res 1998;33:1211–36.

65. Daley J, Forbes MG, Young GJ, et al. Validating risk-adjusted surgical outcomes: site visit assessment of process and structure. National VA Surgical Risk Study. J Am Coll Surg 1997;185:341–51.

66. Hall BL, Hamilton BH, Richards K, et al. Does surgical quality improve in the American College of Surgeons National Surgical Quality Improvement Program: an evaluation of all participating hospitals. Ann Surg 2009;250:363–76.

67. Khuri SF. The NSQIP: a new frontier in surgery. Surgery 2005;138:837–43.

68. Khuri SF, Daley J, Henderson W, et al. The Department of Veterans Affairs' NSQIP: the first national, validated, outcome-based, risk-adjusted, and

peer-controlled program for the measurement and enhancement of the quality of surgical care. National VA Surgical Quality Improvement Program. Ann Surg 1998;228:491–507.

69. Khuri SF, Daley J, Henderson WG. The comparative assessment and improvement of quality of surgical care in the Department of Veterans Affairs. Arch Surg 2002;137:20–7.

70. McLaughlin CG, Normolle DP, Wolfe RA, et al. Small-area variation in hospital discharge rates. Do socioeconomic variables matter? Med Care 1989;27:507–21.

71. Shwartz M, Pekoz EA, Ash AS, et al. Do variations in disease prevalence limit the usefulness of population-based hospitalization rates for studying variations in hospital admissions? Med Care 2005; 43:4–11.

72. Folland S, Stano M. Small area variations: a critical review of propositions, methods, and evidence. Med Care Rev 1990;47:419–65.

73. Bertko JM. Variation in use of medical care services: higher risk or higher consumption? Health Aff (Millwood) 2003;Suppl Web Exclusives:W3-363-5.

74. Fuchs VR. Floridian exceptionalism. Health Aff (Millwood) 2003;Suppl Web Exclusives:W3-357-62.

75. Dettori JR, Norvell DC, Dekutoski M, et al. Methods for the systematic reviews on patient safety during spine surgery. Spine (Phila Pa 1976) 2010;35:S22–7.

76. As nation focuses on reforming healthcare, neurosurgeons release the first evidence-based, multidisciplinary treatment guidelines for brain metastases patients: recent explosion in new technology and increased treatment options led to need for uniform guidance to medical providers. American Association of Neurological Surgeons; 2009. Available at: http://www.aans.org/~/media/Files/Legislative%20Activities/BrainMetastasesTrtGuidelinesNewsRelease102609.ashx. Accessed November 13, 2010.

77. Vachhrajani S, Kulkarni AV, Kestle JR. Clinical practice guidelines. J Neurosurg Pediatr 2009;3:249–56.

78. Groff MW. How to incorporate clinical experience into evidence-based medicine. Clin Neurosurg 2009;56:54–6.

79. Awad IA, Fayad P, Abdulrauf SI. Protocols and critical pathways for stroke care. Clin Neurosurg 1999; 45:86–100.

80. Burke JP. Infection control–a problem for patient safety. N Engl J Med 2003;348:651–6.

81. Gill JM. Use of hospital emergency departments for nonurgent care: a persistent problem with no easy solutions. Am J Manag Care 1999;5:1565–8.

82. Gonzales R, Malone DC, Maselli JH, et al. Excessive antibiotic use for acute respiratory infections in the United States. Clin Infect Dis 2001;33:757–62.

83. Chen LW, Zhang W, Sun J, et al. The magnitude, variation, and determinants of rural hospital resource utilization associated with hospitalizations due to ambulatory care sensitive conditions. J Public Health Manag Pract 2009;15:216–22.

84. Flores G, Abreu M, Chaisson CE, et al. Keeping children out of hospitals: parents' and physicians' perspectives on how pediatric hospitalizations for ambulatory care-sensitive conditions can be avoided. Pediatrics 2003;112:1021–30.

85. Xiao H, Barber J, Campbell ES. Economic burden of dehydration among hospitalized elderly patients. Am J Health Syst Pharm 2004;61:2534–40.

86. Culler SD, Parchman ML, Przybylski M. Factors related to potentially preventable hospitalizations among the elderly. Med Care 1998;36:804–17.

87. American Diabetes Association. Economic costs of diabetes in the US in 2007. Diabetes Care 2008;31: 596–615.

88. Ahern MM, Hendryx M. Avoidable hospitalizations for diabetes: comorbidity risks. Dis Manag 2007; 10:347–55.

89. National healthcare quality report AHRQ 2008. 2008.

90. Beck LA. The life of the Buddha. London; Glasgow (United Kingdom): Collins Clear-Type Press; 1939.

91. Stahel PF, Mehler PS, Clarke TJ, et al. The 5th anniversary of the "Universal Protocol": pitfalls and pearls revisited. Patient Saf Surg 2009;3:14.

92. Ridge RA. Doing right to prevent wrong-site surgery. Nursing 2008;38:24–5.

93. Norton E. Implementing the universal protocol hospital-wide. AORN J 2007;85:1187–97.

94. Wrong site surgery and the Universal Protocol. Bull Am Coll Surg 2006;91:63.

95. Seiden SC, Barach P. Wrong-side/wrong-site, wrong-procedure, and wrong-patient adverse events: are they preventable? Arch Surg 2006;141:931–9.

96. Jhawar BS, Mitsis D, Duggal N. Wrong-sided and wrong-level neurosurgery: a national survey. J Neurosurg Spine 2007;7:467–72.

97. Clarke JR, Johnston J, Finley ED. Getting surgery right. Ann Surg 2007;246:395–403 [discussion: 403–5].

98. Clarke JR, Johnston J, Blanco M, et al. Wrong-site surgery: can we prevent it? Adv Surg 2008; 42:13–31.

99. Catalano K. Have you heard? The saga of wrong site surgery continues. Plast Surg Nurs 2008;28:41–4.

100. van Hille PT. Patient safety with particular reference to wrong site surgery–a presidential commentary. Br J Neurosurg 2009;23:109–10.

101. Shinde S, Carter JA. Wrong site neurosurgery–still a problem. Anaesthesia 2009;64:1–2.

102. Wong DA, Herndon JH, Canale ST, et al. Medical errors in orthopaedics. Results of an AAOS member survey. J Bone Joint Surg Am 2009;91:547–57.

103. Rothman G. Wrong-site surgery. Arch Surg 2006; 141:1049–50 [author reply: 1050].
104. Meinberg EG, Stern PJ. Incidence of wrong-site surgery among hand surgeons. J Bone Joint Surg Am 2003;85-A:193–7.
105. Mody MG, Nourbakhsh A, Stahl DL, et al. The prevalence of wrong level surgery among spine surgeons. Spine (Phila Pa 1976) 2008;33:194–8.
106. Kwaan MR, Studdert DM, Zinner MJ, et al. Incidence, patterns, and prevention of wrong-site surgery. Arch Surg 2006;141:353–7 [discussion: 357–8].
107. Brennan TA. The Institute of Medicine report on medical errors–could it do harm? N Engl J Med 2000;342:1123–5.
108. Mohr JC. American medical malpractice litigation in historical perspective. JAMA 2000;283:1731–7.
109. Gostin L. A public health approach to reducing error: medical malpractice as a barrier. JAMA 2000; 283:1742–3.
110. Cohen FL, Mendelsohn D, Bernstein M. Wrong-site craniotomy: analysis of 35 cases and systems for prevention. J Neurosurg 2010;113:461–73.
111. Gao H, Yang Z, Cao S, et al. Behavior and anti-glioma effect of lapatinib-incorporated lipoprotein-like nanoparticles. Nanotechnology 2012;23:435101.
112. Mitchell P, Nicholson CL, Jenkins A. Side errors in neurosurgery. Acta Neurochir (Wien) 2006;148: 1289–92 [discussion: 1289–92].
113. Devine J, Chutkan N, Norvell DC, et al. Avoiding wrong site surgery: a systematic review. Spine (Phila Pa 1976) 2010;35:S28–36.
114. Shaver K. Hospital changes operation procedure. St Petersburg Times 1995.
115. Lyons MK. Eight-year experience with a neurosurgical checklist. Am J Med Qual 2010;25:285–8.
116. Gawande AA, Zinner MJ, Studdert DM, et al. Analysis of errors reported by surgeons at three teaching hospitals. Surgery 2003;133:614–21.
117. Lingard L, Regehr G, Orser B, et al. Evaluation of a preoperative checklist and team briefing among surgeons, nurses, and anesthesiologists to reduce failures in communication. Arch Surg 2008;143:12–7 [discussion: 18].
118. Lingard L, Whyte S, Espin S, et al. Towards safer interprofessional communication: constructing a model of "utility" from preoperative team briefings. J Interprof Care 2006;20:471–83.
119. Awad SS, Fagan SP, Bellows C, et al. Bridging the communication gap in the operating room with medical team training. Am J Surg 2005;190: 770–4.
120. Studer P, Inderbitzin D. Surgery-related risk factors. Curr Opin Crit Care 2009;15:328–32.
121. Makary MA, Mukherjee A, Sexton JB, et al. Operating room briefings and wrong-site surgery. J Am Coll Surg 2007;204:236–43.
122. Connolly PJ, Kilpatrick M, Jaggi JL, et al. Feasibility of an operational standardized checklist for movement disorder surgery. A pilot study. Stereotact Funct Neurosurg 2009;87:94–100.
123. Stone S, Bernstein M. Prospective error recording in surgery: an analysis of 1108 elective neurosurgical cases. Neurosurgery 2007;60:1075–80 [discussion: 1080–2].
124. Catchpole KR, Dale TJ, Hirst DG, et al. A multicenter trial of aviation-style training for surgical teams. J Patient Saf 2010;6:180–6.
125. Malter L, Weinshel E. Improving handoff communication: a gastroenterology fellowship performance improvement project. Am J Gastroenterol 2010; 105:490–2.
126. Arora VM, Manjarrez E, Dressler DD, et al. Hospitalist handoffs: a systematic review and task force recommendations. J Hosp Med 2009;4:433–40.
127. Catalano K. Hand-off communication does affect patient safety. Plast Surg Nurs 2009;29:266–70.
128. Chu ES, Reid M, Schulz T, et al. A structured handoff program for interns. Acad Med 2009;84:347–52.
129. National Nosocomial Infections Surveillance System. National Nosocomial Infections Surveillance (NNIS) System Report, data summary from January 1992 through June 2004, issued October 2004. Am J Infect Control 2004;32:470–85.
130. DeFrances CJ, Cullen KA, Kozak LJ. National Hospital Discharge Survey: 2005 annual summary with detailed diagnosis and procedure data. Vital Health Stat 13 2007;165:1–209.
131. Martone WJ, Nichols RL. Recognition, prevention, surveillance, and management of surgical site infections: introduction to the problem and symposium overview. Clin Infect Dis 2001;33(Suppl 2): S67–8.
132. Young MH, Washer L, Malani PN. Surgical site infections in older adults: epidemiology and management strategies. Drugs Aging 2008;25:399–414.
133. Fang A, Hu SS, Endres N, et al. Risk factors for infection after spinal surgery. Spine (Phila Pa 1976) 2005;30:1460–5.
134. Pappou IP, Papadopoulos EC, Sama AA, et al. Postoperative infections in interbody fusion for degenerative spinal disease. Clin Orthop Relat Res 2006; 444:120–8.
135. McHenry MC, Easley KA, Locker GA. Vertebral osteomyelitis: long-term outcome for 253 patients from 7 Cleveland-area hospitals. Clin Infect Dis 2002;34:1342–50.
136. Cha KS, Cho OH, Yoo SY. Risk factors for surgical site infections in patients undergoing craniotomy. J Korean Acad Nurs 2010;40:298–305.
137. Labler L, Keel M, Trentz O, et al. Wound conditioning by vacuum assisted closure (VAC) in postoperative infections after dorsal spine surgery. Eur Spine J 2006;15:1388–96.

138. Schuster JM, Rechtine G, Norvell DC, et al. The influence of perioperative risk factors and therapeutic interventions on infection rates after spine surgery: a systematic review. Spine (Phila Pa 1976) 2010;35:S125–37.

139. Inamasu J, Kuramae T, Nakatsukasa M. Does difference in the storage method of bone flaps after decompressive craniectomy affect the incidence of surgical site infection after cranioplasty? Comparison between subcutaneous pocket and cryopreservation. J Trauma 2010;68:183–7 [discussion: 187].

140. Sciubba DM, Lin LM, Woodworth GF, et al. Factors contributing to the medical costs of cerebrospinal fluid shunt infection treatment in pediatric patients with standard shunt components compared with those in patients with antibiotic impregnated components. Neurosurg Focus 2007;22:E9.

141. Attenello FJ, Garces-Ambrossi GL, Zaidi HA, et al. Hospital costs associated with shunt infections in patients receiving antibiotic-impregnated shunt catheters versus standard shunt catheters. Neurosurgery 2010;66:284–9 [discussion: 289].

142. Biyani N, Grisaru-Soen G, Steinbok P, et al. Prophylactic antibiotics in pediatric shunt surgery. Childs Nerv Syst 2006;22:1465–71.

143. Whitehead WE, Kestle JR. The treatment of cerebrospinal fluid shunt infections. Results from a practice survey of the American Society of Pediatric Neurosurgeons. Pediatr Neurosurg 2001;35:205–10.

144. Gruber TJ, Riemer S, Rozzelle CJ. Pediatric neurosurgical practice patterns designed to prevent cerebrospinal fluid shunt infection. Pediatr Neurosurg 2009;45:456–60.

145. Kulkarni AV, Drake JM, Lamberti-Pasculli M. Cerebrospinal fluid shunt infection: a prospective study of risk factors. J Neurosurg 2001;94:195–201.

146. Pattavilakom A, Xenos C, Bradfield O, et al. Reduction in shunt infection using antibiotic impregnated CSF shunt catheters: an Australian prospective study. J Clin Neurosci 2007;14:526–31.

147. Sciubba DM, Stuart RM, McGirt MJ, et al. Effect of antibiotic-impregnated shunt catheters in decreasing the incidence of shunt infection in the treatment of hydrocephalus. J Neurosurg 2005;103:131–6.

148. Wang EE, Prober CG, Hendrick BE, et al. Prophylactic sulfamethoxazole and trimethoprim in ventriculoperitoneal shunt surgery. A double-blind, randomized, placebo-controlled trial. JAMA 1984;251:1174–7.

149. Walters BC, Goumnerova L, Hoffman HJ, et al. A randomized controlled trial of perioperative rifampin/trimethoprim in cerebrospinal fluid shunt surgery. Childs Nerv Syst 1992;8:253–7.

150. Schmidt K, Gjerris F, Osgaard O, et al. Antibiotic prophylaxis in cerebrospinal fluid shunting: a prospective randomized trial in 152 hydrocephalic patients. Neurosurgery 1985;17:1–5.

151. Ratilal B, Costa J, Sampaio C. Antibiotic prophylaxis for surgical introduction of intracranial ventricular shunts: a systematic review. J Neurosurg Pediatr 2008;1:48–56.

152. Kanev PM, Sheehan JM. Reflections on shunt infection. Pediatr Neurosurg 2003;39:285–90.

153. Na'aya HU, Madziga AG, Eni UE. Prospective randomized assessment of single versus double-gloving for general surgical procedures. Niger J Med 2009;18:73–4.

154. Choux M, Genitori L, Lang D, et al. Shunt implantation: reducing the incidence of shunt infection. J Neurosurg 1992;77:875–80.

155. Park JK, Frim DM, Schwartz MS, et al. The use of clinical practice guidelines (CPGs) to evaluate practice and control costs in ventriculoperitoneal shunt management. Surg Neurol 1997;48:536–41.

156. Pirotte BJ, Lubansu A, Bruneau M, et al. Sterile surgical technique for shunt placement reduces the shunt infection rate in children: preliminary analysis of a prospective protocol in 115 consecutive procedures. Childs Nerv Syst 2007;23:1251–61.

157. Rotim K, Miklic P, Paladino J, et al. Reducing the incidence of infection in pediatric cerebrospinal fluid shunt operations. Childs Nerv Syst 1997;13:584–7.

158. Venes JL. Control of shunt infection. Report of 150 consecutive cases. J Neurosurg 1976;45:311–4.

159. Lo CH, Spelman D, Bailey M, et al. External ventricular drain infections are independent of drain duration: an argument against elective revision. J Neurosurg 2007;106:378–83.

160. Leverstein-van Hall MA, Hopmans TE, van der Sprenkel JW, et al. A bundle approach to reduce the incidence of external ventricular and lumbar drain-related infections. J Neurosurg 2010;112:345–53.

161. Wong GK, Poon WS, Wai S, et al. Failure of regular external ventricular drain exchange to reduce cerebrospinal fluid infection: result of a randomised controlled trial. J Neurol Neurosurg Psychiatry 2002;73:759–61.

162. Alleyne CH Jr, Hassan M, Zabramski JM. The efficacy and cost of prophylactic and periprocedural antibiotics in patients with external ventricular drains. Neurosurgery 2000;47:1124–7 [discussion: 1127–9].

163. Holloway KL, Barnes T, Choi S, et al. Ventriculostomy infections: the effect of monitoring duration and catheter exchange in 584 patients. J Neurosurg 1996;85:419–24.

164. Paramore CG, Turner DA. Relative risks of ventriculostomy infection and morbidity. Acta Neurochir (Wien) 1994;127:79–84.

165. Poon WS, Ng S, Wai S. CSF antibiotic prophylaxis for neurosurgical patients with ventriculostomy: a randomised study. Acta Neurochir Suppl 1998;71: 146–8.

166. Rebuck JA, Murry KR, Rhoney DH, et al. Infection related to intracranial pressure monitors in adults: analysis of risk factors and antibiotic prophylaxis. J Neurol Neurosurg Psychiatry 2000;69:381–4.

167. Rossi S, Buzzi F, Paparella A, et al. Complications and safety associated with ICP monitoring: a study of 542 patients. Acta Neurochir Suppl 1998; 71:91–3.

168. Winfield JA, Rosenthal P, Kanter RK, et al. Duration of intracranial pressure monitoring does not predict daily risk of infectious complications. Neurosurgery 1993;33:424–30 [discussion: 430–1].

169. Aucoin PJ, Kotilainen HR, Gantz NM, et al. Intracranial pressure monitors. Epidemiologic study of risk factors and infections. Am J Med 1986;80:369–76.

170. Bogdahn U, Lau W, Hassel W, et al. Continuous-pressure controlled, external ventricular drainage for treatment of acute hydrocephalus–evaluation of risk factors. Neurosurgery 1992;31:898–903 [discussion: 903–4].

171. Clark WC, Muhlbauer MS, Lowrey R, et al. Complications of intracranial pressure monitoring in trauma patients. Neurosurgery 1989;25:20–4.

172. Guyot LL, Dowling C, Diaz FG, et al. Cerebral monitoring devices: analysis of complications. Acta Neurochir Suppl 1998;71:47–9.

173. Mayhall CG, Archer NH, Lamb VA, et al. Ventriculostomy-related infections. A prospective epidemiologic study. N Engl J Med 1984;310:553–9.

174. Rosner MJ, Becker DP. ICP monitoring: complications and associated factors. Clin Neurosurg 1976;23:494–519.

175. Stenager E, Gerner-Smidt P, Kock-Jensen C. Ventriculostomy-related infections–an epidemiological study. Acta Neurochir (Wien) 1986;83: 20–3.

176. Sundbarg G, Nordstrom CH, Soderstrom S. Complications due to prolonged ventricular fluid pressure recording. Br J Neurosurg 1988;2:485–95.

177. Kanter RK, Weiner LB, Patti AM, et al. Infectious complications and duration of intracranial pressure monitoring. Crit Care Med 1985;13:837–9.

178. Khanna RK, Rosenblum ML, Rock JP, et al. Prolonged external ventricular drainage with percutaneous long-tunnel ventriculostomies. J Neurosurg 1995;83:791–4.

179. Prabhu VC, Kaufman HH, Voelker JL, et al. Prophylactic antibiotics with intracranial pressure monitors and external ventricular drains: a review of the evidence. Surg Neurol 1999;52:226–36 [discussion: 236–7].

180. Wyler AR, Kelly WA. Use of antibiotics with external ventriculostomies. J Neurosurg 1972;37:185–7.

181. Pronovost P, Needham D, Berenholtz S, et al. An intervention to decrease catheter-related bloodstream infections in the ICU. N Engl J Med 2006; 355:2725–32.

182. Dasic D, Hanna SJ, Bojanic S, et al. External ventricular drain infection: the effect of a strict protocol on infection rates and a review of the literature. Br J Neurosurg 2006;20:296–300.

183. Classen DC, Evans RS, Pestotnik SL, et al. The timing of prophylactic administration of antibiotics and the risk of surgical-wound infection. N Engl J Med 1992;326:281–6.

184. James BC. Quality improvement in the hospital: managing clinical processes. Internist 1993;34: 11–3, 7.

185. Mirski MA, Chang CW, Cowan R. Impact of a neuroscience intensive care unit on neurosurgical patient outcomes and cost of care: evidence-based support for an intensivist-directed specialty ICU model of care. J Neurosurg Anesthesiol 2001;13:83–92.

186. Chern JJ, Macias CG, Jea A, et al. Effectiveness of a clinical pathway for patients with cerebrospinal fluid shunt malfunction. J Neurosurg Pediatr 2010; 6:318–24.

187. Richards JS, Sonda LP, Gaucher E, et al. Applying critical pathways to neurosurgery patients at the University of Michigan Medical Center. Qual Lett Healthc Lead 1993;5:8–10.

188. Arriaga MA, Gorum M, Kennedy A. Clinical pathways in acoustic tumor management. Laryngoscope 1997;107:602–6.

189. Isla-Guerrero A, Chamorro-Ramos L, Alvarez-Ruiz F, et al. Design, implementation, and results of the clinical pathway for herniated lumbar disk. Neurocirugia (Astur) 2001;12:409–18.

Index

A

Acoustic neuroma
  VORs related to
    in neurosurgery, 212
Adverse events
  in neurosurgery, **157–165**
    data collection related to, 158–159
    errors relationship to, 150
    "never events" and, 159–162
    N2QOD in, 159
    patient safety–related, 144
    relationship to quality improvement, **157–165**
    strategies for reducing, 162–163
Aneurysmal disease
  VORs related to
    in neurosurgery, 212–213

C

Carotid stenosis
  VORs related to
    in neurosurgery, 213
Center for Medicare and Medicaid Innovation (CMMI)
  in relation between quality improvement and national health care policies in neurosurgery, 171
Checklists
  neurosurgical, **219–229**. See also Neurosurgical checklists
Children
  surgical procedures in
    preprocedure time-out, 223
  VORs related to
    in neurosurgery, 213–214
Chordoma(s)
  skull base
    VORs related to
      in neurosurgery, 212
Clinical outcomes
  of neurosurgical procedures
    measuring of, **265–269**
      components in, 267–268
      discussion, 266–268
      future directions in, 268
      introduction, 265–266
      timeline for, 267
Clinical practice guidelines (CPGs)
  defined, 272

evidence-based medicine and, 272–278
general purpose of, 272
in neurosurgery
  concerns related to, 278–281
  critical appraisal of, 278
  development and implementation of, **271–282**
    in evidence-based medicine, 272–278
    introduction, 271–272
  expectations of, 278
  future directions in, 278–281
  history of, 278–281
  limitations of, 278
  potential impact of, 278–281
Clinical registries
  in emerging value-based medicine paradigm, 254–256
  in improving quality of neurosurgical care, **253–262**
    elements in design of, 257
    future directions in, 260–261
    implementation challenges, 261
    introduction, 253
    meeting quality needs of modern neurosurgical practice, 257–260
    N2QOD, 257–258
    N2QOD Lumbar Spine Registry, 258–260
    prospective, patient-centered, longitudinal surgical care registries, 256–257
    STS experience, 256
CMMI. See Center for Medicare and Medicaid Innovation (CMMI)
Comanagement hospitalist services
  for neurosurgery, **295–300**
    candidate selection in, 296
    emergence of, 295–297
    features of, 296–297
    growth of, 295–296
    introduction, 295
    negotiation in, 296
    nonclinical collaboration in, 296–297
    order writing by hospitalist in, 296
    outcomes of, 297–298
    patient experience with, 297
    pitfalls of, 298–299
    success factors in, 299–300
Communication
  in patient safety in neurologic surgery, 145
Cost
  defined, 189

Cost-effectiveness analyses
   in neurosurgery, **189–196**
      areas other than spine, 191
      discussion, 192
      spine-related, 190–191
   in neurosurgical oncology, 192
   principles of, 189–190
Cost-effectiveness research
   in neurosurgery, **189–196**. *See also*
      Cost-effectiveness analyses
      discussion, 192
      introduction, 189
CPGs. *See* Clinical practice guidelines (CPGs)

D

Debriefing
   postoperative, 223–224
Deep brain stimulation
   VORs related to
      in neurosurgery, 214

E

Economics
   in neurosurgery, **197–205**
      assessment of, 198–200
      in comanagement hospitalist services, 298
      perspective on innovations, 201–203
EHR Incentive Program. *See* Electronic Health
   Record (EHR) Incentive Program
Electronic Health Record (EHR) Incentive Program
   in relationship between quality improvement and
      national health care policies in neurosurgery,
      170–171
Electronic medical records (EMRs)
   quality improvement effects of, **245–251**
      early efforts in, 245–246
      HITECH Act of 2009 and, 246–250
      introduction, 245
      quick wins with, 246
      in surgical care, 250–251
      unintended consequences, 246
EMRs. *See* Electronic medical records (EMRs)
Endovascular procedure
   preprocedure time-out for, 220–221
Errors
   in neurosurgery, **149–155**
      adverse events relationship to, 150
      classification of, 149–150
      defined, 149
      epidemiology of, 150–151
      ethical issues in, 152–153
      identification of, 151
      introduction, 149
      patient safety–related, 144
      strategies for reducing, 151–152

Ethical issues
   errors-related, 152–153
EVD insertion. *See* External ventricular drain (EVD)
   insertion
Evidence-based medicine
   CPGs and, 272–278
Evidence-based neurosurgical care
   neurosurgery journals in, **283–294**. *See also*
      Neurosurgery journals, in evidence-based
      neurosurgical care
External ventricular drain (EVD) insertion
   preprocedure time-out for, 220

F

Failure Modes and Effects Analysis (FMEA)
   in quality improvement, 180–182
Fishbone diagram
   in quality improvement, 180, 181
5 why tools
   in quality improvement, 179
Flowcharts
   in quality improvement, 179–180
FMEA. *See* Failure Modes and Effects Analysis
   (FMEA)
Functional disorders
   VORs related to
      in neurosurgery, 214
Functional procedures
   preprocedure time-out for, 221–222

H

HAC Reduction Program. *See* Hospital-Acquired
   Condition (HAC) Reduction Program
Health Information Technology for Economic and
   Clinical Health (HITECH) Act of 2009, 246–250
Health-related quality outcomes
   in neurosurgery
      assessment of, 198
Healthcare science research
   quality improvement projects/research and
      differences between, 185
HITECH Act of 2009. *See* Health Information
   Technology for Economic and Clinical Health
   (HITECH) Act of 2009 Hospital-Acquired Condition
   (HAC) Reduction Program
   in relationship between quality improvement and
      national health care policies in neurosurgery,
      169
Hospital Inpatient Quality Reporting (IQR) Program
   in relationship between quality improvement and
      national health care policies in neurosurgery,
      168
Hospital IQR Program. *See* Hospital Inpatient Quality
   Reporting (IQR) Program
Hospital Value-Based Purchasing (VBP) Program

in relationship between quality improvement and national health care policies in neurosurgery, 168–169

Hospital VBP Program. *See* Hospital Value-Based Purchasing (VBP) Program

Hospitalist services
comanagement
for neurosurgery, **295–300**. *See also* Comanagement hospitalist services, for neurosurgery

I

ICU. *See* Intensive care unit (ICU)

Innovations
in neurosurgery, **197–205**
from economics and quality perspective, 201–203
costly
without improvement in outcomes, 203
decreasing cost and improving quality, 201–202
improving quality but increasing costs, 202–203
reducing costs but leaving quality unchanged, 202

Intensive care unit (ICU) procedures
preprocedure time-out for, 223

Intracranial tumors
VORs related to
in neurosurgery, 207–212
all tumors, 211
subspecialty tumor outcomes, 211–212

M

Meningioma
VORs related to
in neurosurgery, 212

Metastatic brain tumor
VORs related to
in neurosurgery, 211

MFI. *See* Model for Improvement (MFI)

Model for Improvement (MFI)
in quality improvement, 177–179

N

National health care policies
in neurosurgery
quality improvement and
relationship between, **167–175**. *See also* Quality improvement, in neurosurgery, national health care policies and

National Neurosurgery Quality and Outcomes Database (N2QOD), 257–258
in adverse events in neurosurgery, 159

National Neurosurgery Quality and Outcomes Database (N2QOD) Lumbar Spine Registry, 258–260

Neurologic surgery
patient safety in
improving, **143–147**. *See also* Patient safety, in neurologic surgery

Neurological surgery graduate medical education
quality improvement in, **231–238**. *See also* Quality improvement

Neuroma(s)
acoustic
VORs related to
in neurosurgery, 212

Neurosurgery journals
in evidence-based neurosurgical care, **283–294**
future innovations in, 287, 290
introduction, 283–284
knowledge organization in
clinical practice guidelines, 286–289
systematic reviews and meta-analyses, 285–286
peer review in, 287
proliferation of scientific information in, 284
reporting guidelines as tool for literature quality, 284–285

Neurosurgical checklists, **219–229**
effectiveness of, 224
future directions in, 225–226
implementation of, 224–226
introduction, 219–220
postoperative debriefing, 223–224
preprocedure time-out, 220–223
endovascular, 220–221
EVD insertion, 220
functional, 221–222
ICU procedures, 223
pediatric procedures, 223
spine-related, 222–223
tumor removal, 222

Neurosurgical resident education
incorporating quality improvement education into, 234–237

"Never events"
in neurosurgery, 159–162

Nosocomial infections
in neurosurgery
patient safety and quality improvement initiatives related to, 307–309

N2QOD. *See* National Neurosurgery Quality and Outcomes Database (N2QOD)

O

Obesity
VORs related to
in neurosurgery, 214

P

Pain
  VORs related to
    in neurosurgery, 214
Patient safety
  as national problem, 302
  in neurologic surgery
    building program for, 146
    checklists for, 145
    communication and teamwork in, 145
    databases in, 145–146
    economic considerations in, 144–145
    errors and adverse events related to, 144
    improving, **143–147**
    introduction, 143
    modern movement related to, 143–144
    volume outcomes related to, 145
  in neurosurgery
    recent advances in, **301–315**
      implications for, 306–309
        nosocomial infections, 307–309
        surgical errors–related, 306–307
      introduction, 301–302
      local initiatives, 304–306
      national initiatives, 302–304
    technology and simulation in improving,
      239–243
  technology and simulation in improving, **239–243**.
    See also Simulation; Simulator(s)
    discussion, 242
    expansion of training aspects addressed by
      simulators, 240
    introduction, 239
    in neurosurgery, 240
    organized presurgical training models,
      239–240
PDSA. *See* Plan-Do-Study Act (PDSA)
Physician Quality Reporting System (PQRS)
  in relationship between quality improvement and
    national health care policies in neurosurgery,
    169–170
Physician Value-Based Payment Modifier (VBM)
  in relationship between quality improvement and
    national health care policies in neurosurgery,
    170
Physician VBM. *See* Physician Value-Based Payment
    Modifier (VBM)
Pituitary tumors
  transsphenoidal
    VORs related to
      in neurosurgery, 211–212
Plan-Do-Study Act (PDSA)
  in quality improvement, 177–179
Postoperative debriefing, 223–224
PQRS. *See* Physician Quality Reporting System
    (PQRS)

Preprocedure time-out
  indications for, 220–223. *See also* Neurosurgical
    checklists, preprocedure time-out
Public reporting
  in relationship between quality improvement and
    national health care policies in neurosurgery,
    171

Q

Quality analysis, 234
Quality improvement
  curriculum for, 237
  educational principles of, 232–234
    demand for, 232
    quality analysis, 234
    quality improvement, 234
    quality measurement, 232–234
  EMRs and, **245–251**. *See also* Electronic medical
    records (EMRs)
  incorporating education related to in
    neurosurgical resident education, 234–237
  introduction, 231–232
  as national problem, 302
  in neurological surgery graduate medical
    education, **231–238**
    introduction, 231–232
  in neurosurgery, **197–205**
    adverse events relationship to, **157–165**. *See
      also* Adverse events, in neurosurgery
    assessment of, 198–200
    introduction, 197–198
    milestones in, 237
    national health care policies and, **167–175**
      relationship between, **167–175**
        balancing need for big data in, 173–174
        barriers to information exchange in, 173
        CMMI in, 171
        cumulative nature of penalties in, 174
        discussion, 168–171
        EHR Incentive Program in, 170–171
        flaws methodologies in, 172–173
        HAC Reduction Program in, 169
        Hospital IQR Program in, 168
        Hospital VBP Program in, 168–169
        inadequate measures in, 171–172
        insufficient data in, 173
        introduction, 167–168
        ongoing challenges and themes in,
          171–174
        Physician VBM in, 170
        PQRS in, 169–170
        public reporting and transparency in,
          171
        rapid implementation in, 174
        Readmission Reduction Program in, 169

perspective on innovations, 201–203
tools and process in, **177–187**
    fishbone diagram, 180, 181
    5 why tools, 179
    flowcharts, 179–180
    FMEA, 180–182
    introduction, 177
    MDI, 177–179
    PDSA, 177–179
    RCA, 181, 183–185
Quality improvement initiatives
    recent advances in, **301–315**
        implications for neurosurgery, 306–309
            nosocomial infections, 307–309
            surgical errors–related, 306–307
        introduction, 301–302
        local initiatives, 304–306
        national initiatives, 302–304
Quality improvement projects/research
    healthcare science research and
        differences between, 185
Quality measurement, 232–234
Quality of care
    clinical registries in improving, **253–262**. *See also*
        Clinical registries, in improving quality of
        neurosurgical care

R

RCA. *See* Root Cause Analysis (RCA)
Readmission Reduction Program
    in relationship between quality improvement and
        national health care policies in neurosurgery,
        169
Research
    cost-effectiveness
        in neurosurgery, **189–196**. *See also*
            Cost-effectiveness research, in
            neurosurgery
    quality improvement
        healthcare science research *vs.*, 185
Root Cause Analysis (RCA)
    in quality improvement, 181, 183–185

S

Safety
    patient-related. *See* Patient safety
Simulation
    in neurosurgery, 240
        validation of
            proposal for, 240
    in neurosurgery education
        introduction, 239
    in neurosurgery residency

challenges in designing formal curriculum
    using, 240
durotomy repair simulator as training tool,
    240–242
initial use of, 240
Simulator(s)
    durotomy repair
        as model residency training tool, 240–242
    expansion of training aspects addressed by, 240
Skull base chordoma
    VORs related to
        in neurosurgery, 212
Society of Thoracic Surgeons (STS)
    experience with clinical outcomes databases to
        advance quality care in surgery, 256
Spine
    cost-effectiveness analyses in neurosurgery
        related to, 190–191
Spine disorders
    VORs related to
        in neurosurgery, 214
Spine procedures
    preprocedure time-out for, 222–223
STS. *See* Society of Thoracic Surgeons (STS)
Surgical errors
    in neurosurgery
        patient safety and quality improvement
            initiatives related to, 306–307

T

Teamwork
    in patient safety in neurologic surgery, 145
Transparency of public reporting
    in relationship between quality improvement and
        national health care policies in neurosurgery,
        171
Transsphenoidal pituitary tumors
    VORs related to
        in neurosurgery, 211–212
Trauma
    VORs related to
        in neurosurgery, 214
Tumor(s)
    pituitary
        transsphenoidal
            VORs related to, 211–212
Tumor removal
    preprocedure time-out for, 222

V

Value
    defined, 189
Value-based care
    rise of, 253–254

Value-based medicine paradigm
  emerging
    clinical registries in, 254–256
Vascular diseases
  VORs related to
    in neurosurgery, 212–213
Volume-outcome relationships (VORs)
  in neurosurgery, **207–218**. *See also specific
    situations and types, e.g.,* Intracranial tumors,
    VORs related to
    in children, 213–214
    deep brain stimulation–related, 214
    discussion, 214–216
    evolving care paradigms, 215–216
    functional disorders, 214

    intracranial tumors, 207–212
    introduction, 207
    limitations of, 215
    obesity-related, 214
    pain-related, 214
    spine disorders, 214
    trauma-related, 214
    vascular diseases, 212–213
VORs. *See* Volume-outcome relationships
  (VORs)

W

Willingness-to-pay threshold in current practice
  in neurosurgery, 198–200

Moving?

Make sure your subscription moves with you!

To notify us of your new address, find your **Clinics Account Number** (located on your mailing label above your name), and contact customer service at:

Email: journalscustomerservice-usa@elsevier.com

800-654-2452 (subscribers in the U.S. & Canada)
314-447-8871 (subscribers outside of the U.S. & Canada)

Fax number: 314-447-8029

Elsevier Health Sciences Division
Subscription Customer Service
3251 Riverport Lane
Maryland Heights, MO 63043

*To ensure uninterrupted delivery of your subscription, please notify us at least 4 weeks in advance of move.

Printed and bound by CPI Group (UK) Ltd, Croydon, CR0 4YY

03/10/2024

01040366-0011